A–Z of Plastic Surgery

D1579643

PLYMOUTH
HEALTH LIBRARIES

Accession No. _C 2107611_

Class No. _WO 250 / HOD_

Location _Im (Ref)_

A–Z of Plastic Surgery

Andrew Hodges

DISCOVERY LIBRARY
LEVEL 5 SWCC
DERRIFORD HOSPITAL
DERRIFORD ROAD
PLYMOUTH
PL6 8DH

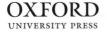

OXFORD
UNIVERSITY PRESS

OXFORD

UNIVERSITY PRESS

Great Clarendon Street, Oxford ox2 6DP

Oxford University Press is a department of the University of Oxford.
It furthers the University's objective of excellence in research, scholarship,
and education by publishing worldwide in

Oxford New York

Auckland Cape Town Dar es Salaam Hong Kong Karachi
Kuala Lumpur Madrid Melbourne Mexico City Nairobi
New Delhi Shanghai Taipei Toronto

With offices in

Argentina Austria Brazil Chile Czech Republic France Greece
Guatemala Hungary Italy Japan Poland Portugal Singapore
South Korea Switzerland Thailand Turkey Ukraine Vietnam

Oxford is a registered trade mark of Oxford University Press
in the UK and in certain other countries

Published in the United States
by Oxford University Press Inc., New York

© Oxford University Press 2008

The moral rights of the author have been asserted
Database right Oxford University Press (maker)

First published 2008

All rights reserved. No part of this publication may be reproduced,
stored in a retrieval system, or transmitted, in any form or by any means,
without the prior permission in writing of Oxford University Press,
or as expressly permitted by law, or under terms agreed with the appropriate
reprographics rights organization. Enquiries concerning reproduction
outside the scope of the above should be sent to the Rights Department,
Oxford University Press, at the address above

You must not circulate this book in any other binding or cover
and you must impose the same condition on any acquirer

British Library Cataloguing in Publication Data

Data available

Library of Congress Cataloging in Publication Data

Hodges, Andrew, 1962-
A-Z of plastic surgery / Andrew Hodges.
   p. ; cm.
ISBN-13: 978-0-19-954657-2 (alk. paper) 1. Surgery, Plastic—Handbooks,
manuals, etc.
   [DNLM: 1. Reconstructive Surgical Procedures—Handbooks. 2. Cosmetic
Techniques—Handbooks. 3. Surgery, Plastic—Handbooks. WO 39 H688a
2008] I. Title: A to Z of Plastic Surgery. II. Title.
RD118.H63 2008
617.9'5—dc22

2008004569

Typeset by Cepha Imaging Private Ltd, Bangalore, India
Printed in Great Britain
on acid-free paper by
Ashford Colour Press, Gosport, Hampshire

ISBN 978-0-19-9546-572

1 3 5 7 9 10 8 6 4 2

To my wife Sarah and
my children Naomi, Sam and Rachel

Preface

Plastic Surgery is an extremely broad subject and the trainee in this specialty is required to assimilate a large amount of information. The *A–Z of Plastic Surgery* has been written as an aid to learning and revising this material and as a reference book. Although it is written in an encyclopaedic format, it does not claim to be a complete text. The concise style should enable subjects to be grasped rapidly. However, this book does not replace, but rather complements fuller chapter-based texts. The primary focus is for Plastic Surgery trainees, but it will also be of value to the specialist as a reference text and to medical workers in allied specialties. In a book of this scope and size there will inevitably be controversy as to what should be included or omitted, and under which heading. In this rapidly changing and expanding specialty, the author would welcome contributions and comments from readers – particularly to augment existing entries or to suggest new entries. These will be incorporated into the second edition.

Andrew Hodges
Consultant Plastic Surgeon
Mengo Hospital, Kampala, Uganda
Andrewhodges3001@yahoo.co.uk

Acknowledgements

I am grateful to the Plastic Surgeons who have inspired and taught me. In particular, I would like to acknowledge Tim Goodacre, who first introduced me to this exciting specialty, and to my consultants in Exeter, Peter Saxby, John Palmer, Vik Devaraj and Chris Stone, who helped me throughout my training and particularly in preparation for the final Plastic Surgery examinations. I am grateful to Oxford University Press and Rose James for their assistance in publishing this book, and for their valuable comments and suggestions.

The publisher is grateful to Lucy Cogswell for her help in reviewing the final manuscript.

How to use this book

- Entries are arranged in alphabetical order. Some subjects are grouped under one main heading (e.g. **burns**).
- Words that are *italicized* and <u>underlined</u> are cross references to other entries.
- Abbreviations have been used to maintain the concise style. A list of abbreviations is available at the end of the book.

Abbé flap

- Useful flap for reconstructing moderate-sized defects (too big to close directly) of the lip.
- Pedicled flap, usually taken from the lower lip to reconstruct a defect on the upper lip, although this can be reversed.
- Blood supply is from the inferior labial artery.
- The flap is positioned so that the width of the vermilion matches the lip segment being replaced.
- The Abbé flap may be quadrilateral, forked or winged to assist closure of the lower lip defect.
- The lower lip can sacrifice 25–35% of its length.
- While pedicle remains attached the patient requires a soft diet.
- Divide the flap in 1–2 weeks.
- A similar principle can be used for upper eyelid reconstruction.

See _Lip reconstruction_. See _Secondary lip and nasal deformities_.

Abdominal wall

Function: Abdominal wall muscles important for posture, standing, walking and bending.

Anatomy:
Muscles:

- _External oblique:_ from lower 8 ribs, inserts into iliac crest and forms inguinal ligament.
- _Internal oblique:_ deep to external oblique. From lumbodorsal fascia, iliac crest and inguinal ligament. Lower fibres form conjoint tendon. Superior fibres insert into linea alba and 7–9 cartilage.
- _Transversus abdominus:_ deep to internal oblique. From lower 6 ribs, lumbodorsal fascia and iliac crest into linea alba and conjoint tendon.
- _Rectus abdominus:_ Longitudinal from symphysis to xiphoid and 5–7 ribs.
- _Pyramidalis:_ small triangular muscle superficial to rectus. From pubis to linea half way between symphysis and umbilicus.

Linea semicircularis or arcuate line lies midway between umbilicus and pubis. Above this the internal oblique splits and half passes deep to rectus. Below this the posterior sheath is only composed of transversus abdominus. Neurovascular structures lie between internal oblique and transversus abdominus.

Blood supply:

- _Superior epigastric artery:_ terminal branch of the internal mammary artery.
- _Thoracic and lumbar intercostal arteries:_ run between internal and external oblique.
- _Deep inferior epigastric artery:_ from the external iliac artery, enters rectus abdominus and supplies it and the overlying skin.
- _Deep circumflex iliac artery:_ from the external iliac artery to the inner ileum and skin.
- _Superficial inferior epigastric artery:_ from the femoral artery, to the skin of the lower abdomen.
- _Superficial circumflex iliac artery:_ from the femoral artery to the lower abdomen.
- _Superficial external pudendal artery:_ from the femoral artery to the skin over the pubis.

Abdominal wall reconstruction
Indications:

- _Trauma._
- _Tumour:_ Desmoid, Dermatofibrosarcoma protuberans.
- _Radiation._
- _Infection:_ Gas gangrene, Necrotizing fasciitis.
- _Iatrogenic:_ Incisional hernia.
- _Congenital:_ Omphalocoele, Gastroshisis, Prune belly syndrome.

Management of acute loss: After aggressive debridement, avoid closure under tension and avoid raising flaps acutely. Cover viscera with synthetic mesh.

Objectives: Cover abdominal contents, prevent herniation and restore the appearance. When direct closure is not possible, closure may be achieved with fascial releases and component separation. If a defect remains, then closure will require alloplastic material or musculofascial flaps for strengths, and skin grafts or flaps for cover.

Procedures:

- *Ramirez Component separation*.
- *Local flaps:* based on vessels supplying abdominal skin. The external oblique can be used as a turn over flap. Rectus can be used.
- *Regional flaps:* pedicled tensor fascia lata (*TFL*), *Rectus femoris*, anterolateral thigh flap. Gracilis is less useful as it only reaches to the perineum.
- *Distant flaps:* omentum, latissimus dorsi.
- *Mesh*: apply over omentum to prevent adhesions. Suture under tension.

Abdominoplasty

An aesthetic procedure which aims to provide a flatter, narrower abdomen by excising skin and fat excess and addressing rectus divarication, generally by using a lower transverse abdominal scar.

Classification:

- *I:* Excess *fat*, liposuction.
- *II: Lax skin infra-umbilical*, resect lower abdo skin.
- *III: Lax skin and muscle with fat* infraumbilical mini-abdominoplasty with muscle plication.
- *IV: Lax muscle*, complete abdominoplasty without umbilical translocation.
- *V: Lax skin and fat*, complete abdominoplasty with umbilical translocation.
- *VI: Circumferential laxity*, circumferential abdominoplasty.

Operation: Mark skin incision with a large ellipse. The lower line passes just above the pubic hairs and is flattened centrally. For a full abdominoplasty, the upper line will be around the level of the umbilicus. Dissect out umbilicus. Elevate flap leaving thin layer of fascia intact. Proceed up to xiphoid if needed. Limit lateral dissection. Tighten aponeurosis. Flex the back. Skin excision should be generous laterally – high-tension abdominoplasty (HTA). Suture flap and find new location for the umbilicus. If there is significant lateral laxity add a vertical component to produce a *Fleur-de-Lys* abdominoplasty.

Complications: Thrombo-embolism, respiratory difficulties, skin necrosis, wound dehiscence, wound infections, haematoma, seroma.

Abductor pollicis brevis

APB: Most superficial muscle of thenar eminence.

Origin: Transverse carpal ligament, palmaris longus and there may also be another slip from abductor pollicis longus.

Insertion: The tendon is adherent to the radial side of the MCP joint capsule. A few fibres join FPB and radial sesamoid. The rest join the extensor expansion.

Nerve supply: Median nerve.

Action: Abduction of the thumb at the carpometacarpal and MCP joint. This is a forward movement in the anteroposterior plane. *See Muscles.*

Abductor pollicis longus

Origin: Dorsum of radius, ulnar and interosseous membrane. It runs obliquely around the radius coursing over the wrist extensors. It runs in the 1st extensor compartment with extensor pollicis brevis and may have several slips.

Insertion: Lateral 1st metacarpal. It gives off a slip to trapezium and another to APB.

Nerve supply: Posterior interosseous nerve.

Action: Abducts the thumb through slip to APB. Extends the thumb and radially deviates the wrist. *See Muscles.*

Absorbable polymers
Synthetic:

- Used for sutures and investigated for other devices such as plates and screws (LactoSorb).
- One class of polymers used is the alpha-hydroxy acids including L-lactic acid, glycolic acid, and dioxanone.
- As polymers these are
  - *PLLA:* poly-l-lactic acid;
  - *PGA:* polyglycolic acid;
  - polydioxanone.
- PLLA and PGA are used together. Breakdown is by hydrolytic scission of the ester bond.
- PGA is degraded more rapidly than PLLA.
- Dexon is pure PGA. Vicryl is 8% PLA, 92% PGA.

Natural:

- Many materials are produced from _Collagen_.
- Haemostatic properties can be reduced by isolating collagen into fibrils.
- The haemostatic properties can also be utilized.

See Alloplasts.

Acanthosis

Hyperplasia of epithelium. _See Skin._

Accutane

Isotretinoin. The synthetic retinoid derivative 13-_cis_-retinoic acid (Accutane) used for severe _Acne vulgaris_. The dose is 1 mg/kg body weight for an initial 4–5-month course of therapy. It reduces sebum excretion and is anti-inflammatory.

Acne vulgaris

- Acne vulgaris is a common skin disorder seen in adolescents and young adults.
- Seborrhoea, small comedones, and inflammatory papulopustules found.
- Acne conglobata is the severe form with deep cysts and sinuses with extensive scarring of face back and chest.

Management:

- Incision of the cystic lesions reduces the inflammation that produces the scarring.
- Dietary control does not appear to be beneficial.
- Topical medications with benzoyl peroxide, topical antibiotics or tretinoin (retinoic acid).
- Skin hygiene and long-term administration of antibiotics, such as tetracycline, has been helpful.
- Ultraviolet rays and superficial X-ray therapy are effective, but with unacceptable long-term effects.
- _Accutane_ is effective for severe acne.
- Dermabrasion, laser resurfacing and collagen injections may help reduce the scarring.
- A facelift procedure may reduce skin laxity, which may improve the appearance of the acne scarring.

Acrochordon

- Common papillomatous lesion occurring in middle adult life.
- Multiple, fleshy, skin-coloured tags.

- Occur mainly on neck, upper chest and axilla.
- The only symptoms relate to local irritation.
- Excise with scalpel or scissors.

See Mesodermal tumours.

Acrosyndactyly

- One of the _Congenital hand anomalies_.
- Fusion of digits distally.
- Mainly sporadic, non-hereditary occurrence.
- Associated with _Constriction ring syndrome_.
- Bilateral in 50%, but asymmetric.
- Also associated with craniofacial syndactyly, such as _Apert's syndrome_, in which it is symmetrical.

Actinic keratosis

Also called senile keratosis and solar keratosis.

- The most frequently occurring premalignant cutaneous condition.
- Due to the cumulative effect of UV exposure.
- Occur on exposed skin and often multiple lesions.
- Lesions may regress if sun exposure is limited.
- They occur in genetically predisposed people.
- Arsenic keratosis occurs secondary to exposure to inorganic arsenic compounds.
- Get well circumscribed, erythematous and maculopapular lesions, red to light brown and scaly.
- Microscopically get hyperkeratosis with dyskaryosis and acanthosis. In the dermis there is an actinic elastosis with inflammatory infiltrate.
- Over time many progress to _SCC_ and 20–25% become invasive. SCCs arising from actinic keratosis rarely metastasize.
- Treat with excision, curettage, liquid nitrogen, 5-fluorouracil (efudex), chemical peel, dermabrasion and photodynamic therapy (_PDT_).

See Cutaneous horn.

Adductor pollicis

See Muscles.

Origin:

- _Oblique head:_ transverse carpal ligament, anterior surface base of 2nd and 3rd metacarpal.
- _Transverse head:_ from anterior surface of shaft of 3rd metacarpal. Two heads join.

The transverse fibres insert mainly into the medial sesamoid and the oblique into the extensor expansion.

Insertion: With the 1st palmar interosseous into medial side of base of proximal phalanx.

Nerve: Deep branch of ulnar nerve.

Action: Adduction of the thumb at the carpometacarpal and metacarpophalangeal joint. This is a backward movement in an anteroposterior plane.

Adipofascial flaps

A flap comprised of fascia and overlying fat. Essentially, the same as a fasciocutaneous flap with the skin dissected away from the flap.

Anatomy:
- Dermal and fascial plexuses exist in subcutaneous tissues. Both gain their blood supply from perforators.
- In adipofascial flaps the tissues are divided between plexuses leaving the dermal and subdermal plexuses to supply the skin and the fascial plexuses are taken with the flap to supply it.
- Three perifascial plexuses are described – sub-, intra- and prefascial plexuses. All anastomose, but only pre- and subfascial plexuses receive branches from perforators. The prefascial plexus (superficial to fascia) is dominant.

Properties: Adipofascial flaps are easy to raise, are more malleable and conform better than fasciocutaneous flaps. They are not so robust and require a skin graft onto the flap.

Indications:
- *Lower limb:* medial flaps use posterior tibial perforators. Usually 2–5 of these, fairly constant. There are usually 4–5 anterior tibial perforators. The perforators to the peroneal artery are less predictable, but usually number 4–5.
- *Upper limb:* small adipofascial flaps can be raised from the dorsum of the finger to cover finger tips or exposed bone.

Adnexal tumours

- In adnexal tumours, the relationship between stromal and epithelial components is maintained though distorted to varying degrees.
- They are classified by the degree and the direction of differentiation to sweat and sebaceous glands, and hair follicles.
- They are also termed organoid or appendageal tumours or *Hamartomas*.
- A tumour with fully developed appendageal structures is called a *Naevus*.
- A tumour with incomplete development of structures is an *Adenoma*.
- A poorly organized tumour is an *Epithelioma*.

Adrenaline

- Extensively used in plastic surgery to produce vasoconstriction, which reduces blood loss during surgery, although there is some concern that this may increase the risk of post-operative haematoma.
- Adrenaline can cause cardiac arrhythmias especially in conjunction with halothane.
- The maximum recommended dose is 10 ml of 1:100 000 (100 µg) over 10 minutes or 30 ml (300 µg) over 1 hour.
- 1 ml 1:1000 in 200 ml = 1:200 000.
- Topical soaks for haemostasis can be 1:10 000.
- The total dose of adrenaline should *not* exceed 500 µg and it is essential not to exceed a concentration of 1 in 200 000 (5 µg/ml) if more than 50 ml of the mixture is to be injected.
- Generally avoided in end arteries, such as digital vessels, although several trials have shown no adverse effects in such situations.

Adson's test

Adson's test arm adducted. A test used in the assessment of *Thoracic outlet syndrome*.
- Patient stands with arm adducted against front of trunk. Feel radial pulse.
- Extend neck and turn chin to affected side. This stretches and tightens the *Scalene* muscles causing neural or arterial compression by scissoring effect.
- Now take a deep breath. This depresses the first rib. Hold breath while traction is applied to arm and feel the pulse. Loss of pulse volume or neurological signs gives a positive result.
- Reverse Adson's test: patient in same position, but patient flexes neck and rotates chin

to contralateral side to shorten the scalenes. Push down with chin against chest to contract scalenes. This may reproduce symptoms when there is scalene hypertrophy.

Advancement flaps

- A local random pattern flap where tissue is advanced to fill an adjacent defect. Examples include
- *Single pedicle:* raised as a square or rectangle with two parallel cuts along the sides of the defect. <u>*Burow's*</u> triangles are excised from the base of the flap to help advancement.
- *Bipedicled advancement flap:* useful for long defects in extremities. An incision is made parallel to the defect and the flap attached at either end is advanced. As there is a blood supply from either end a longer length to width ratio is possible. The donor defect can be grafted.
- *<u>V–Y advancement flap</u>.*
- *<u>Y–V advancement flap</u>.*

Aesthetic unit

Gonzalez-Ulloa in 1956 divided the face into regions or units to aid in the planning of reconstruction. Some principles of reconstruction by units are:

- Patients wish to look normal.
- The normal is defined by regional units, adjacent three-dimensional areas of characteristic skin quality, surface outline and contour.
- The surgeon must restore regional units not fill defects if the normal is the goal.
- The wound may need to be enlarged and normal tissue may be discarded to allow a whole subunit to be reconstructed.
- Scars are best positioned in the borders between units where they will be less apparent.
- Donor material should be chosen for similar quantity and quality.
- Restoring three-dimensional contour not just filling a hole is important for good reconstruction.

Ageing face
Chronology:

- *30s:* redundant eyelid skin, crows feet.
- *40s:* prominent nasolabial folds, forehead furrows.

- *50s:* neck rhytids, jowls.
- *60s+:* skin atrophy with increasing wrinkles.

Retaining ligaments:

- Zygomatic osteocutaneous ligaments.
- Mandibular osteocutaneous ligaments (these two are the most important).
- Platysma-auricular ligaments.
- Anterior platysma-cutaneous ligaments.

Air embolus

Air entering the circulation, usually through the veins. Complication seen in <u>*Neck dissection*</u> and neurosurgery from air entering the internal jugular vein. Air enters the heart and is compressed, rather than expelled. Air froths in the chamber and reduces cardiac output.

Treatment:

- Fill the wound with fluid to reduce further embolisms.
- Lie the patient on the side with head down and aspirate the heart directly or aspirate through a central line.

Albinism

- Characterized by the absence of melanin.
- Due to mutation of genes, which regulate melanin synthesis.
- Equal incidence in sex and race.
- Most are autosomal recessive traits.
- The skin is very sensitive to the carcinogenic action of UVB radiation.

Albright's syndrome

- Polyostotic <u>*Fibrous dysplasia*</u>.
- Pseudohypoparathyroidism.
- Autosomal dominant disorder.
- Deficiency of regulatory protein required to couple membrane receptors to adenyl cyclase.
- Present with:
  - ○ rounded low nasal bridge;
  - ○ short neck;
  - ○ cataracts;
  - ○ short metacarpals and metatarsals;
  - ○ hypocalcaemia with raised phosphate;
  - ○ pigmented skin lesions.

Alexithymia

Lack of words for mood or emotion. Seen in patients with Reflex sympathetic dystrophy (<u>*RSD*</u>).

Alginates
- Derived from seaweed.
- They contain calcium, which activates the clotting cascade when exchanged with sodium in the wound.
- They are very absorbent and become gelatinous upon absorbing moisture.
- They are used clinically for both their haemostatic and absorbent properties.
- Examples include sorbsan and kaltostat.

See Dressings.

Allen's test
- To test the integrity of arterial anastomotis between the radial and ulnar side of the hand.
- Occlude radial and ulnar artery and empty hand by making a fist.
- Release one artery, the hand should fill with blood immediately.
- A similar test can be applied to the finger to confirm the presence of two digital arteries.

Alloderm
An immunologically inert dermis derived from human cadaver.

Allodynia
Marked pain from a usually non-noxious stimulation. *See RSD.*

Alloplasts
An alloplast is a relatively inert foreign body implanted into tissue.

Advantages: No donor site morbidity, quick, unlimited supply, can be prefabricated, selected resorption.

Classification:
- Liquid or solid. The physical form determines whether it will be encapsulated or whether fibrous tissue will penetrate the implant.
- Biological or synthetic.
- Permanent or absorbable.

Properties: Ideal properties of an alloplast are:
- Inert.
- Strong.
- Ability to shape.
- Non-toxic, non-carcinogenic, non-allogenic.

- Sterile.
- Withstands stress.

Goal: To achieve the goal of reconstruction, the implant should be well covered and scars should be concealed.

Liquids:
- *Injectable collagens.*
- *Hyaluronic acid preparations.*
- *Silicone.*

Solids:
Metals:
- *Stainless steel.*
- *Vitallium.*
- *Titanium.*
- *Gold.*

Polymers:
- *Polyethylene.*
- *Polypropylene.*
- *Methylmethacrylate.*
- *Cyanoacrylates.*
- *Fluorocarbons.*

Ceramics:
- *Hydroxyapatite.*
- *Others:* calcium sulphate and calcium phosphate. *Absorbable polymers, sutures.*

Oppenheimer effect.

Fibrous tissue interface: Around an implant there is a dead space into which fibroblasts and macrophages migrate. As a result of this chronic inflammatory response, fibrous encapsulation occurs. This is termed implant bursitis.

Bonding and Osseointegration: Bonding can be mechanical or chemical. Mechanical bonding occurs when there is in-growth into a porous substance. Chemical bonding occurs by molecular adsorption and is poorly understood. Osseointegration refers to bone on an implant surface with no intervening fibrous tissue.

Carcinogenicity: Chromium and nickel are known carcinogens. There are few reports of tumours around implants. Some studies following hip implants have suggested an increase in lymphatic and haemopoietic cancers, but a decrease in breast and colon cancer.

Biomaterial failure: Due to *wear*, e.g. by abrasion and fatigue, or *corrosion*, where the implant is lost by chemical reaction.

Alopecia

- Primary excision with rotation flaps such as the <u>Ortichochea flap</u> are useful to correct defects covering 15–20% of the hair-bearing scalp.
- Also <u>Juri flaps</u>.
- <u>Tissue expansion</u>.

See <u>Hair restoration with flaps</u>. See <u>Burns reconstruction</u>.

Alveolar carcinoma

See <u>Head and neck cancer</u>.
- Third most common site.
- Usually over 50 years.
- Lower jaw is more common than upper jaw, particularly behind the bicuspid teeth.
- Less directly related to tobacco and ethanol.
- Sometimes linked to poor dental hygiene and dentures.
- Commonly present with ulcers without pain.
- Spread is initially lateral. Dental caries can be a site of invasion. If bone is invaded the neurovascular bundle (NVB) is at risk. Direct mandibular invasion is common.
- Regional node metastasis is more common with carcinoma of the lower alveolus than of the upper alveolus mainly to levels I–III.

Treatment:
- For T1N0 lesions, a localized excision with marginal mandibular resection can be accomplished through the mouth.
- More extensive lesions with more significant mandibular involvement require a lip split, cheek flap, and mandibular resection.
- In the upper jaw, a partial maxillectomy is performed through a modified Weber-Fergusson incision. With more invasive lesions that have broken into the maxillary antrum, total maxillectomy is indicated. More extensive involvement (e.g. ethmoid sinus) will require an anterior cranial fossa approach.
- If access to the neck is required for reconstruction, perform a selective neck dissection for an N0 neck. Palpable nodes make this procedure mandatory.

- Small tumours may be treated with external beam irradiation. Osteoradionecrosis may occur if larger tumours are irradiated.
- Large tumours or node positive tumours are irradiated after resection.

Results: Overall 5-year survival rate is 65%.
- *Stage I:* 78%.
- *Stage II:* 65%.
- *Stage III:* 35%.
- *Stage IV:* 15%.

Ambiguous genitalia

See <u>Embryology</u>. In cases of ambiguous genitalia, assign patients sex before the age of 2. Assess by a geneticist and paediatrician. The most common cause is congenital adrenal hyperplasia.

Female pseudohermaphroditism:
- 46XX usually with congenital adrenal hyperplasia.
- Increased androgen production due to a deficiency of the enzyme 21-hydroxylase.
- The appearance of the external genitalia varies from a mildly enlarged clitoris to a normal penis with terminal meatus.
- These children should be raised as female and can be fertile.
- Surgical correction may be necessary. Perform at 3–6 months, clitoral recession and vaginoplasty.

Male pseudohermaphroditism:
- 46XY.
- Have defects in androgen synthesis and other causes of incomplete virilization.
- It may be advisable to raise as a female as there will always be an inadequate phallus. Orchidectomy and vaginal reconstruction will be required. May be due to:
  - enzyme 5-α reductase resulting in decreased testosterone production;
  - testicular feminization syndrome, with absence of androgen receptors.

True hermaphrodite:
- 46XX or 46XY or mosaic karyotype with both testicular and ovarian tissue.
- Very rare.
- Patients have an ovary one side and a testis on the other or bilateral ovotestes.

• Raise as female as they will have an inadequate phallus. Remove the testes.

Mixed gonadal dysgenesis:
• Most have 46XY/46XO karyotype with testes on one side and streak gonad on the other.
• The normal testes has a high risk of developing gonadoblastoma.
• These patients should be raised as female. Perform gonadectomy, clitoral recession and vaginoplasty.

Pure gonadal dysgenesis:
• 45X0, 46XX or 46XY karyotype.
• Usually present with delayed adolescence.
• Bilateral streak gonads. High malignant potential and gonadectomy is recommended.

Ameloblastoma
An aggressive odontogenic tumour thought to form from ameloblasts that do not differentiate to the stage of enamel formation.

Amplitude: of tendon excursion
See _Tendon transfers_. Donor muscles should have similar excursion to that which is replaced.
• Excursion of wrist flexors and extensors is 3 cm, finger extensors is 5 cm, finger flexors is 7 cm.
• Increase amplitude of donors by tenodesis effect and by freeing fascial attachments.

Amputation – upper limb

Digital amputation: Most commonly for complex traumatic injuries. Also vascular disorders, tumours and congenital anomalies. A single finger amputation should usually be terminalized, rather than replanted. The aim is stump coverage with sensate skin and length preservation. Perform bone shortening and trim back tendons. Extensor tendons should not be sutured to flexor tendons to avoid the _Quadriga_ effect. Nerves are cut back and soft tissue opposed without tension. The retracted FDP can pull on the lumbrical giving an intrinsic plus position. This can lead to PIP joint extension with grasp. Treat by partial or complete excision of the lumbrical.

Thumb: Loss of proximal to mid-proximal phalanx results in loss of pinch. Thumb amputations should be replanted if possible though more distal than mid-proximal phalanx will get equivalent function by terminalizing.

Index ray amputation: A racquet incision is made. Divide extensors. Expose metacarpal. Preserve insertions of FCR and ECRL. Cut flexors. Divide NVBs and bury nerves. Similar technique for little finger.

3rd and 4th ray amputation: Either excise metacarpal and narrow the space or transpose ulnar metacarpals to close the cleft. Perform a dorsal longitudinal and volar Bruner incision. Remove the metacarpal and two interossei. Section the border MC and translocate to a central position. Repair deep intermetacarpal ligament.

Wrist disarticulation: Preserves normal pronation and supination 50% of which is transferred to the prosthesis. Progressively more supination and pronation is lost with more proximal amputations. A more distal prosthesis has less padding and is more of a challenge for prosthetics.

Shoulder disarticulation: Amputation through the glenohumeral joint, clavicle acromion and scapula are preserved.

Forequarter amputation: Removal of entire shoulder girdle with clavicle and scapula.

Amyotrophic lateral sclerosis (ALS)
• A type of motor neuron disease with atrophy of skeletal muscles of the body.
• Causes degeneration of motor neurons.
• Patients with ALS have weakness, atrophy and fasciculations.
• Often asymmetric.
• No loss of sensation.
• One-third of patients present with upper limb symptoms.

Anaesthesia
See _ASA classification_, _Local anaesthetics_, _Tumescent anaesthesia_.

Andre-Thomas sign
• In _Ulnar nerve palsy_.
• The deformity of clawing is made worse by an unconscious effort to extend the fingers by tenodesing the extensor tendons with palmar flexion of the wrist.

Aneurysmal bone cyst
- Blood-filled cysts lined with fleshy membrane.
- 50% occur secondary to other tumours.
- 20s–30s.
- Tendency to recur, can be aggressive.

XR: Metaphyseal expansile lesion with a thin rim of reactive bone.

Treatment is bloc bone excision and strut graft.
See *Bone tumours*.

Aneurysms – upper limb
See *Vascular injuries*.
- Most are due to trauma and infection.
- Traumatic aneurysms are most commonly found in the thenar and hypothenar eminence, and the superficial arch.
- True aneurysms contain all layers of the vessel wall. False aneurysms are pulsating haematomas and occur after penetrating injury.
- Most patients complain of a pulsatile mass. It may be difficult to distinguish from a ganglion.
- Arteriography may be useful.

Treatment: Resect and repair pseudoaneurysms. Ligation may be adequate if there is no vascular compromise.

Angel kiss
See *Nevus flammeus neonatorum*. A macular vascular birthmark seen on the upper lip, which fades spontaneously.

Angioblastoma of Nakagawa
See *Tufted angioma*.

Angiofibroma
- Skin lesions usually found on the lower central face.
- Fibrous, erythematous papule 1–3 mm in size.
- When multiple they are associated with the *Tuberous sclerosis* complex (Bourneville's disease), and occur on the cheeks and chin.
- Treatment is by dermabrasion, laser, or excision.
- Peri-ungual angiofibromas (Koenen's peri-ungual tumours) also are often present in this syndrome.

Angiogenesis
- Angiogenesis is the process of forming new blood vessels.
- Platelets secrete PDGF, which attracts macrophages and granulocytes and promotes angiogenesis.
- The macrophage plays a key role in angiogenesis by releasing a number of angiogenic substances, including tumour necrosis factor-alpha (TNF- α) and basic fibroblast growth factor (bFGF).
- *VEGF*, released by keratinocytes is also a potent stimulator of angiogenesis.
See *Wound healing*. See *Cytokines and growth factors*.

Angiosarcoma
See *Sarcoma*.
- Rare vascular neoplasm.
- Aggressive, recurs locally, spreads widely and has a high rate of vascular and lymphatic metastasis.
- 50% occur in the head and neck.
- Male:female, 8:1, elderly.
- Associated with irradiation and some environmental carcinogens.
- Soft violaceous painless compressible mass.
- Treat with wide excision and radiotherapy.

Angiosome
- Manchot studied skin territories in 1889. Salmon expanded this in 1930s, and Taylor and Palmer developed the angiosome concept in 1987.
- An angiosome is a three-dimensional composite block of skin, soft tissues and bone supplied by branches of a single source artery.
- Choke vessels link adjoining angiosomes and may regulate flow between them. The veins do not contain valves and are called oscillating veins as blood may flow in either direction.
- The *anatomic* territory is the area of tissue supplied by an artery before anastomosing with adjacent vessels.
- The *dynamic* territory of an artery is that which stains with fluoroscein.
- The *potential* territory is that which can be included if the flap is delayed.
- Flap principles are that a random flap can support one angiosome. An axial pattern

flap can support another angiosome per-fused via a choke vessel in a random cutane-ous fashion.

Anatomic concepts of blood supply developed by Taylor and Palmer:

- Blood supply detours through muscles.
- Arteries link to form continuous unbroken network.
- The intramuscular territories of arteries and veins match.
- The viability of a muscle flap is depend-ent on the size and number of its vascular territories.
- The vessels hitchhike with nerves.
- The vessels follow connective tissue framework.
- Vessels radiate from fixed to mobile areas.
- There is a direct relationship between mus-cle mobility, and the size and density of the supplying vessels.
- Vessels tend to have a constant destination, but a variable origin.
- The territory of the intramuscular arteries obeys the law of equilibrium.
- Vessel size and orientation are the product of tissue differentiation in the area.
- The muscles are the prime movers of venous return.
- As arterial territories are linked by choke vessels, so the venous territories are linked by oscillating veins, which are devoid of valves.

Angle classification

- System for describing dental occlusion in the anteroposterior plane developed by Edward Angle.
- The upper first molar is the point of refer-ence in describing the anteroposterior rela-tionship of the mandible and maxilla.
- This classification only tells of the relation-ship of mandible to maxilla. It doesn't say which is malpositioned or what the cause is.
- *Class I occlusion:* The mesiobuccal cusp of the maxillary first molar articulates within the mesiobuccal groove of the lower first molar.
- *Class II malocclusion:* the lower first molar is distal to the upper first usually ½ to a full cusp. In II1 the upper anterior teeth are

flared forward, in II2 the anterior upper and lower teeth are retruded with overbite.
- *Class III malocclusion:* the mandibular dentition is positioned mesial to maxillary dentition.

(NB Mesial means situated toward the middle of the front of the jaw along the curve of the dental arch.)

See Orthognathic surgery, Teeth.

Anterior interosseous syndrome

- Anterior interosseous nerve is a branch of the median nerve supplying FPL, FDP (index and middle) and pronator quadratus.
- Compression produces pain in the forearm and a weak pinch grip (O sign).
- Test pronator quadratus by strength of resisted forced supination with elbow flexed to eliminate humeral head of pronator teres.
- EMG may be helpful.
- Incomplete syndromes can occur.
- Distinguish from Parsonage–Turner syndrome.
- Plan to explore if there is confirmation on nerve conduction studies and if there is no improvement after 2–3 months.

Compression points:

- Fibrous bands of pronator teres muscle between the superficial and deep heads.
- FDS bands.
- Gantzer's muscle, an accessory head of FPL.
- Aberrant radial artery.
- Thrombosis of the ulnar collateral vessel.
- As a complication of forearm fracture.
- Accessory bicipital aponeurosis.
- Enlarged communicating veins.

Treatment:

- Surgical exposure as for Pronator syndrome.
- Release the deep head of pronator teres and suture the deep head to the superficial head.
- Interfascicular neurolysis of the anterior interosseus nerve 2–7.5 cm below the elbow is probably warranted if no obvious com-pression identified.

Anterolateral thigh flap

- A fasciocutaneous flap raised from the ante-rolateral aspect of the thigh.
- Supplied by musculocutaneous perfora-tors from descending branch of the lateral

circumflex femoral system through TFL and rectus femoris.

- The perforators reach the skin via intermuscular septum between vastus lateralis and rectus femoris or traverse through the muscle.
- The largest perforator reaches the deep fascia 2 cm inferolateral to the mid point of a line between the ASIS and the superolateral corner of the patella. Occasionally the descending branch is in two parts running parallel to the intermuscular septum.
- Elevate medial edge of flap and fascia. Preserve lateral cutaneous nerve of thigh. Expose the intermuscular septum and look for descending branch.
- This flap can be raised as a proximally or distally based pedicled flap or more commonly as a free flap. It can be raised below the fascia or suprafascially if a thin flap is required. Thinning of the flap has been described.

Apert's hand
See Apert's syndrome.

- All involved portions of upper limb have skeletal unions, incomplete joint segmentation and incomplete separation of rays.
- All hands have skeletal coalitions, distal bifurcation of tendons, nerves and vessels, distal intrinsic insertions and complex syndactylies.
- Shoulder and elbow synostosis may occur especially with type 1 and 2 hands. A discrepancy in size in shoulder may cause reduced ROM with growth. Most have normal elbow motion.
- Hand features are short radially deviated thumb, osseous syndactyly and symbrachydactyly of central 3 rays, simple syndactyly of 4th web and variable syndactyly of 1st web. Carpal coalitions occur, particularly between capitate and hamate, and 4th and 5th metacarpal.
- Ideally treatment is performed bilaterally between 4–12 months of age. Earlier treatment leads to relapse.
- Ideally perform two bilateral releases before the age of 2, mobilize 5th ray, and lengthen and realign thumb when 4–6 years.

Classification: Upton.
- *Type I:* spade hand. Complex syndactyly of digits 2–5 with the thumb and little fingers free.
- *Type II:* spoon or mitten hand. Complex syndactyly of digits 2–5 with simple syndactyly of thumbs or thumbs free.
- *Type III:* rosebud hand. All 5 digits involved in complex syndactyly.
See Apert's syndrome.

Type I:
- Least severe and most common.
- Thumb radial clinodactyly and shallow web.
- Side to side fusion of fingers 2–4 with phalangeal fusion at DIPJ, spade hand.
- Simple syndactyly of 4th and 5th finger.
- Mobile MPJs, stiff IPJs.

Treatment:
- 4–12 months separate index and 5th finger, after 6/12 separate 3rd web. Division of transverse metacarpal ligaments will increase mobility.
- Get frequent tendon, nerve and vessel anomalies.
- Perform osteotomies, which may be through cartilaginous bars of IPJs at time of releases.
- Age 3–5, correct thumb clinodactyly with opening-wedge osteotomy through middle of proximal phalanx. Use bone from iliac crest. Release 4–5th metacarpal synostosis with interposition of dermal graft.

Type II:
- Thumb joined to index in complete simple syndactyly, but have separate nails.
- Central palm gives concave palm, mitten or spoon hand. Conjoined nail. Abnormalies of index proximal phalanx.
- Complete syndacyly between 4th and 5th fingers.

Treatment:
- Release 2nd and 4th web at the same time as 1st web. Need to excise fascial bands between thumb and index.
- If not too tight use 4-flap Z-plasty, otherwise use Y-V. Perform capsulotomy of CMCJ.
- If index finger proximal phalanx is abnormal and radially deviated it may be better to ablate early.

- Later correction of thumb clinodactyly as for type I

Type III:
- Most severe, least common.
- Tight osseous and cartilaginous union between fingers 1–4 with single conjoined nail with index and thumb being indistinguishable, hoof or rosebud hand.
- Thumb radial clinodactyly less severe, but thumb is smaller.

Treatment:
- Perform index ray resection at time of 1st web release. Use dorsal advancement flap, and re-advance with subsequent procedures. Release 4th web at the same time.
- At time of 1st web release perform osteotomy across DIPJs with a transverse K wire, which converts this to a type I hand.

Apert's syndrome

Acrocephalosyndactyly with bicoronal synostosis, Midface hypoplasia, cleft palate, and complex syndactyly. *See Apert's hand.*
- Most are sporadic, but also autosomal dominant inheritance.
- Mutation in *Fibroblast growth factor receptor* 2 (FGFR2).
- Incidence is 1/160 000 live births.
- Only the lambdoidal suture is present. The coronal suture is absent. Possibly primary cranial base synostosis delays the approximation of bones and suture induction doesn't occur.
- The face has a steep forehead and a groove above the supra-orbital ridge. Orbits are shallow with hypertelorism and down slanting of palpebral fissures.
- The mid-third of the face is hypoplastic with a normal mandible.
- The nose is beaked.
- Decreased patency of posterior nasal choanae may result in obstructive apnoea.
- 30% have a cleft palate or uvula.
- Mental retardation is frequent.
- Mirror image abnormalities of hands and feet with an inverse relationship between the severity of craniofacial abnormality and the severity of hand anomalies.
- Syndactyly of fingers 2, 3 and 4 is present and the whole hand may be fused. If the

thumb is free, it is broad and radially deviated. The feet are similarly involved. Acrosyndactyly of hands graded from I–III with increasing severity.
  - *Class* 1: the little finger and thumb are separate;
  - *Class 2:* only the thumb is free;
  - *Class 3:* the whole hand is involved.

See Craniosynostosis.

Aplasia cutis congenita

- Rare, sporadic congenital deformity most often in first-born females.
- Get failure of differentiation of skin ranging from total absence of skin, fat, skull, dura and occasionally underlying brain. Scalp is involved in 60% of cases and ulcers may be multiple.
- Mostly occurs in the midline in the area of the posterior fontanelle.
- Ulcers are sharply marginated with a red base and usually heal rapidly by secondary intention.

Aetiology: May be chromosomal, placental infarcts, amniotic adhesions or pressure necrosis. Also associated with hydrocephalus, facial clefts and spina bifida.

Management:
- May heal with dressings, which should be kept moist.
- For large defects with exposed brain, dura or skull, provide soft tissue cover and reconstruct bone later.
- Use local flaps and possibly tissue expansion. *See Scalp reconstruction.*

Apocrine cystadenoma

- A small, benign, translucent nodule, usually appearing on the face.
- Often pigmented and may contain brownish fluid.
- It may be confused with melanoma or pigmented basal cell naevus.

Apocrine glands

- *Sweat glands* found in axilla and groin.
- They start to function in puberty and give an odour due to bacterial decomposition.
- They have a sympathetic adrenergic nerve supply.

Apocrine tumours
See Apocrine cystadenoma, Syringocystadenoma papilliferum, Chondroid syringoma.

Arachnodactyly
Unusually long slender fingers.

Arcade of Frohse
See Radial tunnel syndrome. A fibrous band on the surface of supinator. One of the structures implicated in compression of the radial nerve at the elbow.

Arcade of Struthers
See Cubital tunnel syndrome. Fascial band above elbow.

Arnez and Tyler classification
Classification for *Degloving injuries.*
- *Type 1:* non-circumferential degloving.
- *Type 2:* abrasion, but no degloving.
- *Type 3:* circumferential degloving.
- *Type 4:* circumferential degloving plus avulsion between deep tissue planes. Requires serial conservative debridement and delayed reconstruction.

Arteriovenous fistulae
Rare in the upper extremity with the exception of high flow *AV malformations* and surgically made AV fistulae. High output failure rarely occurs distal to the elbow. Most become manifest in the first 10 years of life. Most traumatic fistulae are due to penetrating *Vascular injuries.* An arteriogram will help guide treatment. Fistulae with bony involvement are poorly controlled by excision. Diffuse digital masses respond poorly to simple excision. Amputation may be required.

Arteriovenous malformations
- These are the most difficult *Vascular malformations* to treat.
- They can be high flow and haemodynamically active.
- Pure arterial malformations such as aneurysms are rare but they can occur with AVMs.
- The epicentre of an AVM is called the nidus and consists of arterial feeders, micro- and macro-arteriovenous fistulas (AVFs), and enlarged veins.

- AVM is present at birth and can either manifest in infancy, or appear later.
- Intracranial AVM is more common than extracranial AVM, followed in frequency by AVM of the limbs, trunk, and viscera.
- Some may be hormonally active. The fast-flow nature may not be recognized until trauma or puberty stimulate expansion.
- AVMs develop ischaemic skin changes, ulceration, intractable pain, and intermittent bleeding. Low-flow lesions may be associated with skeletal hypertrophy, high-flow with destruction. May present as emergency with haemorrhage or cardiac failure.

Staging: Clinically by Schobinger;
- *Stage I:* blush/stain, warmth and AV shunting.
- *Stage II:* stage I with enlargement, tortuous veins, pulsations, thrill and bruit.
- *Stage III:* stage II with either dystrophic changes, ulceration, bleeding, persistent pain or destruction.
- *Stage IV:* stage II with cardiac failure.

Treatment: See Vascular malformations.

Arthrgryposis
- Greek meaning curved joint.
- Many causes but all have in common immobility of the joints *in utero.*
- This may be due to abnormal muscles, abnormal neurology or crowding due to oligohydramnios, bicornuate uterus etc. *Beal's syndrome* is a contractural arachnodactyly.
- *Findings:* contractures, usually bilateral, adduction and internal rotation of shoulders, fixed flexion or extension of elbows and knees. Club-like hands and wrists, thin waxy skin.
- *Treatment:* dynamic and static splintage, occasionally surgery.

See Congenital hand anomalies.

Arthrodesis hand
Wrist:
- For pain, reconstruction following tumour resection, instability.
- Remove all articular surface, maintain carpal alignment and height, use internal fixation, bone graft and splint until radiological union.

- Optimal position is 15° extension 5° ulnar deviation. If both wrists are being fused place dominant hand in extension and non-dominant in flexion for personal hygiene.
- Use bone graft, bone blocks, intramedullary rods, interosseous wires, external fixators and dorsal plates.

See Proximal row carpectomy.

Limited fusions:

- *Triscaphe arthrodesis (STT):* for rotary subluxation of the scaphoid, non-union, Kienböcks, triscaphe arthritis, DISI.
- *Lunotriquetral arthrodesis:* for lunotriquetral ligament tears and instability.
- *Capitolunate arthrodesis:* mid-carpal degenerative arthritis.
- *Scaphocapitate arthrodesis:* for rotary subluxation of the scaphoid, *Kienböcks*, midcarpal instability.
- *Capitate-lunate-hamate-triquetral (four corner):* for ulnar mid-carpal instability, SLAC, scaphoid non-union.

Fusion across radio-carpal joint gives the greatest loss of movement. A single row fusion gives the least loss of motion.

Small joint arthrodesis:

- *Indications:* pain, instability, deformity and loss of neuromuscular control.
- *Position:* individualize to particular patient.
  - MCP joints cascade radial to ulnar, 25° for the index and add 5° for each digit;
  - PIPJ cascade from 40° in index to 55°;
  - DIPJ fuse in 0° flexion, possibly 5-10° supination for index and middle to achieve pinch grip;
  - thumb, keep length. IPJ fuse in slight flexion (recommended between 0–15°). MPJ 5–15°. CMC fuse with 40° palmar abduction and 20° of radial abduction.
- *Surface preparation:*
  - avoid shortening;
  - cup and cone method enables accurate positioning;
  - remove all the articular cartilage.
- *Fixation:*
  - K wires: crossed;
  - Interosseous wiring: stronger than K wires;
  - Tension band wiring: use for MCP joints and pip joints. Compression is produced by the dorsally placed tension band.

DIPJ: Approach through H incision. Section extensor tension. Flex joint and excise collateral ligaments to increase exposure. Fix with either Herbert screw or interosseous wire and oblique K wire. For the IPJ can use 90-90 wires or if bone stock poor use K wire.

PIPJ: Dorsal longitudinal incision. Split extensor tendon and elevate to either side. Cut central tendon and collaterals. Use 90-90 or tension band wiring.

MPJ: Expose through longitudinal incision in skin and on radial side of finger. Excise collaterals. Fix with mini plate.

Arthroplasty

- *Wrist:* inflammatory, degenerative and post-traumatic arthritis. Arthroplasty most commonly performed in RA. Contraindicated if there are poor wrist motors.
- *PIP joint:* silicone implant arthroplasty may be performed through a palmar, lateral or dorsal approach. For a dorsal approach the extensor mechanism is opened. Collateral ligaments and volar plate are released. The articular surfaces are removed, osteophytes are removed, the medullary canal reamed and the implant inserted. Repair the collateral ligament. Commence active motion immediately. Protect finger from lateral stress.
- *MCP joint: Swanson's arthroplasty.*

Arthroscopy – wrist

Indications: Diagnose and treat pain, tears of ligaments and TFCC. Remove loose bodies.

Portals:

- Named by the extensor compartments, e.g. 3–4 portal is between 3rd and 4th dorsal compartment.
- The 5 used are 1–2, 3–4, 4–5, 6R and 6U – radial and ulna to FCU.
- 3–4 and 4–5 most commonly used, the former for visualization and the latter for instrumentation.
- With 1–2 the nerve and artery are at risk. With 6U dorsal branch of ulnar nerve at risk
- Some surgeons pre-inflate the joint. Lunotriquetral ligament is best seen through 6R.

- *Mid-carpal joint:* three mid-carpal portals – mid-carpal radial (MCR), ulnar (MCU) and scaphotrapeziotrapezoid (STT).

ASA classification
Classification adopted by the American Society of Anaesthesiologists for assessing preoperative physical status.
- *I:* healthy.
- *II:* mild systemic disease.
- *III:* moderate systemic disease, some functional limitation.
- *IV:* severe systemic disease, constant threat to life.
- *V:* moribund patient, unlikely to survive 24 hours.

Aspergillosis
- An opportunistic fungal infection seen in immunocompromised patients, e.g. aplastic anaemia, leukaemia and major burns.
- It is not seen in healthy individuals.
- Invasive aspergillosis usually requires surgical debridement in addition to anti-fungal agents to eradicate infection.
See Fungal hand infections.

Aspirin
- Has an inhibitory effect on platelet aggregation.
- Cyclo-oxygenase is acetylated, which blocks thromboxane A2 production.
See Microsurgery.

Atasoy volar V–Y flap:
- Used in the treatment of *Fingertip injuries.*
- Volar Y–V flap taken from defect down to DIP joint.
- Raise with NVB and free fibrous septa. Tension free closure.
- Also known as Tranquilli–Leali flap.

Ataxia-telangiectasia
See Louis–Bar Syndrome.

ATLS
Advanced Trauma Life Support
A system of trauma care that involves systematic prioritized evaluation and treatment aimed specifically at preventing deaths in the 2nd peak (minutes to hours after trauma) and

minimizing morbidity and mortality in the 3rd peak (days–weeks) by optimizing initial trauma care.
- Prehospital management.
- Triage
- Primary survey:
  - *A:* airway and cervical spine control;
  - *B:* breathing and ventilation;
  - *C:* circulation haemorrhage control;
  - *D:* disability; AVPU – Alert, Vocal stimulus, Painful stimulus, Unresponsive;
  - *E:* exposure and environmental control.
- Resuscitation and repeat primary survey until stabilized.
- Secondary survey.
- Post-resuscitation monitoring.
- Definitive care.

Atypical fibroxanthoma
- A small, firm nodule with crusting. Similar in appearance to a BCC.
- Occurs in the elderly on the head and neck.
- Histologically see atypical spindle and giant cells with a lot of mitoses.
- Treat with simple excision and it rarely recurs.
- If it invades deeply it is called a *Malignant fibrous histiocytoma* and can resemble basal cell epithelioma. Appears on chronically sun-exposed parts of the head and neck, particularly in the pre-auricular area in older persons.
See Pseudosarcomatous lesions.

Axial flaps
A flap raised with a known vessel that increases the length to width ratio available.
- *Direct:* contain a named artery in the subcutaneous tissues. Examples include the *Groin flap* and *Deltopectoral flap.* They may include a random element in the distal portion.
- *Fasciocutaneous flap:* based on vessels running within or near the fascia.
- *Musculocutaneous flaps.*
- *Venous flaps:*

Axilla
Boundaries:
- *Anterior:* pectoralis major, subclavius, pectoralis minor.
- *Posterior:* subscapularis, lat dorsi, teres major.

- *Medial:* 4–5 ribs, serratus anterior.
- *Lateral:* coracobrachialis and biceps.

Nerves:
- *Intercostobrachial nerve:* sensory innervation to upper medial arm.
- *Long thoracic nerve:* to serratus anterior. From C5,6,7. Division cause winging of the scapula.
- *Thoracodorsal nerve:* from posterior cord to lat dorsi.
- *Medial pectoral nerve:* pectoralis major and often wraps around the lateral border of pectoralis minor.

Axillary dissection

Three levels of axillary nodes:
- *I:* lateral to lateral border of pectoralis minor.
- *II:* under pectoralis minor.
- *III:* medial to pectoralis minor muscle.

Make inverted U incision in axilla. Raise skin flaps and stitch back. Define borders of axilla anteriorly and posteriorly. Leave fascia on muscle. Find and preserve long thoracic nerve and NVB to lat dorsi. Having identified these structures and axillary vein, start distally and work proximally from an anterior and posterior front to converge on axillary vein and continue up behind pectoralis minor. Anatomy of axilla.

Axillary nerve

C5, C6 roots from the posterior cord. Supplies deltoid and teres minor.

Axonotmesis

Axonal damage with Wallerian degeneration. *See Seddon classification.*

B Bactigras to Byrd and Spicer classification of fractures

Bactigras

Paraffin gauze impregnated with chlorhexidine.
See Dressings.

Bakamjian

1965: Described the deltopectoral flap.

Baker classification

Classification of capsular contracture (1975).
- *I:* soft.
- *II:* minimal, implant palpable not visible.
- *III:* moderate, palpable and visible.
- *IV:* severe, hard, painful with distortion.
See Breast augmentation, Breast implants.

Balanitis xerotica obliterans (BXO)

- Male genital form of *lichen sclerosis,* which is a chronic, progressive, sclerosing inflammatory dermatosis of unclear aetiology.
- Chronic BXO predisposes to SCC.
- There may be a viral association and HLA association.
- Increased in obese patients.

- Dyskaryosis and inflammatory changes in the early stages lead to fibrosis and skin atrophy.
- The prepuce becomes adherent to the glans with a white stenosing band at the end of the foreskin and a haemorrhagic response to minor trauma leading to phimosis and stenosis.

Treatment:
- Steroid creams for early disease in children.
- Circumcision, meatoplasty.
- Excise advanced disease and apply a buccal mucosal graft in which BXO does not recur.

Balding

See Hair restoration with flaps.

Bannayan syndrome

Microcephaly, multiple vascular malformations and multiple lipomas.

Basal cell carcinoma

- 95% of BCCs occur between 40–80 years, 85% in the head and neck.

- It is the most common malignancy in Caucasians.
- BCCs arise from pluripotential cells of the basal layer of the epithelium or pilosebaceous follicles.
- Directly related to sun exposure.
- Almost never metastasize.

Carcinogens:
- *Ultraviolet radiation (UV).*
- *Ionizing radiation.*
- *Chemicals:* arsenic, psoralens, nitrogen mustard and atmospheric pollutants have been implicated.

Inherited conditions:
- *Xeroderma pigmentosa.*
- *Gorlins syndrome.*
- *Albinism* with increased risk of BCC and SCC.
- *Epidermodysplasia verruciformis.*
- *Muir–Torre syndrome.*
- *Porokeratosis.*
- *Bazex–Dupre–Christol syndrome.*

Types:
- *Nodular:* most common. Usually single on face. Translucent papules. Grow slowly and ulcerate.
- *Superficial:* often multiple, usually trunk, erythematous, scaly.
- *Infiltrative:* also morphoeic, yellow-white, morpheaform, and ill-defined borders. More often recur.
- *Pigmented:* like nodular with pigment.
- *Trabecular: See Merkel cell tumour.*
- *Adnexal:* arise from sebaceous sweat glands. Uncommon and appear as solitary tumours in older patients. No particular features, grow slowly, tend to recur locally and metastasize regionally.

Histology:
- Oval cells with deeply staining nuclei and scant cytoplasm.
- Irregular masses of basaloid cells in the dermis, with the outermost cells forming a pallisading layer on the periphery.
- A fibrous reaction in the surrounding stroma.
- 95% are attached to the epidermis, the rest are attached to a hair follicle.

- *Broder's classification.*

Treatment:
- Surgery:
  - excise with 2–3 mm margin, wider if indistinct;
  - 5% are incompletely excised;
  - Treatment of incomplete excision is controversial between authors; some advise all to be re-excised, others suggest observation as 2/3 don't recur; other than surgery, can use.
- *Radiotherapy.*
- Photodynamic therapy.
- Cryotherapy.
- Curettage.
- *Moh's* micrographic surgery.
- Intralesional interferon or BCG vaccine.

Recurrence: 36% of patients with a BCC develop a second primary within 5 years.
See *Squamous cell carcinoma*. See *Naevus sebaceous.*

Basal osteotomy
For 1st *CMC joint OA.*
- Can provide good stable pain free CMC movement.
- Closing wedge osteotomy.
- 4-cm incision centred on prominence of 1st CMC joint in line with shaft. Retract EPL, expose proximal third of metacarpal.
- Site of osteotomy should be 1 cm from joint. Strip periosteum circumferentially and insert levers. Mark osteotomy – 5 mm wide for 20–30° abduction.
- Wide part of wedge is directed so as to cause abduction on closing the wedge, insert interosseous wire.
- Excise bone wedge keeping far cortex intact. Close wedge. Insert wire and plaster in corrected position for 6/52 (*Journal of Bone and Joint Surgery* 1983;65:179).

Bayne and Klug classification of radial dysplasia
- *I:* short radius.
- *II:* hypoplastic radius.
- *III:* partial absence of radius.
- *IV:* total absence of radius.
See Radial club hand.

Bazex–Dupre–Christol syndrome

- X-linked disorder.
- Follicular atrophoderma, congenital hypotrichiosis, basal cell naevi and _Basal cell carcinomas_.

Beal's syndrome

Contractural arachnodactyly syndrome. Initially thought to be _Marfan's_ with _Arthrgryposis_.

BEAM

Bulbar Elongation and Anastomotic Meatoplasty.

- One stage treatment for _Hypospadias_.
- The whole length of urethra is dissected and advanced to lie at the level of the normal meatus.
- Up to 5 cm advancement can be achieved.

Bean syndrome

See _Blue rubber bleb syndrome_.

Becker's flap

- Based on a fairly constant dorsal branch of the ulnar artery supplying the dorsal ulnar border of the forearm.
- It pierces the deep fascia a few centimetres proximal to the pisiform so it can be used as a distal island flap without sacrificing the ulnar artery.

Becker's naevi

- Acquired pigmented patches.
- Incidence of 1:200, M:F 5:1.
- Appears in adolescence, exaggerated by sunshine.
- Occurs on the upper trunk and arms.
- It gradually spreads, and becomes darker and hairy with acne lesions within it. The melanocytes are excessively active and the epidermis is thickened with enlarged sebaceous glands.
- Q-switched ruby (694 nm) and pulsed dye _Lasers_ (510 nm) may be effective.

See _Naevus_.

Beds – for pressure sores

- Patients are assessed for the risk of developing a pressure sore by using the _Waterlow score_.
- _10+ risk:_ foam mattress such as soft foam premier which contains a contoured insert pad.

- _15+ risk:_ alpha excel has an overlay pressure-relieving mattress.
- _20+:_
  - _dynamic floatation:_ Nimbus 3;
  - _alternating pressure system:_ Pegasus;
  - _air fluidized bead bed:_ Clinitron;
  - _low air loss:_ mediscus, cells inflate and deflate independently.

Belfast regime

- A regime of early active mobilization after flexor tendon repair.
- A dorsal splint is worn, which leaves the fingers free to flex.
- The wrist is held between neutral and 30° flexion. MCP extension limited to 70° flexion. Hyperextension of IPJs is prevented beyond neutral.
- Active mobilization consists of:
  - passive flexion;
  - passive flexion and hold, to maintain muscle function;
  - active flexion, to create tendon glide and limit adhesions.

See _Tendon, Flexor_ repair.

Bell's palsy

- Paralysis of the facial nerve.
- Described by Charles Bell in 1814.
- Originally referred to facial nerve paralysis from any cause.
- Now refers to idiopathic facial nerve paralysis.
- A diagnosis of exclusion.
- It may be a viral infection with swelling of the nerve in the tight intratemporal course.
- 80% recover full function, which begins within 4 weeks.

See _Facial nerve_

Bell's phenomenon

- Upward movement of eye with closure of eyelid.
- Test by holding upper lid open, while patient attempts gentle closure of the eye.

See _Ptosis_.

Below knee amputation

See _Skew flap_, _Long posterior flap_.

Benelli mastopexy

- Treatment for mastopexy with excision of peri-areolar skin.
- Concentric skin excision around the areolar, which moves the nipple superiorly. Dimensions may be up to 14 cm vertically and 12 cm horizontally.
- Breast may be sutured to periosteum and crisscross flaps may help increase projection.
- Tendency for the scar to stretch is combated with a non-absorbable purse string suture, as well as nylon cross sutures to reduce areolar herniation.
- It may help in the constricted or tuberose breast with mild to moderate laxity.
- Three problems may occur:
  - ○ the areola may enlarge;
  - ○ the scar may be hypertrophic;
  - ○ breast contour may be flattened.

See Mastopexy.

Bennet's fracture

Intra-articular fracture-subluxation of base of thumb metacarpal. Oblique fracture through volar beak, which is held by beak ligament. APL pulls metacarpus radially causing subluxation. Reverse Bennet's fracture occurs in the base of the 5th metacarpal.

Bernard operation

- Used for Lip reconstruction with significant-sized defects.
- Advances full thickness flaps with triangular excision to allow proper mobilization.
- May have diminished sensation and mobility which may be lessened in Webster modification.

Biers block

- Intravenous regional anaesthesia which lasts 90 minutes.
- Cannula placed in arm which is exsanguinated and a tourniquet applied.
- 4–6 mg/kg of 0.5% lignocaine without adrenaline (not bupivicaine, which is cardiotoxic) is injected slowly.
- The tourniquet should be on for at least 25 minutes to reduce the risk of generalized spread of lignocaine.
- If tourniquet pain is a problem, inflate a second more distal.

Bilhaut–Cloquet operation

- Used to correct distal Thumb duplication.
- Both elements of the duplicated thumb are reduced and joined.
- Nails are removed, the outer segments approximated and the nail bed repaired.
- It can be modified by taking unequal portions of each finger. This avoids the central longitudinal nail bed repair and reduces the risk of susequent nail irregularities.

Bilobed flap

- A transposition flap with 2 lobes 50° apart.
- The first lobe is the same size as the defect and the second is half the size. The defect left by the second lobe is closed directly. The angle of rotation of each flap should be 50°.

Principles:

- No more than 50° for each lobe.
- Excise a triangle of dog-ear between defect and flap pivot point before the flap is rotated.
- Make the first lobe the same size and thickness as the defect and undermine to enable it to inset without pin-cushioning.
- For the nose it can be used for a defect up to 1.5 cm.

See Nasal reconstruction.

Binder's syndrome

- A congenital malformation with nasomaxillary hypoplasia.
- M = F, most sporadic but there may be a hereditary component.
- It may be due to an inhibition of the ossification centre that would have formed the lateral and inferior borders of the piriform apertures.
- The nose appears pushed in with malocclusion.

Treatment:

- Le Fort 3 osteotomies with advancement of maxilla until teeth occlude.
- Gaps are filled with bone chips.
- Augmentation rhinoplasty with costal cartilage grafts can be performed.

Biobrane

- A dressing used for partial thickness wounds.
- A bilaminate semi-permeable silicone membrane bonded to a thin layer of nylon fabric

which is bound to modified porcine dermal collagen.

- It is available as a glove, which allows active movement during healing.
- It can't be used for deeper or full thickness wounds.

Biological skin substitutes

- Allograft: _Cadaver skin_.
- _Xenograft_: pigskin. Less expensive, doesn't last as long, and doesn't cause wound bed vascularization.
- _Biobrane_.
- _Human amniotic membrane_.
- _Transcyte_.
- _Integra_.

See _Burns_. See _Transplant immunology_.

Biomaterials
See _Alloplasts_.

Bites

- _Human:_ aerobic pathogens include _Staph. aureus_ and epidermidis, and _Strep._ Anaerobic bacteria include _Peptostrep. peptococci_, _Eikenella corodens_ and bacteroides.
- _Animal:_ dogs and cats also have _Pasteurella multocida_. Only 20% of dog bites get infected, whereas 80% of cat bites get infected due to the depth of the wound.

Blauth classification for thumb hypoplasia
See _Thumb hypoplasia_.

Blauth and Gekeler classification of symbrachydactyly

- _Short finger:_ four short stiff coalesced fingers, normal thumb.
- _Oligodactylic:_ central aplasia and cleft.
- _Monodactylic:_ aplasia of all fingers, thumb preserved.
- _Peromelic:_ transverse absence of all digits at metacarpal level.

See _Symbrachydactyly_.

Blepharochalasis

- A rare inherited condition with recurrent episodes of eyelid oedema.
- This results in ptosis due to an attenuated levator aponeurosis.

- Eyelid skin remains excessive.
- The term _Dermatochalasis_ should be used for involutional skin excess.

Blepharomelasma
Dark discolouration of eyelid skin.
See _Blepharoplasty_.

Blepharopachynsis
Thickening of eyelid skin.
See _Blepharoplasty_.

Blepharophimosis
Congenitally small palpebral fissures caused by a triad of _Ptosis_, _Epicanthal folds_ and _Telecanthus_.
See _Ptosis – eyelid_.

Blepharoplasty
The procedure to shape the appearance of the eyelids and create lid creases. Usually skin, some muscle and excessive orbital fat is removed.

Assessment: Ask whether the patient wears contact lenses, suffers from dry eyes or diplopia.

Examination: Assess position of the eyebrow, eyelid pathology, fat pads, lagophthalmos, position of eyelid in relation to the eye.

- Tests:
  - _compensated brow ptosis:_ as the patient opens the eyes the eyebrow moves up;
  - _snap test:_ distract eyelid, >1 second to return is abnormal;
  - _distraction test:_ lax if the lower lid can be pulled more than 7 mm from the globe;
  - _fat pads:_ push on globe and look for herniation;
  - lateral herniation may be lacrimal gland;
  - _Bell's phenomenom_;
  - _enopthalmos:_ look at position of globe from above;
  - visual fields;
  - visual acuity.

Operation:

- _Upper blepharoplasty:_ while patient is supine design upper eyelid incisions. Elevate the eyebrow manually. Make caudal incision first. In the crease in younger patients, 1 mm above in older patients. Gently stretch the skin. Pinch the skin and mark the upper incision. Extend the upper mark laterally and medially.

Examine and mark the fat pads. Excise skin with orbicularis if required. Incise orbital septum to expose the pre-aponeurotic fat pad and remove with careful haemostasis. Inject with local anaesthetic to reduce the oculocardiac reflex. If the lacrimal gland is prominent it may need to be elevated. A lateral canthopexy may be required.

- *Lower blepharoplasty:* incise just inferior to the lid margin. Stop before the punctum. Dissect orbicularis leaving the pretarsal portion attached to the tarsus. Continue submuscularly until the orbital rim is reached. Here, incise septum to expose and remove the fat. Gently press the globe to asses the amount of fat excess. Drape the skin back and pull downwards to simulate gravity. Excise 2–3 mm skin with orbicularis.
- *Transconjunctival lower blepharoplasty:* this enables fat pads to be excised without an external incision. Skin excess may be address with laser resurfacing.
- *Compensated brow ptosis:* If the resting position of the brow has dropped, frontalis contracts to elevate brow and lid. Lid resection allows relaxation of frontalis and the position of the eyelid remains unchanged. A brow lift may be required prior to performing a blepharoplasty.

Complications:
- *Immediate:*
  - loss of vision;
  - retrobulbar haematoma – if this occurs decompress as an emergency; acetazolamide and mannitol can be given;
  - injury to inferior oblique muscle;
  - wound dehiscence.
- *Late:*
  - over or under correction;
  - dry eye syndrome;
  - epiphora,

Blepharoptosis
Drooping of the upper lid.
See *Ptosis – eyelid*.

Blisters – in burns
The management of burns blisters is controversial. Some advocate leaving blisters intact to provide sterile wound coverage. However, blisters are rich in prostaglandins, particularly thromboxane, which may increase burn wound depth by increasing the zone of stasis.

Blood flow
Muscular tone of vessels is controlled by:
- *Sympathetic nerve supply:* these regulate flow by:
  - increasing arteriolar tone and precapillary sphincter tone which decreases blood flow;
  - decreasing AVA tone enabling blood to bypass the capillary bed.
- *Pressure:* an increase in intraluminal pressure results in vasoconstriction and a decrease causes vasodilatation. This is the explanation for hyperaemia after releasing the tourniquet.
- *Humeral factors:*
  - adrenaline and noradrenaline cause vasoconstriction;
  - histamine and bradykinin cause vasodilatation;
  - low O_2, high CO_2 and acidosis result in vasodilatation.
- *Temperature:* increase in temperature produces cutaneous vasodilatation and flow, which bypasses the capillary beds.

Blood supply to skin
Six layers of vascular plexuses
- *Subfascial plexus:* small plexus under the fascia.
- *Prefascial plexus:* larger plexus, prominent on limbs, predominantly supplied by fasciocutaneous vessels.
- *Subcutaneous plexus:* in superficial fascia. Predominant in torso, supplied by musculocutaneous vessels.
- *Subdermal plexus:* main plexus supplying skin.
- *Dermal plexus:* arterioles, important for thermoregulation.
- *Subepidermal plexus:* contains small vessels without muscles. Predominantly nutritive and thermoregulatory.

Blood supply to upper limb
- *Radial artery*.
- *Ulnar artery*.
- *Dorsal carpal arch*.

- *Superficial palmar arch*.
- *Deep palmar arch*.

Blood vessels
Anatomy:
- The inner layer consists of basement membrane with endothelial cells sitting on it.
- The next layer is the intima composed of elastin.
- Next is the media made of collagen and smooth muscles.
- The outer layer is the adventitia with the vasa vasorum.

Injury and repair:
- After injury endothelium is regenerated from endothelial cells from the edge.
- At an anastomosis get healing of all layers.
- Initially platelets aggregate on exposed collagen, but by the end of a week the endothelium proliferates and sutures are covered by 2 weeks.

Blue naevus
- Round, solitary bluish naevus.
- Found on dorsum of extremities or buttocks and often present at birth.
- Female: Male 2:1.
- Very low malignant potential.
- Due to arrested migration of melanocytes bound for the dermo-epidermal junction.
- Naevus of Ota occurs in area of 1st and 2nd trigeminal nerve.
- Naevus of Ito occurs in the dermatome of the upper chest.
- Current treatment is excision though lasers should be effective.

See *Naevus*. See naevus of *Ota* and *Ito*.

Blue rubber bleb nevus
- Sporadic combination of cutaneous and visceral VMs.
- The skin lesions are soft, blue and nodular; they can occur anywhere, but are typically located on the hands and feet.
- The gastrointestinal lesions are best seen by endoscopy.
- Recurrent intestinal bleeding can be severe, requiring repeated transfusions.

See *Venous malformations* (Bean syndrome).

Body dysmorphic disorder (BDD)
- Preoccupation with an imagined defect in one's appearance.
- If a physical anomaly is present, the person's concern is markedly excessive. Patients with BDD have a high risk of committing suicide.
- The most common preoccupation is with the nose.
- Surgery tends to increase the preoccupation and the dissatisfaction.
- Patients turned down for surgery may attempt DIY surgery.
- BDD begins in adolescence.
- Men and women show differing concerns for different body parts.

See *Psychology and plastic surgery*.

Body Mass Index (BMI)
Measured by body wt (kg) divided by height^2 (m)

- Normal   20–25 kg/m^2
- Overweight   25–30 kg/m^2
- Obese   30–35 kg/m^2
- Morbidly obese   35–55 kg/m^2
- Super morbidly obese   >55 kg/m^2

See *Obesity*.

Bolan case
Bolan versus Freean Hospital Management Committee 1957: by this ruling, doctors defending negligence actions could rely on evidence of opinion from colleagues to justify their actions even if there is a body of opinion that would take the contrary view.

- 'I myself would prefer to put it this way, that he is not guilty of negligence if he has acted in accordance with a practice accepted as proper by a responsible body of medical men skilled in that particular art ... Putting it the other way round, a man is not negligent, if he is acting in accordance with such a practice, merely because there is a body of opinion who would take a contrary view.'

See *Ethics*.

Bolitho case
Bolitho versus city and Hackney Health Authority, 1997. Based on a case of a child admitted for observation with respiratory difficulties.

The registrar did not come when called and the medical experts were divided on whether it would have made any difference.

- *Basic premise:* the body of opinion relied upon must be logical, and the judge must be satisfied that the experts have considered the question of comparative risks and benefits, and reached a defensible conclusion.
- *In other words:* it is no longer enough for the defence to put up experts to say they genuinely believe a doctor's actions conformed with accepted practice. The defence now has to show a logical basis for the opinion.

See Ethics.

Bone

To maintain function, bone must regenerate.

Anatomy: Bone is generated by osteoblasts. They are surrounded by their matrix and they are trapped. Once trapped they become smaller and become osteocytes.

- *Enchondral* bone (long bones) starts as cartilage, which ossifies.
- *Membranous* bones in the facial skeleton lay down bone directly. Membranous bones are more vascular but less strong.
- *Cortical* bone has concentric lamellae around Haversian canals containing blood vessels.
- *Cancellous* bone has large and small units of bone – trabeculae and spicules. Also have osteocytes, though not as compact as cortical bone. Bone is only 8% water. The matrix is 98% collagen (type I).
- *Blood supply:* of long bones from a primary nutrient artery, proximal and distal metaphyseal vessels and the periosteum. Though the endosteal circulation is dominant in undisplaced fractures, in displaced fractures, the main blood supply is derived from the periosteum.

Healing:

- *Primary healing:* if bone is rigidly fixed. Get restoration of normal bone structure without the inflammatory and proliferative phase. Callus is not formed. Osteoclasts first cross the fracture line followed by osteoblasts.
- *Secondary healing:* occurs if fragments are not rigidly fixed or if there is a gap. If the fracture is widely displaced or mobile then scar tissue bridges the gap forming a non-union.

In more favourable conditions, new bone formation occurs.

Phases of healing:

- *Haematoma*
- *Inflammation*: osteoclasts remove debris. Associated with pain.
- *Cellular proliferation:* periosteal and endosteal.
- *Callus formation:* immature woven bone, osteoid laid down by osteoblasts and mineralized with hydroxyapatite.
  - *Soft callus:* neovascularization mainly from periosteum. Precursor cells differentiate into fibroblasts, chondroblasts, and osteoblasts. These produce collagen, cartilage and osteoid that makes up callus. Mainly type II collagen.
  - *Hard callus:* soft callus is mineralized. 3–4 weeks after injury. Osteoclasts remove all dead bone and type II collagen is replaced by type I collagen. Calcium hydroxyappatite is deposited. Initially get woven bone.
- *Remodelling:* cortical structure and medullary cavity are restored. Fibres are reorientated along stress lines (Wolf's law). Woven bone is remodelled into lamellar bone.

Guided bone regeneration: Controlled stimulation of new bone into a defect by osteoconduction, osteo-induction or osteogenesis. Periosteum provides a source of osteoprogenitor cells and blood supply. The periosteum may also provide a barrier to the in-growth of fibrous tissue. Other membranes have been tried in place of periosteum. PTFE sheets have been used. Resorbable barriers are being evaluated.

See Ilizarov.

Bone graft
Source:

- *Autogenous:* preferred due to improved take. Autogenous grafts contain cells and growth factors. Cancellous bone has these in greater amounts. Cortical bone provides bulk. Grafts can be vascularized or free, inlay or onlay.
- *Allogenic implants:* bone transplanted between individuals. As the cells are killed it is not an allograft, but an implant. Less

predictable than autografts. Get delayed vascularization, resorption and poor osteogenic capacity.

- *Xenogenic transplant:* first performed in 1668 when a Dutch surgeon put pig calvaria into a Russian soldier. The Russian church demanded its removal 2 years later during which he died. Xenogenic grafts are presently not performed.

Heal by:

- *Osteogenesis:* formation of new bone by surviving cells in the bone graft. This only occurs in vascularized bone grafts.
- *Incorporation:* graft adheres to the host tissue.
- *Osseoconduction:* cells migrate from the bone ends into the graft, which acts as a scaffold.
- *Osseoinduction:* precursor cells are stimulated to become osteocytes, which move into the graft. Osseo-induction is controlled by bone morphogenic proteins (*BMPs*).

Graft survival:

- *Systemic factors* are similar to those affecting *Wound healing*.
- *Intrinsic graft factors:* grafts with intact periosteum and membranous bones undergo less absorption.
- *Graft placement factors:* particularly if in a normal bone site, quality of bed, graft fixation.

Bone substitutes: *Polymethylmethacrylate*, *Polytetrafluoroethylene*.

Bone morphogenetic proteins (BMPs)

- BMPs are responsible for bone regeneration
- Multiple BMPs exist. 15 have been identified, and all apart from BMP-1 belong to the TGF-β family.
- Bone produced at non-bony sites may be caused by the presence of BMPs.
- There are pathological and oncological concerns about the presence of BMPs, which may limit clinical use.

Bone tumours

Hand bone tumours account for 5% of bone tumours and 2% of malignant bone tumours.

- *Aneurysmal bone cyst*.
- *Chondroblastoma*.
- *Chondromyxoid fibroma*.
- *Chondrosarcoma*.
- *Enchondroma*.
- *Ewing's sarcoma*.
- *Fibrous dysplasia*.
- *Giant cell tumour of bone*.
- *Histiocytosis*.
- *Osteochondroma*.
- *Osteogenic sarcomas*.
- *Osteoid osteoma*.
- *Osteoblastoma*.
- *Unicameral bone cyst*.
- *Metastatic carcinoma*.
- *Myeloma*.
- *Non-ossifying fibroma*.

Classification: *Enneking's system*.

Clinical presentation: pain is a common symptom. Family history is important for some diseases with a high association with tumours.

Investigations:

- Hypercalcaemia is common.
- Alkaline phosphatase is elevated in 50% of patients with osteosarcoma.
- Lactate dehydrogenase is elevated with Ewing's sarcoma.
- Perform plain XRs. Assess the bone, the tumour and the matrix. Bone scans are not very useful.
- MRI is useful to assess intramedullary extent.
- CT is useful to detect matrix calcification. CT of the chest is important.
- USS differentiates cystic from solid masses.
- PET is useful for some carcinomas such as hepatic carcinoma and melanoma.

Principles: Without surgery, the tumour will recur. The options for resection are intracapsular, marginal, wide (intracompartmental) and radical (extracompartmental). The aim is to cure the patient of the tumour, preserve the limb and preserve function if possible.

- *Biopsy:* a tissue diagnosis is important. Perform an incision longitudinally over the tumour closest to the skin within one compartment. Frozen section may be used to ensure a good sample of the tumour has been taken. FNA and core biopsies can be used if the pathologist is confident. The incision or core tract will require complete excision at the time of definitive surgery.

- *Curettage:* this is not curative and is reserved for recurrent or stage 3 tumours. The cavity can be filled with bone cement or treated with liquid nitrogen. Bone graft or allograft can be used to fill the defect.
- *Resection/amputation:* most primary tumours are located in the metaphysis and require sacrifice of the joint.

Bonnet–Dechaume–Blanc
Telangiectatic facial birthmark with intracranial AVM.
See *Vascular malformations.*

Boss – carpometacarpal
- Bony prominence usually arising at the base of the second and third metacarpal.
- The joint becomes hypertrophic with an overlying bursa, and tendons may bowstring over the swelling.
- Possibly secondary to trauma.
- *XR:* use a carpal boss view taken in 30–40° supination and 20–30° ulnar deviation.

Treatment:
- Conservative with splint, NSAIDS and steroid injection, surgery if symptoms persists.
- Excise the boss through a longitudinal or transverse incision. Retract extensors. Make a longitudinal incision over the boss. Expose the boss subperiosteally. Elevate part of ECRB from the bone. Excise the boss with an osteotome until normal cartilage is seen. Inadequate excision results in persistent pain and swelling, so the entire boss needs to be excised, exposing the CMC joint. A ganglion at this site will require excision of the ganglion and the boss.

Botulinum toxin
- Botulin was first used clinically to attenuate extra-ocular muscle in the 70s and also used for blepharospasm.
- *Clostridium botulinum* produces eight serologically distinct exotoxins. These release acetylcholine at the neuromuscular junction resulting in flaccid paralysis.
- Type A toxin is the only one available. It is supplied dry in vials containing 100 MU. It is unstable and must be kept in a freezer. It is dissolved in 2 ml of saline.

- paralysis appears within 24–48 hours of injection.
- Botox can be used for hyperhidrosis, rhytids, facial asymmetry and focal hand dystonia when EMG may be useful in helping to locate the muscle.

Bouchard's node
Osteophyte developing at the PIP joint.

Boutonnière deformity
- Flexion of the PIP joint and extension of the DIP joint.
- Due to a disruption of the extensor mechanism. The central slip is often disrupted and the lateral bands move volarly and become flexors of the PIP joint. The FDS tendon now has nothing to resist it and unopposed flexion occurs. With time the lateral bands contract and their pull on the oblique retinacular ligament (ORL) pulls the DIP joint into hyperextension. The MCP joint also moves into hyperextension.

Assessment:
- Active and passive ROM of DIP joint and PIP joint.
- Check tightness of ORL by extending PIP joint and assessing tension at DIP joint.

Classification:
- *Stage 1:* dynamic, passively correctable.
- *Stage 2:* established deformity which cannot be passively corrected.
- *Stage 3:* established deformity with secondary PIP joint changes.

Treatment:
- Acute central slip divisions should be repaired.
- Stage 1 and 2 problems should be splinted to stretch volar structures, lateral bands and the ORL.
- Stage 3 problems are difficult to correct. Joint release may be performed. Central slip reconstruction, lateral band release, arthrodesis or arthroplasty may be required.

Bouvier's manoeuvre
- A test for *ulnar nerve palsy.*
- When hyperextension is passively prevented by dorsal pressure, EDC can extend the middle and distal phalanx.

Bowen's disease
- *Squamous cell carcinoma in situ*. 10% become invasive after many years with 1/3 of these developing metastatic disease.
- Seen in older patients in sun exposed and covered areas.
- Found on skin or mucous membrane (*Bowen's of mucous membranes*). Most are solitary with a long clinical course.
- More common in men than women.
- Appearance of sharply defined erythematous reddish scaly plaque with pruritus and superficial crusting.
- Histologically see hyperkeratosis and acanthosis with disordered epithelium and frequent mitoses, but no dermal invasion.
- Treat with excision or curettage.
- *There is also a relation between Bowen's disease and internal malignancies.*

Boyes sublimis transfer
For *Radial nerve palsy*.

• PT	→	ECRB
• FDS middle	→	EDC 2–5
• FDS ring	→	EPL, EIP
• FCR	→	APL, EPB

Bra
See *Cup size*.

Brachial plexus – anatomy
- *5:* nerve roots (C5–T1).
- *3:* trunks (upper, middle, lower).
- *6:* divisions (3 posterior, 3 anterior).
- *3:* cords (lateral, medial and posterior).
- *4:* major nerves (median, ulnar, radial and musculocutaneous).
- *Dorsal root:* sensory afferents, cell bodies in the dorsal root ganglion.
- *Ventral root:* motor efferents (relay in anterior horn cells).
- Dorsal and ventral roots combine to form spinal nerves which split into anterior and posterior rami. The major plexuses are formed from the anterior rami. The posterior rami become the posterior intercostal nerves.

Roots: C5–T1, variably C4 and T2. lie behind scalenus anterior.

Trunks: Upper, middle, lower between the anterior and middle scalenes. Cross lower part of posterior triangle.

Division: Anterior and posterior. Each trunk divides at the lateral edge of first rib. Lie behind clavicle.

Cords: Lateral, medial and posterior. Formed by the combinations of divisions and named in relation to the axillary artery. The anterior division of lower trunk continues to become the medial cord, the posterior divisions join to become the posterior cord and the anterior division of lower joins with anterior division of upper to become the lateral cord.

Nerves: Commence at the lateral border of pectoralis minor.

Examination based on anatomy
C5 and C6 roots and upper trunk:
- *Dorsal scapular nerve supplies rhomboids:* squeeze shoulder blades and palpate.
- *Long thoracic nerve supplies serratus anterior:* push wall.
- *Suprascapular nerve supplies supra- and infraspinatus:* look at muscle bulk and test for external rotation of the shoulder.
- *Third branch joins middle trunk to form axillary nerve:* test abduction of shoulder, palpate deltoid.
- *Lateral pectoral nerve:* clavicular head of pectoralis major, don't examine.
- *Musculocutaneous nerve:* biceps and sensation lateral arm
- *Upper trunk contribution to median nerve:* supplies FCR and pronator teres. Test FCR with wrist flexion and palpation. Test PT with pronation against force at 90°.

C7 root:
This is like examining the radial nerve with subscapularis.
- *Assess internal rotation and latissimus dorsi:* push down on hips and palpate.
- Axillary nerve has already been tested.
- Final branch is radial nerve. Brachioradialis and ECRL/B are supplied by C6, EPL and EDC supplied by C7 and 8. Test sensation.

C8–T1 root:
- *Medial pectoral nerve:* supplies pectoralis major.

- *Medial cutaneous nerve of the arm and forearm:* test sensation.
- Contribution to median nerve supplying FDS, FDP index and middle, FPL, APB.
- Terminates as ulnar nerve.

Also note pain, fractures, phrenic nerve palsy and *Horner's syndrome*.

Brachial plexus injury
Obstetric brachial plexus palsy

Incidence 1:1000. Most recover, 10% are severe.

Aetiology:
- Lateral distraction of the head from shoulder with injuries to upper roots.
- C5 has strong dural attachment so ruptures.
- C6 and C7 will avulse at the roots.
- C8 and T1 are usually only injured once the other roots are completely avulsed.
- However, Klumpke's is lower root due to hyperabduction in breech delivery.

Classification: by *Narakas*.

Prognosis:
- Any partial lesion has a better prognosis.
- Good grasp at 8/52 is likely to recover well.
- No recovery by 6/12 is unlikely to improve much.
- Breech delivery gives the most severe injuries.

Indications for operation:
- Groups 1 and 2 with no recovery in 3/12.
- Group 3 no biceps recovery in 3/12.
- Group 4 lesions.

Management:
- Once the diagnosis is made, assess at 6 weeks then every 6 weeks after. Maintain supple joints. Explore:
  - complete injuries.
  - C5 and C6 injuries, where there is evidence of phrenic nerve palsy.
- If no biceps and wrist extension by 3 months. This is controversial and some may observe for longer.

Surgery:
- Nerve repair: direct or with grafts, or intra-plexural or extraplexural neurotization.
- Secondary surgery may be required, e.g. to improve external rotation.

Injury:
Most occur in birth or are post-traumatic most commonly from RTAs. Obstetric palsies have a functional deficit and a growth deficit.

Diagnosis:
- *History:* the nature of the force. The position of head and arm. Shoulder abduction will suggest lower root injury. If the arm is pulled down it is more likely to involve upper roots. Traction will cause a central C7 injury.
- *Examination:* look for muscle atrophy. Wasting of paraspinal muscles indicates high cervical nerve avulsion injury.
- *Electrodiagnostic studies:* Repeat 6 weekly and if there is no recovery after 3 months and no evidence of root avulsion, explore surgically:
  - low amplitude potentials suggest re-innervation;
  - diminished fibrillations and sharp waves and activated muscle units suggest re-innervation, but don't correlate with function;
  - sensory nerve action potential (SNAP) and normal conduction velocity indicate root avulsion with a preserved dorsal root ganglion.
- *Neuroradiology:*
  - CT myelograms can be helpful to diagnose root avulsions;
  - MRI can reveal the roots beyond the spinal foramina. So CT for proximal, MRI for distal lesions;
  - angiogram may also be required.

Classification: *Millesi.*
Timing:
- For acute trauma, re-establish blood supply and examine.
- Some advocate early repair if possible, others wait for 4–6 weeks to allow for Wallerian degeneration, which helps identify the level of injury.
- Closed injuries should be explored before 2 years after. Preferably from 6 weeks to 3 months.

Priorities: Aim is to restore use and prevent amputation.

- *Shoulder:* stabilizing the shoulder prevents subluxation – by neurotization of the suprascapular nerve with intraplexus nerve donor or accessory nerve.
- *Elbow:* flexion is the first priority. Musculocutaneous nerve is restored with intraplexus donors or extraplexus donors such as intercostals.
- *Sensation:* median nerve neurotization from sensory intercostals or cervical plexus.
- *Hand function:* priorities are finger flexion and extension, then intrinsics and thumb opposition and abduction.

Prognosis: Determined by the type of lesion, age, denervation time, degree of root involvement, surgical technique and patient compliance.

Operative procedures: The final diagnosis can only be made at exploration. After an extensive exploration, perform intra- and extraplexus ipsilateral and contralateral neurotizations with nerve grafts and free-functioning muscle transfers.

- *Microneurolysis:* either perform epineuriotomy or interfascicular dissection. Use methylene blue to delineate the fascicles. Use palpation to assess the extent.
- *Direct nerve repair:* usually only possible for a fresh cut.
- *Nerve grafting:* the graft can be split into fascicles to increase the chance of survival. Also free vascularized nerve grafts such as ulnar nerve can be used.
- *Neurotization:* aims to reconstruct the peripheral nerve when the stump is unavailable e.g. in root avulsion. Examples of donors are intraplexus donors, intercostal nerves, spinal accessory nerve, cervical plexus, phrenic (partial), hypoglossal, contralateral pectoral, contralateral C7. May be end-to-end or with nerve grafts. Contralateral C7 provides a powerful motor donor and is useful for global avulsions.

Secondary reconstruction: These are necessary as only partial recovery will occur with the above procedures.

- *Shoulder:* aim for abduction and external rotation with tendon transfers such as latissimus dorsi for external rotation and trapezius advancement for abduction. Free

muscle transfer can be used, e.g. gracilis and adductor longus on a single pedicle.
- *Elbow:* pedicled latissimus dorsi can restore elbow flexion. Use local muscles first before free flaps. Forearm flexors have been moved proximally to act on the elbow. Free transfers used are lat dorsi, gracilis (but not very strong), vastus lateralis and rectus femoris for biceps.
- *Wrist:* fuse in global avulsion as restoration of wrist function is not feasible.

Brachioplasty

Many patients seeking improvement in arm contour have significant skin excess. This will leave a scar from axilla to elbow. This is a significant disadvantage as the scar is very visible. Most patients have therefore had marked weight loss with severe skin excess.

Brachioradialis

See *Muscles*.

Origin: Proximal 2/3 of lateral supracondylar ridge of humerus and intermuscular septum proximal to ECRL. It lies on the radial aspect of forearm, crossing ECRL and PT.

Insertion: Styloid process of radius and antebrachial fascia. The latter is divided if the tendon is used as a tendon transfer.

Nerve supply: Radial nerve.

Action: Flexes elbow joint, supinates the pronated forearm, weak pronator of supinated forearm.

Brachydactyly

Unusually short fingers.

Brachytherapy

- Radiotherapy treatment by implantation of radioactive material.
- Originally radium needles were used but now iridium 192 is implanted in wires.
- Plastic tubes are inserted at the time of operation.
- These are then loaded with radioactive seeds. This can be performed manually or it can be automated to reduce radiation exposure to the technicians.
- Useful in tongue and mouth lesions.

- May be preferable for posterior 1/3 of tongue tumours, which cross the midline which would otherwise require a debilitating total glossectomy.
- High risk of osteoradionecrosis.

See Radiation.

Bracka repair

This is a modification of the original Cloutier operation for *Hypospadias* repair.

First stage: Aims are to correct chordee, excise the urethral plate and apply a FTSG. Perform at 3 years. Place penis on board. Tourniquet to root of penis. Horton erection test. Excise urethral plate well laterally (1.2–1.5 cm width). Excise chordee down to corpus cavernosum. At glans/shaft junction split glans transversely to correct glandular tilt. Split glans to level of new meatus. If foreskin is present take graft from inner surface, leave the rest of the foreskin intact. Meticulously suture on graft with fine absorbable suture to floor of shaft, not to edge of skin. Use quilting sutures particularly at shaft/glans junction. Catheterize. Once well sutured roll jelonet and tie over with 3 firm 4/0 nylon. Take tourniquet off. Post-op remove dressing and catheter at 5 days.

Second stage: Aims to tubularize the skin graft to form a neo-urethra. Perform when the graft is well healed and softened. Tourniquet, glans stitch, catheterize, penile board. Incise around graft at a width adequate to create tube around size 8 Foley catheter. Mobilize minimally and suture over catheter with fine absorbable suture. Incise around corona lifting skin and preputial fascia with dorsal veins off shaft. Dissect out a preputial flap and pedicle over suture line as a waterproofing layer. Achieve haemostasis then suture the skin.

Results: Fistula rate of 5% reported by Bracka, but 15% by trainees in the same unit.

Branchial cysts

- Branchial cleft anomalies are the most frequently occurring masses in the lateral neck.
- They occur because of failure of maturation of the first and second branchial arches. The remnant remains trapped in the neck.
- Between the arches are clefts. The 2nd, 3rd, 4th clefts are usually obliterated by the 6th week. If they persist they become a sinus or cyst.
- They occur along the anterior border of the sternocleidomastiod.
- May occur at any age, usually present by 8 years of age.
- Cysts are soft non-tender.
- They often become infected which should be treated prior to excision.
- Require imaging prior to surgery.

Cysts:

- *First branchial cleft cysts:* very rare. Get dimple or tract close to parotid, associated with facial nerve.
- *Second branchial cleft cysts:* more common. Occurs at the junction of middle and lower thirds of sternocleidomastiod in the direction of the tonsillar fossa between internal and external carotid artery.
- *Third branchial cleft cysts:* rare.
- *Fourth branchial cleft cysts:* runs behind the internal carotid artery then beneath the subclavian artery on the right and aortic arch on the left, opening into upper oesophagus.

See Head and neck embryology.

Branemark implant

See Osseointegration.

BRCA

- *BRCA1* and *BRCA2* are tumour suppressor genes present in all women.
- Mutations in these genes increase the risk of developing *Breast cancer*.
- 1:300 women are carriers of mutations of *BRCA1* gene.
- Autosomal dominant.
- Present in 2% of women with breast cancer.
- 85% risk of developing breast cancer and 65% risk for ovarian cancer.

Breast

Anatomy:

- The breast develops from ectoderm. The milk line forms in the 5th week of gestation. Incomplete involution of the milk ridge produces accessory nipples.
- At adolescence the breast grows and differentiates with ptosis developing after the age

of 16. At menopause glandular involution occurs.

- The breast is mainly fibrous with around 15 main ducts running through to drain at the nipple. Each duct drains a lobe and lobes are separated by fibrous septae. The ligaments of Astley Cooper attach deep fascia to skin and provide support.

Boundaries: 2nd to 7th rib, sternal edge to anterior axillary line overlying the pectoral fascia and serratus anterior, external oblique, and rectus abdominus.

Blood supply:
- *From perforating branches of the internal thoracic artery (60%):* medial portion.
- *The lateral thoracic artery:* lateral portion.
- *Highest thoracic artery.*
- *Lateral branches from the 3rd, 4th and 5th posterior intercostal arteries:* lower outer portion.
- Veins follow arteries.

Lymphatics: Parallel the venous system, though most is to the axilla. The internal thoracic may carry 3–20% of lymph.

Nerve supply: Sensory innervation from:
- The supraclavicular nerves of the 3rd and 4th branches of the cervical plexus.
- The anterior cutaneous nerves from the 2nd–6th intercostal nerves.
- The anterior branches of the lateral cutaneous nerves from the 3rd–6th intercostal nerves. Sensation to the nipple is from the lateral cutaneous branch of the 4th intercostal nerve.

Shape:
- The shape varies but in the mildly ptotic breast, most of the fullness is in the inferior half.
- The nipple to inframammary fold distance measures 5–6 cm in the 'ideal' breast.
- The nipple-areolar complex is the point of maximum projection and measures 35–45 mm in diameter.

Accessory breast tissue:
- Due to failure of regression of ectoderm or mesoderm along the mammary line. <2% of children.
- M:F 1:2.
- Accessory nipples are confused with pigmented naevi and breast tissue with lipomas.

- May develop the same pathological diseases as breast.

Breast augmentation:
History:
- Czerny transplanted a lipoma in 1895.
- Cronin and Gerow inserted a silicone prosthesis in 1962.

Incisions:
- *Peri-areolar:* with good scar, but possibly nipple paraesthesia.
- Inframammary with good exposure but more noticeable scar.
- Axillary with no scar on the breast but decreased exposure.
- Endoscopic placement through umbilical or axillary route.

Position:
- *Subglandular:* below breast tissue, above fascia.
- *Submuscular:* below pectoralis and rectus abdominus.
- *Subpectoral:* below pectoralis major superiorly and subglandular inferiorly.

Infection: Incidence is 2.2%, most commonly with *Staph. epidermidis.* Prophylactic antibiotics are required.

Complications:
- Nerve injury to _Nipple_ with decreased sensation in 15%.
- _Capsular contracture_.
- *Rupture:* around 2% per year, but less with newer implants.
- *Autoimmune disease and cancer:* no evidence of increased risk.

Breast cancer:
- *Incidence:* 1:8. The most common cancer in women. 25 000–33 000 new cases per year in Britain.
- *Risk factors:* Age, family history, DCIS, First pregnancy >40 years, early menarche and late menopause.
- *Inheritance* Linked to _BRCA_ carriers.

Pathology: WHO classification – non-invasive and invasive.
- *Non-invasive:*
  ○ ductal carcinoma *in situ* (DCIS):
    ▪ dysplasia in the epithelial cells of the mammary ducts;

- 10% bilateral. 20% multicentric. 30% become invasive;
- Small, local excision; larger, mastectomy;
  - lobular carcinoma *in situ* (LCIS):
    - a marker of breast cancer;
    - 40% bilateral, 60% multifocal;
    - 1% chance per year of developing invasive breast cancer;
    - treat by observation or bilateral mastectomy.
- *Invasive:*
  - ductal, lobular, medullary, tubular, papillary, mucinous, adenoid cystic;
  - 75% are ductal, 10% are lobular.

Classification:
- *TNM:*
  - *T* is: *in situ* carcinoma
  - *T1:* <2 cm;
  - *T2:* 2–5 cm;
  - *T3:* >5 cm;
  - *T4:* tumour invades skin and chest wall;
  - *N1:* ipsilateral mobile lymphadenopathy;
  - *N2:* ipsilateral fixed;
  - *N3:* internal mammary;
  - *M0:* no metastasis;
  - *M1:* supraclavicular nodes or distant metastases.
- *Staging:*
  - Stage 0: TisiN0M0;
  - *Stage 1:* T1N0M0;
  - *Stage 2a:* T1N1M0, T2,N0M0;
  - *Stage2b:* T2N1M0, T3N0M0;
  - *Stage 3a:* T0N2M0, T1N2M0, T2N2M0, T3N1M0, T3N2M0;
  - *Stage 3b:* T4 any N any M, any TN3;
  - *Stage 4:* any T, any N M1.

Survival rates:
- *Stage 1:* 85%.
- *Stage 2:* 66%.
- *Stage 3:* 41%.
- *Stage 4:* 10%.

Investigation:
- *Mammography:*
- FNA:

Treatment:
- T1 and T2 disease may be treated with lumpectomy, axillary node sampling and radiotherapy.
- Larger tumours or in a small breast may require quadrantectomy, mastectomy,

subcutaneous mastectomy or oncoplastic breast surgery.
- *Tamoxifen:* an anti-oestrogen. Affects recurrence free and overall survival. Greater benefit over 50s, and oestrogen receptor positive tumours.
- *Chemotherapy:* affects disease-free and overall survival. Greater benefit under 50s and combination therapy. CMF (cyclophosphamide, methotrexate, and 5 fluorouracil) is the best combination.

Recurrence: In breast, lymph nodes and distant metastasis to any site, especially lung, liver, bone.

Breast implants
Types:
- *Shell composition:*
  - Silicone;
  - textured or smooth which affects contracture;
  - polyurethane-coated implants had a low rate of capsular contracture but have been withdrawn due to carcinogenic concerns.
- *Contents composition:* silicone – cohesive or liquid gel, saline, hydrogel, trigylceride, hyaluronic acid. Only silicone and saline are currently used.
- *Shape:* round or shaped. Also expandable which can also be round or shaped. Shaped implants are fuller inferiorly, but may not make a lot of difference once they are inserted.
- 1st generation implants were smooth and thick walled, 2nd generation were smooth and thin, 3rd generation were textured and thick, 4th generation are cohesive gel.

Complications:
- Infections, haematoma, scar, lactorrhoea, asymmetry, rupture.
- *Contracture:* Baker classification:
  - contracture rate for silicone implants varies from 58% for smooth implants to 8% for textured implants (Coleman, Foo, Sharpe, BJPS 1991);
  - saline implants have a 5% contracture rate;
  - the cause is not known, but may result from episodes of subacute infection with *Staph. epidermidis*;
  - get a fibroblastic foreign body reaction.
- *Rupture:*
  - Robinson APS 1995 found a 63% rupture rate but implants were up to 25 years old

with only 50% intact at 12 years, but implants have changed.

- *Implants and breast care:*
  ○ implants are radio opaque and microcalcification in capsule can confuse; one study suggests a delay in detection of ca with implants;
  ○ Berkel looked at 11 000 women with implants; there was no increase in incidence of breast cancer with an implant.
- *Implants and breast milk:* a suggestion that implants cause oesophageal motility problems in children. However, there is no increase in silicon in breast milk with an implant though silicon from the environment is in breast and bottled milk.
- *Silicon controversy:*
  ○ *1962:* first implant inserted.
  ○ *1982:* Van Nunen linked implants to connective tissue disorders (CTD).
  ○ *1992:* cosmetic implants were banned in USA, France, and Spain.
  ○ *1994:* a class action settlement of $4.25 billion for any of 10 CTD developed within 30 years.
  ○ Sanchez-Guerro looked at 90 000 women in a nurse health study. 1% had implants and there was no increase in CTD.
  ○ Independent review group UK – www.silicone-review.gov.uk.

See Breast augmentation.

Breast reconstruction:

Survival: No evidence that breast reconstruction adversely affects survival. No increase in local or distant recurrence with skin sparing mastectomy.

Immediate vs delayed: Immediate – may have better cosmetic result, fewer procedures, less psychological morbidity. Delayed – more scar tissue, skin loss, but more time to think about the options. 20% incidence of skin necrosis in smokers with skin sparing mastectomy.

Symmetry: In a small breast, implants may give reasonable symmetry, in a large breast autogenous tissue gives a better result. Consider contralateral mastopexy, reduction, or augmentation. A TRAM flap gives the best breast shape.

Radiation: Prior radiation increases the risk of problems from reconstruction. Tissue expanders are more problematic with poor quality skin and increased infection rate. Flaps also have a higher complication rate. Delay reconstruction if radiotherapy is likely to be given.

Surgical options:

- *Oncoplastic surgery:* for immediate reconstruction after quadrantectomy. Use techniques learnt from breast reduction surgery and reduce the contralateral breast.
- *Implants:* without prior expansion there is an increased risk of capsular contracture, wound breakdown, infection and loss of the implant.
- *Tissue expansion:* used to address the problem of skin loss. Difficult to achieve symmetry. Used in thin patients, not wishing a flap reconstruction and the elderly. Leaves less scarring and normal skin. Complications include skin necrosis, infection, implant failure, subcutaneous adipose tissue and muscle atrophy. Radiotherapy is a contraindication to tissue expansion. Place subpectorally. Place permanent prosthesis after 3–6 months.
- *TRAM* flap: partial flap loss 6–30%, hernia 0.3–13%.
- *SGAP.*
- *Latissimus dorsi flap:* usually with an implant. Also described without an implant by making a fleurs-de-ly skin incision. This leaves a poor donor site with high donor complication rate (14.5%). Small breasts can be matched with an extended latissimus dorsi flap taking fat as well as muscle. If the incision is high, place flap in lower incision to recreate inframammary fold. Failure rate 5%, seroma 9–33%.

Breast reduction:

Indications: Neck and back pain, painful breasts, embarrassment, asymmetry.

History:

- *1669:* by Durston.
- *1930:* de-epithelization was performed to improve nipple survival.
- *1950s:* Wise described the keyhole pattern.

Other modifications include:
- *Virginal hypertrophy:* rarer than macromastia. The prepubertal or pubertal breast develops

unilateral or bilateral gigantomastia. Due to end organ sensitivity. Treat surgically. Tamoxifen may help.

Techniques:
- The large variety of techniques differ in the way the pedicle is preserved and the technique for reducing the skin envelope. Some of the many techniques are:
  - *Regnault B*;
  - *Aries–Pitanguy:* inferior pole of the breast resected;
  - *Strombeck:* horizontal bipedicled technique with an inverted T closure;
  - *McKissock:* vertical bipedicled flap;
  - *Weiner:* superior pedicle technique;
  - *Balch:* central mound technique;
  - *Ribeiro:* inferior pedicle technique. Also Robbin;
  - *Lejour:* popularized the vertical scar technique described by Lassus;
  - *Benelli:* circumareolar reduction;
  - *Marchac:* short inverted T scar.
- Also can use liposuction and ultrasound-assisted liposuction which are controversial.
- *Breast amputation:* this can produce well-shaped breasts. Sensation and nipple projection is lost. Particularly indicated for very large reductions and when there is a pedicle of over 15 cm. The markings are similar to a vertical pedicle technique. Remove the nipple. Raise superior flaps and retain inferior breast to be covered by the skin flaps. Fix this inferior mound to pectoralis. Replace the nipple as a free graft.

Breast feeding: 70% of inferior pedicle patients can breast feed.

Breast cancer: The incidence in 5000 reduction specimens was 0.4%. 25% were detected preoperatively, 25 % intra-operatively and 50% on histology.

Mastopexy:
Ptosis is related to the quality of the skin envelope and volume loss. Volume loss occurs from weight loss, post-partum and post-menopausal. Gravity stretches the skin. *Classification: Regnault*.

Aim: Reverse ptosis by moving the NAC and breast mound and restoring the shape and contour.

Disadvantages: Scars, temporary benefit, poor-quality skin, upper pole flatness requires an implant, may result in a smaller breast.

Technique:
- Mild ptosis may just require augmentation. Can lead to double bubble.
- The same markings as for reduction can be used. Elevate NAC to the level of the inframammary fold. Redundant breast is suspended and attached to the chest wall.
- *Benelli mastopexy:* Flattens the central breast and reduces projection. This may be advantageous with a *Tuberous* breast.

Breslow thickness
- For histological staging of *Malignant melanoma*.
- The distance measured is the distance between the granular layer of the epidermis to the deepest part of the melanoma.
- This avoids the confounding effect of the variable thickness of the reticular dermis seen in *Clark's levels*.
- More precise at predicting the risk of metastatic disease and survival.
- The groupings for prognosis are 1, 2 and 4 mm Brewerton's view.
- XR view for demonstrating involvement of metacarpal heads in RA.
- Profile second to fifth MCP joint with no overlapping of cortical surfaces.
- Reveals early erosions and occult fractures of metacarpal heads.

Broder's classification
Histological grading of tumours:
- *Grade 1:* well differentiated.
- *Grade 2*: moderately differentiated.
- *Grade 3*: poorly differentiated.
- *Grade 4*: anaplastic.

Brow lift
Anatomy:
- *Blood supply:* internal and external carotid via the temporal, supratrochlear and orbital arteries.

- *Nerve supply:* the supratrochlear and orbital nerves.
- *Muscles: Frontalis* is opposed by corrugator supercilii, procerus and orbicularis oculi.

Indications:
- Ptosis of the forehead.
- Transverse lines.

Surgical procedure: Plane of dissection is between galea and pericranium.
- *Supraciliary eyebrow lift:* gives a good lift, but leaves a visible scar. Mark the upper border of the eyebrow in the hairline. Close the eyes and push up the brow to estimate the amount to excise. Excise skin, frontalis and orbicularis down to periosteum. If there is a 7th nerve palsy, suture dermis to periosteum with non-absorbable sutures. If functioning, preserve the frontal nerve.
- *Midforehead lift:* incision placed centrally in a forehead crease. Divide frontalis and elevate eyebrows. Leaves a visible scar.
- *Bitemporal lift:* elevates lateral brow through paired incisions. Concealed scar. For younger patients with lateral hooding.
- *Bicoronal incision.*
- *Hairline incision:* may become visible if there is a receding hairline. A zig-zag incision allows the scar to be hidden by hair growth; hair-bearing skin is excised. The forehead is therefore raised, which is useful in patients with short foreheads, but undesirable if the hairline is already high. Largely superseded by endoscopic lift.
- *Endoscopic forehead lift:* make several small incisions, extensive subperiosteal dissection, release of corrugator and procerus, preserve nerves and elevate forehead and attach with screws or drill hole in outer table. There is no scalp resection, less scarring, less bleeding. Good with alopecia.

Complications: Usually transient. Haematoma, numbness, hair loss, scars.
See *Forehead flap*.

Buccal mucosa cancer
- A disease of the elderly.
- Common in tobacco and betel nut-chewing areas. Also teeth trauma and leucoplakia. In other areas tends to be slow growing.

- Verrucous carcinoma is a well differentiated SCC and rarely spreads. The lesions begin as flat, erythematous, roughened areas, later becoming ulcerated.
- The submandibular nodes become involved, but there may also be direct spread to the jugulodigastric, preparotid, and mid-jugular nodes.

Treatment:
- T1 and T2, excision and radiation therapy are equally effective.
- Large, indurated lesions may require full-thickness resection of the cheek with a variety of flap reconstructions.
- Bone involvement will require maxillectomy or mandibulectomy.
- Radical neck dissection for positive nodes or in the N0 neck involved in the primary.
- Radiation with palliative surgery or stage III or IV disease.

Results: 5-year survival rates:
- *Stage I:* 92%.
- *Stage II:* 86%.
- *Stage III:* 65%.
- *Stage IV:* 15%.
See *Head and neck cancer*.

Buerger's disease
Thrombo-angiitis obliterans.
- An idiopathic segmental inflammatory recurrent occlusive disease of small- and medium-sized arteries and veins in the extremities.
- Mostly seen in young male smokers.
- More common in Asia.
- A high percentage of patients have immune reactivity to collagen.
- Usually begins before 40 years.
- Get trophic changes, ischaemic pain at rest and venous thrombosis. Progression is slowed by cessation of smoking.
- Surgery is required for debridement and wound care.
- Sympathectomy may help, but neither cessation of smoking or sympathectomy will reverse the arterial changes.
See *Vascular injuries*.

Buncke
- *1966:* performed a hallux to hand transfer in a monkey.

- *1972:* performed the first successful clinical composite free tissue transfer, a free omental flap to cover a large scalp defect.

Bunnell test

- For intrinsic tightness.
- Full passive flexion of IPJ with MPJ flexion, but not in MPJ extension indicates intrinsic tightness.

Bupivicaine

<u>*Local anaesthetic:*</u> Maximum dose is 2 mg/kg, with or without adrenaline, e.g. 60 kg woman with 0.5% marcaine = $60 \times 2 \times 2/10 = 24$ ml.

Burns

Epidemiology: Burns occur to the very young, the very old, the very unlucky and the very careless. Domestic burns are mainly scalds in children, occurring mainly in the kitchen or the bathroom.

Skin function:
- Barrier to heat loss, evaporative loss mechanical injury and infection.
- Dermal layer provides skin appendages and elasticity.
- Loss of the barrier leads to hypothermia, fluid loss, infection which is exacerbated by immunosuppresion.

Pathophysiology:
Local response:
- Degree of injury relates to temperature and duration of exposure most tissue is lost from heat coagulation of protein.
- *Jackson* described three zones of injury.
- Final tissue loss is progressive and results from release of local mediators, change in blood flow, oedema and infection.
- Get initial vasoconstriction followed by vasodilatation and oedema.
- Get activation of complement and coagulation systems with thrombosis, and release of histamine and bradykinin.
- Get capillary leak and vasoconstriction.
- Get release of inflammatory cytokines.
- Chemotaxis to neutrophils, which degranulate and increase injury.
- Only fluid resuscitation has been shown to have a clear benefit in reducing the injury occurring during this local response.

Systemic response:
Fluid loss and cytokine release lead to a characteristic systemic response.
- Hypovolaemia, vasoconstriction and possibly cardiac dysfunction mediated by TNF.
- In burns, over 20–30% TBSA the zone of oedema is not just limited to the burned area, but includes the whole body. This is due to systemic increased microvascular permeability. It can be thought of as if Jackson's zone 3 involving the entire body.
- RBCs may be lost due to membrane fragility.
- Hypothermia from evaporative loss.
- Acute respiratory failure.
- Marked catabolic response.
- *Bacterial translocation:* get intestinal villous atrophy, particularly if nutrition is not supplied enterally. The atrophy with capillary leak can lead to translocation of bacteria into the portal circulation. This can alter hepatic function and cause sepsis and multisystem organ failure.
- *Immune consequences:* all elements of the immune system are suppressed and sepsis is a major cause of death in large burns. Get reduced neutrophil function, skin and mucosal barrier disrupted.

Criteria for referral:
- Inhalational injury.
- Burn >10% in adults or 5% in children.
- *Burn involving special area:* hands, perineum, face.
- Full thickness burns greater than 5%.
- Electrical and chemical burns.
- Circumferential burns.
- Other illnesses and associated trauma.
- Social reasons (e.g. child abuse).

Resuscitation:
- Get burn oedema. In burned tissue there is a transient decrease in blood flow followed by arteriolar vasodilatation resulting in oedema. The rate and amount of oedema formed depends on the degree of thermal injury and fluid resuscitation. In a large wound, oedema is usually maximal at 18–24 hours post-burn. Oedema also occurs in unburned tissue. This has classically been attributed to a generalized increase in microvascular permeability with thermal injury in excess of 25% to 30% TBSA.

- *Parkland formula* most commonly used resuscitation formula. Also Muir and Barclay.
- *Protein:* after the first 24 hours of endothelial leak, protein can be replenished with 0.5 ml/kg/% TBSA of 5% albumin. Only for burns >30%.
- Urine output as >30 ml/hour or 0.5–1 ml/kg/hour in adults and 1–2 ml/kg/hour in children.
- Hypertonic saline may be considered to minimize the amount of fluids given and reduce oedema
- Give maintenance fluids for children of:
  ○ 100 ml/kg/24 hours for first 10 kg;
  ○ 50 ml/kg/24 hours for next 10 kg;
  ○ 20 ml/kg/24 hours for next 10 kg.

Clinical response:

- Get cardiovascular instability due to the microvascular and cell membrane changes. The function of the cell membrane as a semi-permeable barrier is lost in burn tissue. To restore plasma volume, extracellular space also needs to be restored.
- Myocardial depression occurs with burns of >40%.
- RBC destruction in large burns may be up to 40% of the circulating volume. 15% is destroyed by the initial burn and a further 25% by decreased survival time.
- There may be glucose intolerance secondary to catecholamine release.
- Outcome varies with percentage burn and age.

Assessment:

- Map percentage of burn using *Lund and Browder chart*, or *Wallace* rule of 9s or palm of hand (1% TBSA). In extensive burns subtract unburned skin from 100%.
- Other factors affecting mortality and morbidity include age, inhalation injury, other injuries and other medical problems.

Burn depth:

- *Superficial* (1st degree) epidermis only.
- *Partial dermal:* heal within 3 weeks (2nd degree).
- *Deep dermal:* take longer than 3 weeks to heal. The presence of blisters is the hallmark of a partial thickness burn. To produce blisters there must be at least some element of

viable dermis. Capillary return and sensation also suggest partial thickness.
- *Full thickness:* involves all of epidermis and dermis (3rd degree).

Pain: Important to control. Patients with good pain control have a more stable BP and heart rate, and are less hypermetabolic with less long-term post-traumatic stress disorder. Morphine given in small frequent doses is good for the initial resuscitation period. PCAs are useful.

PE: The incidence in burns patients is very low and, therefore, prophylactic heparinization is not justified.

Burns dressing: See *Integra*, *Biological skin substitutes*. Three functions:

- *Protective:* physical barrier is lost. Dressings can isolate the wound reducing the number of organisms.
- *Metabolic:* occlusive dressings reduce evaporative heat loss and minimizes cold stress and shivering.

Topical antimicrobials: Topical antimicrobials provide a high concentration of drug at the wound surface. Prophylactic therapy aims to delay and then minimize colonization. 10^4 organisms/g suggests invasive infection.

- *Silver sulphadiazine*.
- *Mafenide acetate*.
- *Silver nitrate*.
- *Cerium nitrate-silver sulphadiazine*.

GI bleeding: This can adequately be prevented by using H2 antagonists.

Infections:

- Burn patients have a large area of tissue where infection can enter, as well as a lot of invasive procedures.
- They are immunocompromised and may not exhibit normal signs of infection.
- The principle organisms are:
  ○ bacteria: *Pseudomonas aeruginosa* and *Staphylococcus aureus*;
  ○ fungal: *Candida*;
  ○ viral infections present, but of unknown significance.
- Give IV antibiotics with sepsis.

Paediatric burns:
- Mainly scalds.
- A child with a 95% scald has a 50% chance of survival.
- Prone to hypoglycaemia and hyponatraemia.
- Consider NAI.
- Differences between adults and children:
  - *A:* airway narrower, prone to laryngo-malacia;
  - *B:* diaphragmatic respiration – may need escharotomy;
  - *C:* hypovolaemia hard to assess, need higher urine output;
  - *D:* neurology difficult to assess;
  - *E:* lose heat rapidly;
  - *F:* Parkland formula and maintenance fluid;
  - *Long term:* emotional needs, growth retardation.

Surgery:
Timing:
- *Immediate:* escharotomy and tracheostomy.
- *Early:* early excision and grafting within 72 hours may produce better results.
- *Intermediate:* when depth difficult to determine. If there is little healing after a week grafting can be performed.
- *Late:* more than 3 weeks after the burn.

Escharotomy:
- Circumferential burns can prevent swelling leading to raised pressures and impaired tissue perfusion.
- In the chest, ventilation can be restricted.
- Escharotomy should be performed to maintain distal flow.
- Usually can be performed under local anaesthetic.
- Perform midlateral.
- Fasciotomies may be required with large burns or electrical burns.
- In chest perform in anterior axillary line and if bleeding is still restricted, then join incisions with a chevron-shaped incision over the costal margin.
- An occlusive dressing of cotton gauze and the biological dressings minimizes water vapour loss.
- Comfort: superficial burns are sensitive to air currents and deep burns become more sensitive as the nerves regenerate.

Excision:
- *Tangential:* excise in layers and stop when healthy tissue is found.
- *Fascial excision:* for big or deep burns as it limits the amount of bleeding.

Skin grafting:
- *Meshed graft:* can cover large areas and hae-matoma can be released, but gives a honey-comb appearance.
- *Full-thickness grafting:* mainly for secondary burns reconstruction. However, more durable and contract less.
- *Non-autograft options:*
  - *live-related allograft:* from family members;
  - *live-unrelated allograft:* freshly harvested during organ retrieval;
  - *Cadaveric* allograft;
  - *Skin* substitutes.
- *Alexander technique:* meshed allograft is laid over widely meshed autograft. Useful in patients with limited donor sites.
- *Cuono technique:* take biopsy from unburned skin and culture. Place allograft. After 10 days remove the epidermis and apply the sheets of keratinocytes. The dermal elements of allograft may survive as rejection is mediated by Langerhans cells.

Upper limb:
- Excise and graft all wounds, which will take >2 weeks to heal to enable early movement.
- Use a tourniquet, but don't exsanguinate as pooled blood helps guides excision.
- Use adrenaline swabs and pressure dressing to reduce haemorrhage.
- Lay meshed grafts. Use thick grafts on the palm and maintain first web space.
- For deep burns. Use pedicled or free flaps such as radial forearm fascial or fascio-cutaneous, lateral arm temporalis fascial flap.
- Up to 30% of patients develop compression neuropathies. Intrinsic muscles may need decompression.
- Tendon rupture and adhesions are common, particularly of extensors. They require good-quality tissue cover.
- Heterotopic calcification occurs in 10% of patients with burns of the upper extremity, particularly around the elbow.

Inhalation:

- Inhalation is the most serious complication of thermal injury.
- It increases mortality by 40%.

Assessment:

- *Symptoms:* shortness of breath, brassy cough, hoarseness, wheezing.
- *Signs:* circumoral soot, soot in the mouth, singed nasal hair, increased ventilatory effort, stridor, altered consciousness.

Investigations: Blood gases, CO levels, CXR, bronchoscopy.

Action: Divided into three broad areas:

- *Carbon monoxide inhalation*: CO intoxication. Also *Hydrogen cyanide* toxicity.
- *Direct thermal injury* to the upper aero-digestive tract – oedema and acute respiratory swelling. Due to the dissipation of heat energy to the tissues of the larynx and pharynx. Diagnosis by direct visualization. If there is swelling, soot or erythema, intubate. Extubate when swelling decreases.
- *Inhalation of products of combustion:* with respiratory failure:
  - chemical pneumonitis due to products of combustion, treat with PEEP and suction; view with bronchoscopy;
  - bronchoconstriction and bronchorrhoea – ciliary function may be depressed;
  - the chemical injury may lead to pulmonary oedema and adult respiratory distress syndrome with a mortality of 60%;
  - secondary infection occurs after 72 hours.

Management:

- Intubate early.
- 100% oxygen.
- Pulmonary lavage.
- Treat infection and monitor fluids.

Electrical injuries:

- Two mechanisms:
  - Joule heating: current-generated heating with a thermal burn;
  - electrical denaturation of cell membrane;
  - protein and lipids leading to electroporation – creation of large pores.
- Muscles carry most of the current.
- Entrance and exit wounds are at points of contact.

- Minimal voltage for injury depends on the frequency, type and magnitude. AC current can be less than DC to produce VF. >10 mA will not allow the arm to let go, due to direct flexor contraction, and respiratory muscle contraction will cause respiratory arrest.
- High voltage is >1000 V and may arc before mechanical contact.

Treatment:

- Resuscitation.
- Treat compartment syndrome and *Myoglobinuria* and acute renal failure.
- Fluid load for diuresis, and mannitol and sodium bicarbonate.

Surgery:

- *Scalp and skull:*
  - may get exposed skull and brain injury;
  - cover early – dead bone can remain as a graft;
  - split calvarial grafts or methylmethacrylate.
- *Lip and oral commissure:*
  - the commonest site in children;
  - treat with splints;
  - commissure reconstruction.
- *Extremities:*
  - decompression;
  - amputation may be necessary.

Long-term sequelae:

- Cataract formation after electrical injury to the head and neck.
- *Peripheral neuropathy:* possibly due to progressive microvascular occlusion and fibrosis.
- Personality changes and post-traumatic stress.

Chemical injuries:

- Injury is by a chemical reaction that may have a thermal component.
- Broadly classified into acids and alkalis. In general, although alkalis cause more destruction as acids cause coagulative necrosis with precipitation of protein, alkalis cause liquefaction enabling greater depth penetration. Alkalis dissolve and unite with proteins, which are soluble and cause further destruction. Organic solutions will disrupt lipid membranes. More accurately, they act by:
  - *reduction:* agents bind free electrons in tissue proteins, e.g. HCL;

o *oxidation:* oxidized on contact with proteins leading to toxic products, e.g. sodium hypochlorite;

o *corrosive agents:* denature tissue proteins, e.g. phenols;

o *protoplasmic poisons:* bind or inhibit calcium and other ions, e.g. HFl;

o *vesicants:* produce ischaemia with necrosis, e.g. mustard gas;

o *dessicants:* dehydrate and release heat, e.g. H_2SO_4.

First aid:

• Remove clothing and agent, irrigate for 1–2 hours.

• Over resuscitate.

• Don't use water for elemental sodium, potassium and lithium which will ignite. Use a fire extinguisher or sand and cover with cooking oil.

• Don't use water for phenol, which penetrates more in a dilute solution. In the eye use normal saline if available. Manually hold the eye open as they will have blepharospasm.

Specific chemicals:

• *Tar and grease:* petroleum jelly dissolves the tar and grease. Long exposure may cause pulmonary, renal and hepatic failure.

• Hydrofluoric acid.

• Sulphuric acid.

• *Lye:* in many cleaning products – an alkali.

• *Cement:* composed of calcium carbonate, silicon dioxide, aluminium oxide, magnesium carbonate, sulphuric acid and iron oxide.

• *Ammonia:* a strong alkali base, can cause severe injury to skin, eyes, GI tract with liquefaction necrosis. One of the most devastating chemicals to injure the eye. May get rapid blindness. Distinct odour and irritant with cough. Affects upper airways only as it is very water soluble. Treat with irrigation.

• *Anilines:* from the dye industry. They cause superficial burns often violet or brown in colour. May get systemic toxicity. Get methaemoglobinaemia. Treat this with methylene blue IV 1–2 mg/kg.

• *Bleach solutions:* (sodium or calcium hypochlorite). Strong oxidizers. They are stabilized by adjusting pH and are maintained at a pH of >10. Prolonged contact may cause burns. If acid is added, chlorine gas may escape. Chlorine is a respiratory tract irritant. May produce laryngeal oedema.

• *Phosphorus:* phosphorous ignites spontaneously on exposure to air and is rapidly oxidized to phosphorous pentoxide. It is extinguished by water. Particles of phosphorous continue to burn. Treat with water irrigation followed by removal of any particles. Wash with 1% copper sulphate to form black particles, which can be seen and removed.

Extravasation injuries:
See Chemical weapons.

Metabolism and nutrition:
Hypermetabolic response:

• Increased cardiac output, ventilation, temperature, and decrease nitrogen balance.

• Response proportional to burn size. Burn over 50% has a metabolic rate of twice resting.

• Maintaining temperature is important to reduce energy expended.

• The metabolic rate begins to return to normal when wounds are closed, but doesn't fall to normal until wound remodelling is complete.

• Caloric requirements can be calculated with:
  o the Curreri formula, this is not very accurate;
  o the Harris–Benedict equation.

• The protein content can be estimated by using a calorie to nitrogen ratio of 100–150:1. The normal diet is 300:1. Also require fats, micronutrients.

• Weight should be monitored closely and should not fall below 10% of the ideal body weight.

Mediators: Catecholamines. Also increased glucagons and cortisol. All organs involved, get early hypofunction and later hyperfunction.

Nutritional support:

• Aim to provide adequate calories and protein.

• Will be required for >20% burns.

• Start as soon as possible, preferably by the enteral route. This helps maintain mucosal integrity.

- May need NGT or feeding jejunostomy Most patients with burns of over 20% get an ileus of upper GI tract, but the small bowel is usually functioning so enteral feeding should be possible. It usually resolves in 72 hours.
- Avoid TPN if possible as there is an increase of sepsis.
- Measure nitrogen balance by 24-hour urinary measurements.
- Give vitamin and micronutrient supplements.

Secondary reconstruction:
Scar management:
- Hypertrophic scar will affect recovery.
- It is more common in children and in areas of stretch and motion.
- Reduce with early wound closure, scar management and surgical treatment.
- Pressure garments aim to provide 25 mmHg of pressure. Also silicon sheets and steroids.

Scalp: Tissue expand larger defects.

Face:
- Decide whether to graft by 7–10 days.
- For forehead a single high-quality STSG is used.
- Use neurosurgical halo to immobilize the grafts.
- Produce a face mask to wear after the halo is removed.
- Cheek can be reconstructed with flaps or tissue expansion.
- The whole face can be reconstructed with one large FTSG.
- Also use a very large scapular flap with two pedicles.

Neck:
- Scar bands are best corrected with local flaps or Z-plasties.
- Tissue expansion for moderate defects, using lateral skin is the first option.
- Free tissue transfer for large defects and pre-expanded scapular or groin flaps can give thin pliable skin.
- Intubation may require fibre optic endoscope or emergency release or tracheotomy.

Eyelids:
- SSG directly onto orbicularis.
- If the eyelids are destroyed, the conjuntiva can be mobilized and covered with skin graft.

- *Contractures:* use skin grafts, using good-quality skin such as post-auricular for lower eyelid and thicker skin for upper. Don't do upper and lower at the same time. Extend release beyond the medial and lateral canthi.

Eyebrows:
- Tattooing or make-up may be sufficient.
- Free scalp composite grafts, micrografts and island flaps on superficial temporal artery.
- Graft success was higher in free than in islanded grafts.

Ear:
- Aim to prevent suppurative chondritis – use *Mafenide*.
- If suppurative chondritis occurs, debride immediately and treat with systemic antibiotics.
- *Pseudomonas* is the most common organism. *See* ear *Reconstruction*.

Nose:
- Nasal ectropion is best treated with composite grafts or turn-over flaps with a FTSG.
- Stenosis requires grafts and splints.

Lip and mouth:
- Oral *Commissure* must be symmetrical. wait for scars to mature and over-correct compared with opposite side.
- The commissure is not triangular in shape, but has a vertical component.
- Converse described a flap to reconstruct this.
- Hair-bearing upper lip can be reconstructed with a pedicled scalp flap.
- Lower lip can be resurfaced with full thickness skin grafts and the downward pull can be counteracted with a fascia lata sling. Free flaps can be used to resurface entire subunits.

Axilla:
- For minor defects use Y–V-plasty.
- Moderate contractures will need a latissimus dorsi flap designed to conform to the shape of the axilla.
- This is preferable to SSGs with improved post-operative mobilization and quicker recovery.

Abdomen:
Tissue expansion.

Burow's triangles

The excessive skin at the base of an advancement flap.

Byrd and Spicer classification of fractures

1985, classification based on the mechanism of the trauma and bone and soft tissue injury.

- *Type I:* low-energy oblique or spiral fractures, clean laceration <1 cm.
- *Type II:* medium-energy trauma; displaced or comminuted fracture, laceration >2 cm and soft tissue contusion.
- *Type III:* high-energy trauma; severely displaced or comminuted fracture; segmental fracture or bone defect, laceration >2 cm, soft tissue loss.
- *Type IV:* high-energy bursting trauma; crushing or avulsion, arterial damage requiring microvascular repair.

See *Lower limb reconstruction.*

C Cadaveric skin to Cytokines and growth factors

Cadaveric skin

- Used as a temporary wound cover, usually for extensive burns when there are not enough donor sites from which to harvest a graft.
- Provides good vascularization of the wound bed.
- Lasts 2–3 weeks or even longer in burn patients who may be immunocompromised.
- Expensive and there are concerns about the transmission of viral infections.
- Skin can be:
  o cryopreserved at –80ºC, which may contain some viable cells;
  o glycerol preserved, which has a longer lifespan and can be stored in a normal fridge; the European bank uses glycerol preserved skin;
  o Cuono technique involves placing cultured keratinocytes on allograft dermis which is less immunogenic.

See *Biological skin substitutes,* See *Burns.*

Café au lait macules

- Pigmented benign lesions that can occur in isolation or associated with *Neurofibromatosis* when 5 or more should be present.
- Removal may be requested.
- Dermabrasion, salabrasion and excision can be used, but may leave scarring and permanent pigmentary changes.
- *Lasers* including Q-switched Nd:YAG (532 nm), pigmented dye laser (510 nm), and the

Q-switched ruby laser (694 nm) may be effective.

- They may recur. Some lesions darken initially with treatment.

Calcifying epithelioma of Malherbe

See *Pilomatrixoma.*

Calcinosis

- Hard whitish superficial areas especially over elbows knees and fingers.
- May discharge chalky substance.
- May require excision.
- Seen in *Scleroderma*, dermatomyositis, hyperparathyroidism, tumours and parasitic infections.
- No medical treatment. Colchicine may reduce the inflammation associated with calcinosis.

Calvarial flap

- Vascularized calvarial bone may be raised with temporoparietal fascia.
- This may be used for zygoma reconstruction.
- Place the template over parietal calvarium. Additional filler is obtained by folding the superficial temporal fascia around the bone graft. Pass the flap through a subcutaneous tunnel via a facelift excision to the zygomatic defect.

Calvarial graft

- Outer table of calvarium can be split from inner and used as a bone graft.

- Donor site morbidity is minimal and the graft can be moulded to fit the defect.
- The parietal skull is the usual site of harvest as there are no underlying venous sinuses.
- Two techniques to harvest:
  - the *in vivo* technique where the outer table is split from the inner;
  - the *ex vivo* technique, where a craniectomy is performed, the tables split and the outer table is replaced with the inner table being used for graft.

See *Cranium reconstruction*.

Camper's chiasm

The decussation of FDS distal to where the FDP tendon pierces the two slips of FDS.
See *Flexor tendons*.

Camptodactyly

- Flexion deformity of PIP joint, most commonly of the little finger.
- It typically presents between growth spurts which occur between age 1–4 and 10–14.
- All structures crossing the volar aspect of the finger has been implicated. The most common causes are an abnormal lumbrical insertion and an abnormal FDS insertion.
- Assess whether there is extensor lag or block, the severity, whether it is progressive, the age and how many digits.
- Treat a contracture >50°, where conservative treatment has failed and progressive contracture.

Classification: Benson classification.
- *I:* unilateral or bilateral PIP joint contracture, otherwise healthy.
- *II:* seen in adolescence.
- *III:* other associated anomalies; usually more severe with multiple digits.

Treatment:
- Splint.
- Difficult to correct surgically. Especially if there is a narrow joint space, indented neck, flattened head of proximal phalanx. Options are explore and release, angulation osteotomy or arthrodesis.
- Total anterior tenoarthrolysis (TATA) described by Saffar, involves releasing the entire flexor apparatus and the interphalangeal volar plates through a lateral incision with volar subperiosteal dissection.

Capillary malformation

See *Port wine stain*.

Capitate – fracture

- Rare.
- *Classify:* isolated or part of a perilunate injury.
- May get a fragment rotating 180° when the perilunate dislocation is reduced – scapho-capitate syndrome.
- Usually due to force transmitted through 3rd metacarpal to capitate.
- A dorsal fracture can be associated with CMC fracture/dislocation.
- If non-displaced treat with a cast, if displaced, operate.
- Reduce through a dorsal approach. Hold with a K wire or screw. Consider bone graft.

Capsaicin

- Depletes neurones of substance P.
- Application in *RSD* appears to cause desensitization to inflammatory agents.

Caput ulna syndrome

- End-stage destruction of the distal radio-ulnar joint.
- Get ulnar-sided wrist pain, dorsal ulnar prominence and decreased rotation.
- *Piano keyboard sign:* prominent ulnar head is volarly depressed and springs back. This should be performed gently as it can be painful.
- Ulnar prominence can lead to rupture of ulnar-sided extensors (Vaughn–Jackson syndrome).

Carbon monoxide

- Odourless, tasteless gas which binds preferentially to Hb, 210× stronger than O_2.
- This displacement is the major pathogenic effect.
- If it enters the cell's cytochrome system, it impairs oxygen utilization – *Sick cell syndrome*.
- >5% COHb indicates *Inhalation*, >20% toxic, >60% fatal.
- The half-life of carbon monoxide on room air is 4 hours and on 100% oxygen is 45 minutes. So treat with 100% oxygen, change when COHB levels are <10%.

Carpal tunnel

- Roof formed by _Transverse carpal ligament_ spanning from scaphoid tubercle and crest of trapezium to pisiform and hamate.
- Traversed by 10 structures – FDS(4), FDP(4), FPL and median nerve.

Carpal tunnel syndrome (CTS)

- Caused by an acute intermittent or persistent increase in the pressure in the carpal tunnel.

Causes:

- _Congenital:_ anomalous muscles, hypoplastic carpal bones.
- _Traumatic:_ fractures and dislocations, haematoma.
- _Inflammatory:_ rheumatoid tenosynovitis and nodules.
- _Infective:_ pyogenic tenosynovitis.
- _Neoplastic:_ lipofibroma of median nerve, lipoma.
- _Degenerative:_ OA of 1st CMC joint.
- _Endocrine:_ DM, hypothyroidism, acromegaly, pregnancy, menopause.
- _Metabolic:_ obesity, amyloidosis, haemodialysis, gout.
- _Vascular:_ haemangioma, median artery thrombosis, coagulopathy.

Most are idiopathic or multifactorial. No proven association between CTS and manual activities. Not a prescribed disease.

80% patients are >40 years old, female to male 4:1, 50% bilateral.

Symptoms: Pain, paraesthesia feeling of swelling in distribution of median nerve.
Worse at night or when elevating hand. Loss of grip, clumsiness.

Signs: Decreased sensation, wasting of APB, _Tinel's_, _Phalen's_ wrist flexion and _Durkan's_ compression test.

Investigations: NCS – often not needed, not very sensitive. Assess response to steroid. Image if lesion suspected.

Management:

- _Steroid injection:_ 25 mg of hydrocortisone. For reversibly CTS.
- Futoro splint particularly at night.
- Longitudinal incision to release _Transverse carpal ligament_. External neurolysis.

- Endoscopic release.

Complications: Persistent symptoms, 7–20%, usually incomplete release especially distally. May be due to compression more proximally (double crush), painful scar 'pillar pain', bleeding and infection (rare), nerve damage and recurrence.

Carpenter's syndrome

- Autosomal recessive inheritance.
- Rare disorder craniosynostosis of various sutures leading to an asymmetric head with differing shapes depending on the sutures involved. Ranges from brachycephalic to turricephalic.
- Partial syndactyly usually of the 3rd and 4th digits and pre-axial polysyndactyly of the feet.
- Low-set ears and lateral displacement of the inner canthi are also prominent features.
- Mental deficiency may be present.
- Congenital heart defects have been reported in as many as 33% of the cases.

See _Craniosynostosis_.

Carpue

1814: Reintroduced the forehead flap for nasal reconstruction taking 15 minutes. It had been reported in the _Gentleman's Magazine_ in 1794.

Carpus

- _Stability:_ determined by bony architecture, ligaments, TFCC and balanced musculotendinous forces.
- _Ligaments:_ extrinsic, intrinsic and collaterals.
- _Space of Poirier:_ a fenestration in the capitolunate articulation where a capsular tear occurs with a lunate dislocation.
- _Assessment:_ take a history and examine. Palpate for tenderness. Perform provocative tests:
  - _Watson test:_ scaphoid shift test;
  - _Reagan ballottement test:_ for lunotriquetral ligament;
  - _Masquelet's test;_
  - _Kleinmann shear test._
- _Investigations:_
  - _XR:_ AP, lateral, grip and radial and ulnar deviation of both wrists;

○ *other:* arthrography, distraction XR, bone scan, USS, CT, MRI, arthroscopy.

Dorsal Intercalated Segmental Instability/Volar Intercalated Instability (DISI/VISI)
Dislocation:
• either volar or dorsal caused by high energy.
• 4 stages of ligamentous injury in a perilunate injury. The wrist is forced into dorsiflexion, ulnar deviation and intercarpal supination.
   ○ *Stage I:* scapholunate ligament injury;
   ○ *Stage II:* capitolunate disruption;
   ○ *Stage III:* lunotriquetral joint disruption;
   ○ *Stage IV:* volar dislocation of the lunate. If the lunate fossa is empty then the lunate has dislocated volarly. However, in volar or dorsal perilunate dislocation the lunate remains in the lunate fossa of the radius and the carpus is displaced.

Treatment: Dislocation should be reduced early. Varying opinion regarding open or closed treatment but results appear better for open treatment with ligamentous repair.

Carpal instability: Dissociative is the relationship between bones in a row.
• *Carpal instability dissociative (CID):* instabilities include scapholunate and lunotriquetral ligament disruptions.
• *Carpal instability non-dissociative (CIND):* the bones maintain their normal relationships in rows but the radiocarpal and midcarpal joints are disrupted.
• *Carpal instability complex (CIC):* describes greater or lesser arc injuries with lunate dislocation or fracture.

Arc injuries:
• *Greater arc:* perilunate with fracture of one or more carpal bone.
• *Lesser arc:* involves only the ligaments.
• *Inferior arc:* are spread from the radiocarpal joint with volar and dorsal radiocarpal ligament rupture with radial or ulnar styloid. Can get a pure radiocarpal dislocation.

Scapholunate instability:
• Abnormal alignment of the scaphoid.
• Terry Thomas sign, or increase scapholunate angle of >45° due to excessive volar flexion of the scaphoid.

• *May get a cortical ring sign:* axial view forms a round projection.
• *Treatment:* options are splints, scapholunate repair, capsulodesis to prevent palmar flexion of the scaphoid, intercarpal arthrodesis (4 corner, STT or scaphocapitate), proximal row carpectomy or total wrist arthrodesis.

Lunotriquetral instability:
• Isolated instability is rare.
• Most have perilunate injury.
• *Treatment:* options include primary repair, soft tissue reconstruction using ECU, LT arthrodesis or 4 corner arthrodesis for severe cases.

Mid-carpal instability:
• Some mobility that can be marked in young females.
• Trauma can destabilize the joint.
• If conservative treatment fails, perform limited intercarpal arthrodesis, total wrist fusion, reefing of dorsal and volar ligaments or radius osteotomy if there is malunion.

Axial instability:
• Rare injuries with dissociation of bones of the distal carpal row.
• The forces are axial and dissipate around the capitate with diastasis and possibly fractures.
• Fractures may be multiple, compartment syndrome.
• *Treatment:* often open and require debridement, fasciotomies and nerve decompression.

Ulnar translocation of the carpus:
• Rare extrinsic ligament injury with ulnar migration of the carpus.
• The lunate then sits on the ulna.
• Ligament repair gives unpredictable results and total wrist arthrodesis may be required.

Fractures:
• Scaphoid fracture 80%.
• Triquetral fracture 15%.
• Trapezium 2–5%.
• The rest 1–2%.
• Trapezoid is the least common.

Cartilage
• Hyaline (e.g. joints), elastic (e.g. ear) and fibrocartilage (e.g. intervertebral disc, tendon attachments). Hyaline cartilage dissipates loads, fibrocartilage transfers loads.

- Consists of chondrocytes in an extracellular matrix composed of proteoglycans, collagen and water. Chondrocytes are not very metabolically active and divide slowly.
- *Collagen:* type II in hyaline cartilage, type I in fibrocartilage.
- Get proteoglycans rich in chondroitin sulphate.
- Cartilage has no blood supply or lymphatic vessels.
- Nutrition is by diffusion.

Injury:
- Generally it has a limited response.
- The inflammatory response usually results in scarring.
- Cartilage regeneration can only occur if bone is injured.
- Get fibrocartilage forming, which eventually becomes hyaline cartilage

Cat-scratch disease
- Infection caused by the intracellular parasite *Bartonella henselae*, characterized by indolent, occasionally suppurative regional lymphadenitis occurring after being scratched by a cat. *Bartonella clarridgeiae* also implicated.
- The primary lesion is a raised slightly tender non-pruritic papule covered by a vesicle or eschar.
- Unilateral lymphadenopathy follows in a few days to weeks after.
- Systemic symptoms are mild with headache, fever and malaise lasting a few days.
- Diagnose with a skin test, which is positive after 30 days.
- No treatment is required and there is a good prognosis.

Cauliflower ear
- Particularly in pugilists.
- Direct blows, haemorrhage and fibrosis with loss of contours.
- Evacuate haematoma acutely.
- In chronic cases, carve and excise thickened tissue.
See Ear reconstruction.

Causalgia
- *Minor causalgia:* injury involving a purely sensory nerve in the distal portion of the extremities.

- *Major causalgia:* partial injury to a major mixed nerve in the proximal part of the extremity, often by high-velocity missiles. The pain is in the distal extremity, but not necessarily in the distribution of the injured nerve. They may benefit from sympathectomy with a response rate of 70–100%.
See RSD.

Cellulite
- Dimpling of the skin of the buttocks and lower limbs. Mainly in women.
- It results from hypertrophy of the superficial adipocytes.
- The superficial layer of fat is interspersed with connective tissue which attaches the skin to the superficial fascia. These areas do not distend as the fat hypertrophies giving the dimpled appearance.
- Cellulite may also occur due to skin laxity and can be seen in weight loss. The underlying mechanism is gravity pulling on the fibrous septa. This can be corrected by tightening the skin.
See Fat anatomy.

Cephalocoele
- A herniation of intracranial contents through a cranial defect.
- If it contains meninges it is a meningocoele. If meninges and cerebral tissue are present it is a meningoencephalocoele.

Classification: Based on anatomic location.
- Sincipital (frontal), parietal, basal and occipital.
- Sincipital encephalocoeles have a great geographic variation being more common in Africa and Southeast Asia.

Cephalometrics
- The science of skull measurement. Provides a quantitative method for describing dento-facial patterns.
- Useful for diagnosis, growth prediction and surgical treatment objective.
- Analysis performed using a standard lateral view of the skull. For a standard cephalogram the distance from object to XR should be 60 inches. The distance from object to film is 6 inches. The central beam is perpendicular to the ear. The head is held.

This gives 10% magnification. Tracing is then performed.

- *Landmarks:* a cephalometric plane connects three or more standardized points. Cephalometric analysis is composed of skeletal, profile and dental analysis.

Skeletal analysis:

- Used to classify facial types and establish the anteroposterior relationship of the basal arches.
- So SNA refers to maxillary position and SNB the mandibular position. The ANB gives the relation between maxilla and mandible.
- Measure in vertical plane. Total face height, upper and lower (100%, 45%, 55%).
- Measure anterior maxilla to cranial base, posterior maxilla to cranial base and the mandibular plane angle:
  - ○ S = sella, centre of pituitary fossa;
  - ○ N = nasion;
  - ○ A is the deepest mid-point of the maxillary alveolar process;
  - ○ B is the deepest mid-point of the mandibular alveolar process.

Dental analysis: Indicates the anteroposterior position of the teeth in relation to the bones.

Profile analysis:

- Assesses the soft tissue overlying the bones.
- Ricketts' aesthetic plane is a line drawn from nose tip to chin. The lower lip lies on this plane, the upper lip 2 mm behind.
- *Holdaway ratio:* orthodontic method to evaluate lip retrusion/prominence. Relates prominence of mandibular incisor and pogonion to the NB line. The lower incisor should be 4 mm in front of NB line and therefore so should the chin.
- Progress can be analysed by superimposing images.

Ceramics

- Three-dimensional arrays of positively charged metal ions and negatively charged non-metal ions, often oxygen.
- Probably the most chemically inert implant material.
- Low strength and brittleness limit their applications.

See Alloplasts.

Cerebrospinal fluid

- In trauma, if CSF leakage is suspected check for double ring.
- Collect nasal drainage on paper towel. If blood separates then other component may be present. If so then blood is internal and CSF is external.
- Tau protein is only found in CSF so its presence as detected by electrophoresis is diagnostic of CSF leakage.
- Also dye can be placed in the CSF at a lumbar puncture.

Cerium nitrate-silver sulphadiazine

- Cerium, an element has antimicrobial activity and is relatively non-toxic.
- The efficacy may be due to its affect on the immune function with improved cell-mediated immunity.
- Methaemoglobinuria is rare problem.

See Burns.

Cervical radiculopathy

- Most commonly caused by spondylosis.
- Get degeneration of the cervical disc with osteophytes and impingements on spinal roots.
- Get pain in lateral neck radiating to scapula, occiput, arm or hand.
- May have sensory signs.
- May develop muscle wasting.
- XR show loss of joint space, subluxation and MRI may demonstrate reduced foramina.

Cervicofacial flaps

- A rotation flap involving the cheek and neck used to reconstruct cheek defects.
- Raised inferomedially or inferolaterally
- Not totally reliable high on the cheek as the transverse branch of the superficial temporal artery is divided.
- It can be raised in the subcutaneous plane or to improve reliability in the deep plane beneath SMAS. It may extend beneath platysma.
- Preserve branches of facial nerve.
- Place anchoring sutures along the anterior aspect of the zygomatic arch and inferolateral orbital rim.

- The weight of the flap can give an ectropion.
- Anteriorly based flaps are useful for pre-auricular lesions.
- Primary delay can give more reliability. The base can include platysma. The lower level of the flap may be in the neck or below the clavicle.
- A larger defect may require a cervicopectoral flap based on the anterior perforators of the internal thoracic artery. It is elevated deep to platysma and to pectoral fascia. The incision extends behind the anterior trapezius border to prevent a hypertrophic scar.

See _Cheek reconstruction_.

Charles operation

- Radical excision of lymphoedematous tissue.
- Remove skin, subcutaneous tissue and deep fascia.
- Graft muscle.
- High morbidity, grafts are injured easily and scar extensively.
- FTSGs give a more durable result but still have significant complications.

See _Lymphoedema_.

Cheek advancement flap

- Used in _Nasal reconstruction_ for defects of the lateral nose.
- When the inferior border of the incision is placed along the alar crease, the paranasal skin is advanced onto the nasal wall to reach the midline.
- A compensatory Burow's triangle is excised from the alar base and the nasolabial area.
- Can be used for lateral nasal defects, particularly in elderly patients.
- Up to 2.5 cm of skin from the paranasal and cheek area can be used with primary closure.
- They cause loss of the nose/cheek angle which may need correcting as a secondary procedure.

Cheek reconstruction

Surgical anatomy:

- SMAS and superficial muscles (orbicularis oculi, depressor anguli oris, zygomaticus major and minor, risorius) form a superficial fascial layer.
- Over parotid SMAS is adherent to parotid gland.

- The superficial mimetic muscles of midface are responsible for facial expression, and nose and mouth.

Aesthetic units: Three overlapping zones.
- Suborbital.
- Pre-auricular.
- Buccomandibular.

Zone 1:

- Bounded by the nasolabial line, anterior sideburn, gingival sulcus and lower eyelid. It can be split into subunits.
- Below the eye there is a risk of ectropion. FTSGs are preferred to SSGs.
- _Rhomboid flaps_ can be used, with the donor site scar in the relaxed skin tension line (RSTL).
- _Cervicofacial flaps_ are used for more extensive zone 1 defects.
- Tissue expanders have been used.

Zone 2:

- From superolateral junction of helix and cheek, crossing medially across the sideburn to the malar eminence and then inferiorly to the mandible. It includes all tissues over the parotid/masseteric fascia.
- This area is often used as a skin graft donor site.
- Larger defects can be resurfaced with anteriorly based _Cervicofacia flaps_.
- Also deltopectoral flaps, cervicohumeral flaps, _Trapezius_ flap, pectoralis major and latissimus dorsi.
- Free flaps, such as scapular flaps may be better than pedicled flaps.

Zone 3:

- Lower anterior cheek and reconstruction may require lining as well.
- Some flaps can be folded and split including the DP flap, pectoralis major and trapezius.
- Also use a combination of flaps.
- Free flaps have replaced many pedicled techniques and can be composite, e.g. including palmaris longus.

Cheek rotation flap

- Can be used anywhere on the face based inferiorly or superiorly.
- The optimal design places the scars at the borders of aesthetic subunits.

- It can be used for lower eyelid reconstruction with the *Mustardé flap*.
- Elevate beneath the SMAS.
- The defect can be closed primarily or by using a post-auricular flap.

Chemical peels

- Multiple fine and course facial rhytids, and uneven skin pigmentation are not effectively treated surgically.
- They can be treated with chemical peeling *Dermabrasion* and *Laser*.
- They affect the epidermis and superficial dermis, smoothing irregularities and altered skin pigmentation.
- *Phenol peels.*
- *Trichloro-acetic acid peels.*

Chemical weapons
Mustard gas:

- Used in World War I is still the most frequently used chemical agent.
- Decontamination of the wound within 2 minutes is the only way to decrease the effects of mustard gas.
- Irrigation with dilute hypochlorite and water. Open bullae and irrigate.
- After this, treat like a burn.
- Get erythema at 4–8 hours, vesiculation at 2–18 hours.

Lewisite:

- An arsenical vesicant similar effect as mustard gas.
- Effects start in seconds. Irrigate as with mustard gas.

Phosgene oxime:

- A corrosive agent that causes severe pain.
- Erythema, urticaria and ulceration develop.
- Effects are immediate. Irrigate, but damage is irreversible due to rapid absorption.

White phosphorus:

- Used in many anti-personnel weapons and ignites when exposed to air.
- Wounds develop from ignited clothing.
- Treat as standard burn.
- Particles embedded in skin need to be debrided.

See Chemical injuries.

Chemotherapy

- Wound healing and tumour growth share many pathways.
- Nine different classes of drugs are used to treat cancer. All attenuate the inflammatory phase of healing by interfering with the vascular response.
- The fibroblast is the primary cell affected.
- If chemotherapy is delayed by a couple of weeks after surgery then healing is not normally affected.
- The most significant effect occurs when they are used pre-operatively. Particularly alkylating agents, anti-metabolites, anti-tumour antibodies and steroids.

Cherubism

- Familial fibrous dysplasia.
- Multiple areas of *Fibrous dysplasia* in the mandible and maxilla.
- They may occur as early as the first year.

Chest wall reconstruction
Anatomy:

- *Inspiratory muscles:* include sternocleidomastoid and scalene.
- *Expiratory muscles:* attach to the lower part of the rib cage. Include rectus abdominus, inferior and exterior oblique.
- A flail segment with paradoxical breathing will occur with >4 neighbouring ribs are excised or >5 cm of chest wall.

Indications:

- Trauma.
- Tumour.
- Radiation.
- Infection: *Median sternotomy infection.*
- Congenital: *Poland's syndrome*, *Pectus excavatum*, *Pectus carinatum*, *Ectopia cordis*, *Sternal cleft*.

Principles:

- Debride, obliterate dead space, fix skeleton, soft tissue cover, aesthetics.
- *Soft tissue:* muscle flaps most commonly used to reconstruct, usually pedicled, *Pectoralis* major, *Trapezius*: *latissimus* dorsi rarely free. Mobilize pedicles extensively so that they are completely free.
- *Skeleton:* stabilization is necessary to maintain protection and function if over four

ribs resected. Can use rib grafts with muscle flaps or mesh or composites, such as _Methyl methacrylate_ and mesh.

Chondroblastoma

- Benign tumour of chondroblastic germ cells in the epiphysis.
- Pt <25 years old.
- Patients present with soft tissue swelling and pain with loss of range of motion.
- On XR these lesion have a thick reactive rim of bone.
- Treat by extended bone grafting or cementation.

See Bone tumours.

Chondrodermatitis nodularis helicis (CDNH)

- A painful condition affecting the ear.
- Occurs on a prominent aspect and is probably a pressure sore.
- Histological examination reveals nodular hyperplasia, fibrinoid necrosis of collagen and perichondritis.
- The condition is seen in patients who can only sleep on one side.
- Often treated surgically to exclude malignancy.
- The mainstay of treatment is relief of pressure.
- Other treatments include resection, curettage, and laser, but recurrence is high.

Chondroid syringoma

- Mixed tumour of skin, salivary gland type.
- It has both epithelial and mesenchymal tissue components – sweat gland elements (syringoma) and cartilage-like elements (chondroid).
- They are deep to the epidermis and benign.
- Simple excision is performed for diagnosis.

Chondromyxoid fibroma

- Rare cartilaginous lesions that occur most commonly in the metaphyseal bone about the knee.
- They form near the anterior tibial cortex.
- The cartilaginous component is fibrocartilage not the hyaline seen in enchondromas.

See Bone tumours.

Chondrosarcoma

- Second most frequent primary malignant tumour of bone.
- Typically a low-grade malignant neoplasm with malignant chondrocytes producing cartilaginous matrix.
- Neoplastic bone is never seen.
- Primary and secondary:
  - primary occurs in previously normal bone, usually in older patients in the axial skeleton and shoulder;
  - secondary occurs in benign cartilage tumour, such as _Enchondroma_ or _Osteochondroma_.
- Histologically, it is difficult to distinguish benign from malignant and the diagnosis is made based on the history and the imaging. Three variants:
  - _clear cell chondrosarcoma_, rare is the malignant version of the chondroblastoma, it is low grade;
  - _dedifferentiated chondrosarcoma_ is low grade with areas of high grade, they have a poor prognosis;
  - _mesenchymal chondrosarcoma_ is high grade with islands of mature cartilage, the prognosis is better than dedifferentiated.
- CT is very helpful.
- Treatment is aggressive surgical resection. Radiotherapy and chemotherapy are not effective.

See Bone tumours.

Chordee

- Downward curvature of penile shaft.
- Mainly seen associated with _Hypospadias_.
- The ventral penile structures distal to the hypospadias are not normal.
- The mesenchyme which would have formed these structures does not differentiate normally. Instead, it becomes a layer of inelastic fibrous tissue that extends in a fan shape from the meatus to the glans. This tethers the penis and causes downward curvature with erections.

Causes:

- _Congenital:_ fibrosis of corpus spongiosum, skin tethering, deficiency of Buck's fascia, hypoplastic urethra, differential corporal growth. >90% are due to skin shortage.

- *Acquired:* Peyronie's disease, peri-urethral fibrosis associated with stricture.

Treatment:
- Correct by making an incision around the coronal sulcus and retract the skin to the base of the shaft.
- The urethra is mobilized away from the corporal bodies and the bands resected.

Cierny and Mader classification
Staging of osteomyelitis.

Anatomic type:
- *Stage 1:* medullary osteomyelitis.
- *Stage 2:* superficial osteomyelitis.
- *Stage 3:* localized osteomyelitis.
- *Stage 4:* diffuse osteomyelitis.

Physiological class:
- *A host:* normal host.
- *B host:*
  - Bs, systemic compromise;
  - Bl, local compromise;
  - Bls, systemic and local compromise.
- *C host:* treatment worse than disease.

Circumduction
Of the thumb, measured as the angle of the 2nd and 3rd MC to 1st and 2nd MC. Usually around 130°.

Clark's levels
For measuring depth of invasion of <u>Malignant melanoma</u>.
- *Level 1:* tumour confined to epidermis.
- *Level 2:* tumour extending to papillary dermis.
- *Level 3:* tumour extending to junction of papillary and reticular dermis.
- *Level 4:* tumour extending into reticular dermis.
- *Level 5:* tumour extending into subcutaneous fat.
See <u>Breslow</u>.

Clasped thumb
- Congenital condition with the thumb metacarpal held adducted and the proximal phalanx flexed.
- Treat by splinting in extension for 6 months.
- If there is significant adduction contracture, perform 1st web space release.

- Tendon transfers or joint fusions may be required.

Claw hand
- Seen in <u>Ulnar nerve palsy</u> due to intrinsic paralysis.
- The intrinsics pass volar to MCP joint and dorsal to PIP joint.
- They prevent hyperextension of the MPJ.
- With extension of the MCP joint, they are placed under tension causing extension of the PIP joint.
- Paralysis leads to weakened MCP joint flexion and unopposed extension.
- As the MCP joint hyperextends flexors are placed under tension and cause unapposed PIP joint flexion. This is the *intrinsic minus position.*
- Wrist flexion worsens the clawing through tenodesis effect.

Cleft hand
Typical:
- Familial, bilateral, usually middle ray absent, maybe index.
- V defect. Radial side more affected.
- Syndactyly of the 1st and sometimes 4th web space.
- Autosomal dominant.
- Associated with other musculoskeletal abnormalities.
- Patients have good function.

Atypical:
- <u>Symbrachydactyly</u>.

Treatment:
- Surgical techniques involve reconstruction of the transverse metacarpal ligament.
- The Snow–Littler technique involves raising a dorsal flap from the cleft and transposing radially to the first web.
- The 2nd metacarpal is then transferred to the 3rd metacarpal.
See <u>Congenital hand anomalies</u>.

Cleft lip and palate
History:
- *390 AD:* reported in China.
- *Yperman (1295–1351):* used a needle and wax suture with a figure of 8 stitch.
- *Paré (1575):* used an obturator.

- *Tagliocozzi (1597):* used mattress sutures.
- *Dieffenback (1828):* closed the hard palate.
- *Langenbeck (1859):* used bipedicled flaps.
- *Lip repairs:* LeMesurier (1949), Tennison (1952) and Millard (1958).

Incidence:
- Fogh-Andersen (1942) established the incidence of CL/P in Denmark as 1:700 live births.
- Caucasians 1:1000, Asians 1:500, Africans 1:2500.
- CLandP 45% CP 30% CL 20%.
- Lt:Rt:bilateral 6:3:1.

Embryology:
Aetiology:
- Failure of fusion of the frontonasal, two lateral maxillary, and two mandibular segments.
- Or failure of mesenchymal penetration.
- Relate to genetic factors, smoking, possibly nutritional.

Epidemiology: Cleft lip and palate (*CL/P*) different from cleft palate (CP).

CL/P:
- More common in males.
- Not often other syndromes – *Van de Woudes* syndrome is one of the few to be associated with CL alone.

CP:
- More common in females.
- May be associated with foetal alcohol syndrome, anti-convulsants, maternal diabetes, retinoic acid, folate deficiency.
- Often associated with other abnormalities as part of a syndrome. Associated with *VCF*, *Treacher Collins*, *Stickler's*, *Apert's*, *Crouzon's* Down's, *Pierre Robin*.

Genetics: CL/P variable expressivity or multifactorial. Suggests a threshold over which the cleft phenotype is expressed. Genetic or environmental factors may carry one over the threshold:

	CL/P	CP
1 sib	4%	2%
1 parent	4%	6%
1 sib, 1 parent	15%	15%

Syndromic clefts: 3% of clefts, classified as major mutant gene e.g. Treacher Collins, chromosomal aberrations, e.g. trisomies and teratologic syndromes related to drugs and alcohol.

Classification: Kernahan classification.

Timing of repair:
- Cons are:
  - better psychologically;
  - better wound healing;
  - but technically more difficult as smaller;
  - logistically difficult;
  - anaesthetic difficulties particularly with post-op airway obstruction.
- *Conventional repair:*
  - lip and anterior palate 3 months;
  - remaining hard and soft palate 6–9 months.
- *Delaire* technique.
- *Schweckendiek* technique.

Cleft alveolus:
Grafting of the maxilla was first performed in 1900, but not routinely carried out until 1955. It is now an accepted part of the cleft management.

Indications:
- *Stabilization of the maxillary arch:* prevents the collapse of the lesser segment behind the greater segment in unilateral and the greater segments behind the premaxilla in bilateral clefts.
- *Elimination of the oronasal fistula:* prevents regurgitation into the nose.
- *Odontogenic bony support:* aids tooth eruption.
- *Nasal bony support:* provides a platform for nasal correction.

Nomenclature:
- Previously this has been described by age as primary (<2 year), secondary (2–5) and late secondary (5–12).
- More helpful to describe primary before palate repair and secondary after palate repair.

Operations:
- *Primary bone grafting:* fit obturator to align the maxillary segments. By 9–12 months when they are abutting, mucosal flaps are raised and turned over to create a palatal lining. A small rib graft is taken from the lateral chest around the level of the inframammary

fold, sectioned longitudinally and the cortical half is onlaid over the labial surface. The inner half is broken up and packed into the space between onlay graft and palatal flaps. Dissection is limited and the midface growth region of the premaxillary-vomerine suture is avoided.

- *Secondary bone grafting.*

Cleft lip:

Abnormality of the primary palate. This lies anterior to the incisive foramen and consists of lip, alveolus and hard palate.

Anatomy:

characterized by the following:

- Discontinuity of skin and soft tissue.
- Vertical deficiency.
- Abnormal lip muscle attachment to alar base and nasal spine.
- Alveolar cleft at level of canine.
- Hard palate defect anterior to incisive foramen.
- *Nasal deformity.*
- Also *Simonart's band*, *forme fruste*.

Unilateral cleft lip:

Surgery:

- Evolved in five stages from simple closure to refined skin repair followed by muscle repair addressing the bony platforms and nasal repair.
- Various principles can be summarized as:
  - lengthen shortened vertical height;
  - bring in lateral tissue;
  - retain normal Cupid's bow;
  - rotation-advancement;
  - muscle reconstruction;
  - bony platform;
  - nasal anatomy.

Techniques:

- *Straight line*:
  - *Rose and Thompson*: slight length increase was achieved by curving the incision;
  - *Mirault–Blair–Brown* increased the lip length by introducing a flap from the lateral lip. However, the importance of the Cupid's bow being in the medial lip was not realized.
- *Lower lip Z-plasty*:
  - *Le Mesurier–Hagedorn* provided a quadrangular flap to recreate Cupid's bow;

- *Tennison–Randall* provided the same with a triangular flap. So both these brought tissue from laterally and recreated Cupid's bow.
- *Upper lip Z-plasty*:
  - *Millard* introduced the concept of rotation-advancement, placing incision under the nose where they are more hidden;
  - Mohler brings the incision into the columella to achieve a more rectangularly-shaped philtrum;
  - the importance of realigning the muscle was realized. A number of different techniques are suggested to bring them in a more anatomic position. The bone is affected variably. The lateral incisor may be missing, small, duplicated or rotated. Correction may require repositioning of the alveolar segments or bone grafting in the mixed dentition period. Primary nasal tip plasty has been shown to give lasting results and consists of wide nasal undermining.
- *Upper and lower lip Z-plasty:*
  - Skoog and Trauner.

Operative repair (Millard):

- Medial markings cupid bow and C flap with small back cut on vermilion margin for small Tennison flap.
- Excise mucosa. For lip-only incision of C flap passes around nasal floor to meet lateral incision.
- Mobilize muscle.
- On lateral lip incise along mucosa with small flap. Excise mucosa. Mobilize muscle.
- Incise in buccal sulcus and mobilize periosteum off bone to piriform fossa. Mobilize periosteum around nasal floor.
- Do McComb on lateral nose.
- For repair start with nasal floor then alar base. Put stitch in vermilion equidistant to pull down lip.
- Suture mucosa to close to red line.
- Suture muscle at lower end using overlapping stitch. Suture upper end then those in-between. Tie all sutures after all are placed. Make sure the very upper end is sutured.
- Suture skin starting at vermilion junction and Tennison flap then the rest including insetting C flap. Suture vermilion making Z-plasty to line up red line.
- Finally, put bolster stitch to nose.

Bilateral cleft lip:
Analysis of the defect:
- Complete or incomplete.
- Note widened alar bases, shortened columella, obtuse nasolabial angle, hypoplastic prolabium, short upper lip particularly centrally, protrusion of premaxilla, absence of sulcus in premaxilla, absence of muscle in premaxilla, absence of Cupid's bow, abnormal white roll.
- *Premaxilla:* normally a premaxillary-maxillary growth suture is not present so anterior growth is restricted. The cleft acts like a suture allowing abnormal forward projection. This gives a vertically long maxilla, absent nasal spine, short columella and blunted nasal tip.

Timing and principles:
- Variable timing as some surgeons perform initial lip adhesion followed by lip repair.
- The central lip is formed from prolabium. Muscle is required to come from the lateral elements into the prolabium. The prolabium is thinned to prevent the over wide central lip.
- *Premaxilla:* protrusion can be controlled by non-operative means with a head cap, tapes or acrylic plates or operative means, such as fixed pin traction, lip adhesion or surgical setback.

Operations:
- *Lip adhesion:* for wide lips, over 1 cm distance between cleft.
- *Manchester repair:* uses the prolabium vermilion to which the lateral lip elements are attached. The muscle is brought across the midline.
- *Millard repair:* prolabium marked and elevated. Vermilion turned down to create sulcus. Lateral flaps are elevated as forked flaps. Lateral lip segments come to midline bringing white roll to the prolabium. Muscle brought to midline.
- *Mulliken repair:* makes a much narrower prolabial flap. Intercartilaginous incisions are made to superiorly advance the lateral alar cartilages before suturing them overlapped with the upper lateral cartilages. The alar base flaps are medially transposed.

- *Noordhoff repair:* as for Millard, but the alar cartilages are freed via an intercartilaginous incision originating from the piriform aperture and secured together at the domes and to the upper lateral cartilages. The buccal mucosal flaps are then sutured into the inferior intercartilaginous incision to increase length for the nasal floor reconstruction.
- *Columellar lengthening:*
  ○ may not be required in Mulliken's procedure;
  ○ Cronin procedure involves a V–Y advancement of banked forked flaps;
  ○ produce tip projection by intercrural or interdomal sutures.

Cleft nose:
- Slumping of alar dome.
- Lateral displacement of lateral crus.
- Shortening of medial crus.
- Loss of continuity of piriform aperture and bony platform.
- Displacement of septum.
- Loss of overlap of upper and lower lateral cartilages.

Operation:
Correction of the nose may be performed at the time of lip repair or delayed until nasal growth is complete. Delayed correction usually involves an open rhinoplasty in the late teenage years.
- *McComb technique:* performed at the time of lip repair. The skin is separated from cartilage and bolster sutures are inserted to lift the alar cartilages.
- *Tajima:* a reversed U incision is used to gain access to the alar cartilages, which are sutured.
- *Matsuma splints:* come in different sizes and aim to mould the nasal cartilage.

Cleft palate:
- *A failure of the palatal shelves to fuse:* the secondary palate consisting of the soft and hard palate.

Embryology:
- In the 7-week old embryo, the two palatal shelves lie vertically.
- The neck straightens, the tongue drops posteriorly, and the shelves rotate superiorly to horizontal.

- They fuse from anterior to posterior by 12 weeks.
- In rodents the right rotates before the left. This may explain the higher incidence of left-sided clefts.

Anatomy:
- The incisive foramen behind the incisors is the point where the lateral maxillary bones meet the premaxilla.
- The primary palate refers to structures in front of the incisive foramen and are the structures involved with cleft lip.
- The secondary palate, which refers to the hard and soft palate.
- The hard palate is composed of palatal process of maxilla anteriorly and palatal bones posteriorly.
- The soft palate contains five muscles:
  - *tensor veli palatine:* originates around Eustachian tube and passes around the hamular process of the pterygoid plate to insert into palatine aponeurosis;
  - *Levator veli palatini:* originates around the Eustachian tube and descends down to insert into the palatine aponeurosis; important for velopharyngeal closure; there may be an isolated failure of fusion of levators in submucous cleft palate;
  - *muscularis uvulae:* lies within the uvula at the centre of the palate; it may be small or absent in submucous CP, and thickens the centre of the soft palate;
  - *palatoglossus;*
  - *palatopharyngeus:* pulls the soft palate posteriorly.
- The greater palatine artery passes anteriorly and medially from the greater palatine foramen situated at the posterolateral border of the palate.
- In unilateral cleft palate, the vomer is attached to one palatal shelf. In bilateral cleft palate it is attached to neither shelf.

Aetiology:
- Genetic. Some syndromes such as Stickler's, velocardiofacial, foetal alcohol syndrome, DiGeorge syndrome and trisomies.
- The most common associated anomaly is Pierre Robin sequence.

Principles and timing:
- Separate oral from nasal layer.
- Reposition the soft palate muscles.
- Minimize growth disturbance.
- Palate repair may help Eustachian tube function, which decreases serous otitis media.
- Timing is a balance between speech, growth and safety of operation.
- Most surgeons perform palate repair at 6–9 months when the child has grown, is no longer an obligate nasal breather and before early speech development has commenced. *See Cleft lip and palate* for other timing options.

Operations:
- *Von Langenbeck's repair:* bipedicled flaps are raised to enable closure. Each flap receives its blood supply from the greater palatine vessels.
- *Medial Langenbeck flaps:* bipedicle flaps based medially to the artery to attempt to reduce growth disturbance, but have a high fistula rate.
- *No flaps:* may be possible to oppose across the midline without raising flaps. Particularly if the anterior palate or soft palate has been closed at the time of lip repair.
- *Bardach's repair:* single pedicle flaps based on the greater palatine artery.
- *Veau–Wardill–Kilner repair:* with 4 flaps, 2 close off the region of the incisive foramen, and 2 are pushed back to lengthen the palate.
- *Furlow technique:* attempts to lengthen the palate with a Z-plasty. Used for primary repair and also for velopharyngeal incompetence.
- *Intravelar veloplasty:* to reposition the muscles of the soft palate.
- *Sommerlad radical intravelar veloplasty:* wide dissection of the soft palate musculature to enable them to lie at the posterior aspect of the soft palate.

Velopharyngeal insufficiency:
Secondary lip and nasal deformities:
Assessment: Nose.

Unilateral cleft lip:
- *Assessment:* look at lip symmetry, length discrepancies, Cupid's bow and white roll alignment. Assess dynamic lip function asking the patient to purse the lips.

- *Vermilion asymmetry:* due to scar, poor alignment of muscle or vermilion. Treat with local tissue transposition procedures:
  - white roll mismatches can be corrected with Z-plasty or excision;
  - superficial notching can be corrected with a simple V–Y advancement;
  - if more severe a series of Z-plasties may be needed;
  - reduction or augmentation on one side may be required;
  - severe deficiencies may require re-operation.
- *Short upper lip:* with asymmetry in the vertical lengths of the repaired cleft lip segments. Due to poor planning or scar contracture. In either case the treatment is re-operation.
- *Constricted upper lip:* vertical and horizontal deficiency. Usually due to too much tissue resection, but may be tissue hypoplasia. Requires re-operation.
- *Long upper lip:* due to poor planning. Re-operate. May require full thickness lip reduction.
- *Muscular diastasis:* requires resuturing of muscle layer.
- *Mucosal anomalies:* Z-plasties.
- *Loss of Cupid's bow:* triangular skin excision above the mucocutaneous line. The excision is then is closed horizontally.

Bilateral cleft lip:

- *Assessment:* problems relate to the size, shape and positioning of the premaxillary and prolabial segments, which are generally hypoplastic and anteriorly displaced. The buccal sulcus narrow.
- *Whistle tip deformity:* soft tissue deficiency in the central portion of lip vermilion, but with an adequate prolabium:
  - small defects are treated by local mucosal V–Y flaps or Z-plasties;
  - moderate deformities use <u>*Kapetansky flaps*</u>;
  - *severe deformities:* re-operate or use an <u>*Abbé flap*</u>.
- *Short upper lip:* reflects a composite central lip deformity. The cause is the hypoplastic lip. First re-operate that allows correction of prolabial width, reorientation of muscle and scar resection. This can be accompanied by lateral vermilion advancement.

- *Constricted upper lip:* with vertical and horizontal deficiency. Reconstruct with an <u>*Abbé flap*</u>.
- *Long upper lip:* This can be corrected by using a curved elliptical excision below the nasal sill.

Unilateral cleft nose:

- *Assessment:* the tip is asymmetrical with a depressed dome. The alar cartilage is laterally displaced and widened. The septum is deviated toward the non-cleft side. Get hypoplasia of the maxillary structures.
- *Operation:* straighten septum, address alar cartilage with a vertical septal cartilage graft, adjust cartilage with sutures and shield grafts. Perform an osteotomy. A V–Y columellar advancement may be required.

Bilateral cleft nose:

- *Assessment:* columella is short, the tip is flattened due to alar separation. The hypoplastic maxilla is symmetrical.
- *Operation:* plan to increase columellar length, augment tip projection and narrow the alar base. Perform in two stages:
  - at 18/12 perform the Cronin columellar lengthening procedure;
  - in mixed dentition period, perform open rhinoplasty and add septal and shield grafts to increase projection and support. Perform V–Y columellar lengthening.

Cleland's ligaments

- These originate from the digital skeleton and pass laterally to attach to the digital skin.
- The major bundles are around the PIP joint. They arise from the distal third of the proximal phalanx and the base of the middle phalanx, diverging away from the joint to be attached to the skin.
- The minor bundles are short strong fibres originating from the lateral aspect of the DIP joint and insert into the skin laterally and dorsally.
- They all pass dorsal to the neurovascular bundles.

See <u>*Grayson's ligament*</u>. See <u>*Retinacular system*</u>.

Clinodactyly

- Inherited condition (usually autosomal dominant).

- The finger deviates in the radial-ulnar plane.
- Most often bilateral little fingers.
- Usually caused by a delta phalanx of the middle phalanx so called because it is triangular (Δ) – a longitudinal bracketed epiphysis.
- The growth plate is C-shaped.
- Worsens with growth.
- Associated with mental retardation.
- Surgery is not usually indicated for functional reasons though if performed should be with a wedge osteotomy – closing wedge if long and opening wedge if short. In the immature skeleton, physiolysis can be performed which aims to remove the tethering on the short side of the bone by inserting a fat graft.

CMC joint arthritis thumb
- Two key ligaments are palmar (ulnar) ligament (beak ligament) that holds trapezium to MC and dorsal intermetacarpal ligament which holds 1st metacarpal to 2nd.
- Ligaments stressed in opposition and pinch. Once the ligaments are disrupted arthritis will follow.
- Hypermobility leads to early OA.

Assessment:
- Get pain and weakness.
- One-third of patients with CMC OA also have carpal tunnel syndrome. Tenderness over joint. Locate with 1st MC in adduction.
- *Torque test (grind test):* axial rotation in distraction and compression.
- *Crank test:* axial loading while passively flexing and extending the metacarpal base. Prominent MC base and laxity with crepitus.
- *Swan neck deformity:* get radial subluxation leading to adduction contracture. Compensatory MCPJ hyperextension occurs to allow adequate thumb positioning during grasp.
- *XR changes: Eaton/Glickel classification*.

Treatment:
- *Non-operative:* splints, steroid injection, analgesia.
- *Operative:*
  ○ reconstruct UCL: Eaton–Littler uses FCU.

Surgery:
- *Basal osteotomy*
- *Trapeziectomy*.

Coagulation cascade
- Essential for haemostasis. Results in the formation of fibrin clot.
- Coagulation factors circulate as inactive precursors (zymogen). These are converted into enzymes that activate the next zymogen causing amplification to finally produce thrombin and then fibrin.
- The classic description is of an extrinsic pathway stimulated by injury and exposure of tissue factor and an intrinsic pathway activated when blood contacts a foreign surface.
- Probably tissue factor and factor VII in the intrinsic pathway are the main factors, which start clotting, and the intrinsic pathway maintains clot.
- Intrinsic clotting cascade begins with factor 12. Extrinsic cascade starts with factor 7. Both converge on factor 5 and then have a common pathway.
- Protease inhibitors regulate the pathway, e.g. anti-thrombin III, which is enhanced by heparin. Protein C and protein S are also anticoagulants. Deficiencies in these factors increases thrombosis.

Cocaine
- First local anaesthetic discovered.
- A crystalline alkyloid derived from coco leaves, first isolated in 1860.
- Local anaesthetic, vasoconstrictive and sympathomimetic.
- It blocks reuptake of norepinephrine and epinephrine centrally and peripherally.
- Most commonly used for topical anaesthesia, particularly in nasal surgery and laceration in children.
- The safe maximum dose for nasally administered 4% cocaine solution is 1.5 mg/kg. Each drop of 4% cocaine solution has approximately 3 mg cocaine.

See Local anaesthetics

Cold intolerance (TICAS)
Or *TICAS:* trauma-induced cold-associated symptoms.
- A collection of acquired symptoms resulting in an aversion to cold with:
  ○ pain/discomfort;
  ○ stiffness;

o altered sensibility;

o colour change.

• Half of patients experience these at the time of injury, the rest after a 4-month lag period once the cold weather comes.

• Symptoms generally improve after 2 years.

Collagen

• Makes up 30% of total body protein.

• Collagen can withstand a static load of 20 kg per 1 mm fibre.

• Procollagen is produced by fibroblasts. This is excreted from the cell and forms tropocollagen. They wrap around each other in a triple-helix conformation. Each chain is 1000 amino acids long.

• Two unique amino acids are hydroxyproline and hydroxylysine. Get cross-linking of 3 polypepeptide chains in a left-hand helix. These then wind in a right-hand coil.

• Collagen formation is inhibited by colchicine, penicillamide, steroids, vitamin C and iron deficiency.

• There are 13 types of collagen.

• Normal dermis mainly composed of type I collagen (90%). Type III collagen is produced by the foetus and in early stages of wound healing. By week 2 type I collagen is again produced. During remodelling type III collagen is replaced by type 1.

• Collagen production in a healing wound peaks at 6 weeks though accumulation is maximal at 3 weeks. Rates of synthesis remain elevated for up to a year. Reduced scar strength is due to lack of organization not lack of quantity.

• Collagen type by tissue:

o *type 1:* in skin, bone, tendon;

o *type 2:* hyaline cartilage and cornea;

o *type 3:* healing tissue, foetal wounds;

o *type 4:* basement membrane;

o *type 5:* also basement membrane.

See *Wound healing*, *Foetal wound healing*, *Skin*.

Collagen: injectable

• Injectable collagens shrink as they extrude water and biodegrade.

• Primarily type I collagen.

• Bovine collagen was developed in 1981 and has the antigenic peptide end regions removed.

• The main concern with injectable collagens is the immune response so perform skin testing first.

• Cross-linkage with glutaraldehyde gives a longer lifespan.

• Re-injection required up to 6 monthly.

Types of injectable collagen:

• *Zyderm 1:* bovine collagen, 35 mg/ml. For fine wrinkles.

• *Zyderm 2:* as above, but 65 mg/ml. For more coarse wrinkles.

• *Zyplast:* cross-linkage of collagen with glutaraldehyde. Firmer than the above and used for coarse wrinkles.

See *Alloplasts*.

Collar-button abscess

• An infection commencing superficially between skin and palmar fascia.

• It erodes through the fascia and then spreads quickly in the underlying loose space.

• A poor understanding of the anatomy may lead to incomplete drainage.

Collateral ligament

• True collateral ligament of phalanges arises from condyle of proximal bone and inserts into palmar third of distal bone.

• Accessory collateral ligament inserts into lateral margin of volar plate distally.

See *PIPJ*, *MCPJ*.

Coloboma

• A notch or cleft of the eyelid of varying degree.

• In a *Tessier* 3 cleft they are found medial to the punctum of the lower eyelid.

Commissure reconstruction

• Converse described the three-flap mucosal technique:

o a triangular wedge of scar is excised with the apex at the desired point for the commissure;

o three flaps of oral mucosa are created the centre of which is everted laterally to form the small vertical component of the commissure;

o the superior and inferior mucosal flaps are folded outward to fill the defect of the upper and lower lateral lip elements.

- Z-plasties, double opposing Z-plasties, vermilion transposition flaps and bilobed mucosal flaps have been described.

See Lip reconstruction.

Common peroneal nerve

- L4–S1.
- Winds round head of fibula then enters peroneal compartment.
- The deep peroneal nerve supplies tibialis anterior, extensor digitorum longus, extensor hallucis longus, extensor digitorum brevis and the skin to the 1st web space.
- The superficial peroneal nerve supplies peroneal muscles and sensory supply to lateral lower leg and dorsum of foot.
- Compression leads to foot drop and paraesthesia but not usually pain.

Compartment syndrome

- Vascular compromise and tissue necrosis in a compartment resulting from sustained rise in intracompartmental pressure.
- Normal pressures 0–8 mmHg.
- Perform fasciotomy if tissue pressure rises to within 10–30 mmHg of diastolic pressure, or over 30 mmHg for over 8 hours.
- In one study all patients with pressures over 55 mmHg had neuromuscular problems.
- Recommendation is that pressure over 30 mmHg with clinical symptoms require fasciotomy.
- Increase compartment pressure raises venous pressure. Capillary flow is reduced leading to ischaemia. When compartment pressure exceeds venous pressure there is no perfusion.

Aetiology:

- Most common is fracture.
- Decrease of compartment size, e.g. constrictive dressings, casts and burns.
- Increase fluid content, e.g. crush, reperfusion, bleeding, electrical injury venopuncture.

Diagnosis:

- Clinical diagnosis is the best method. Pain, exacerbated by passive stretching.
- Loss of distal perfusion is a late sign.
- Pressure measurement with a Stryker device or a Wicks catheter.

- Untreated compartment syndrome results in *Volkmann's ischaemic contracture*.
- Beware rhabdomyolysis.

Upper limb:
Forearm:

- *Three compartments:* volar, dorsal and mobile wad. The compartments are interconnected so they can be decompressed by releasing the volar compartment though the dorsal compartment may also require decompression.
- *Volar forearm:* should include release of carpal tunnel. Carry incision towards the ulnar border then centrally. This avoids injury to radial artery and median nerve, and the radial flap covers the tendon. Incise fascia. Examine superficial and deep compartments. The deeper compartments should be particularly examined in electrical injuries as the most injured muscles are adjacent to bone.
- Complete release will usually also release mobile wad and dorsal compartment. If they remain tense then incise dorsally.

The hand:

- *Ten separate non-communicating compartments:* 4 dorsal interossei, 3 volar interossei, hypothenar, thenar and a separate compartment for adductor pollicis. Each must be released separately. Test by abducting and adducting the fingers. The finger has tight fascia which can cause a localized compartment syndrome.
- Release interossei through two dorsal incisions along 2nd and 4th MC.
- Incise over thenar and hypothenar muscles. Debride necrotic muscle.
- Digital decompression is indicated if blood supply is compromised. Mid-axial incision, ulnar side of index, middle, and ring and radial side of little finger.

Lower limb:

- Four compartments in the lower leg, anterior, lateral and deep and superficial posterior. Two incisions are required to decompress.
- Incise 2 cm medial to tibial border to release anterior and deep compartments.
- Incise 2 cm lateral to tibial border to release lateral compartment.

Complex combined vascular malformations
- Include CVM, CLM, CLVM, and CLAVM.
- They are often associated with soft tissue and skeletal hypertrophy.
- Like the 'pure' _Vascular malformations_, complex-combined anomalies can be categorized as either slow flow or fast flow.

Slow-flow complex-combined malformations:
- _Klippel–Trenaunay syndrome_.
- _Proteus syndrome_.

Fast-flow complex-combined anomalies:
- These anomalies are uncommon.
- CAVM, CAVF or CLAVM correspond to the old term _Parkes Weber syndrome_ (capillary, arterial, venous and lymphatic malformation).
- Cutaneous warmth, bruit, and thrill are pathognomonic.
- MRI or arteriography in young children usually shows only diffuse hypervascularity of the limb; multiple AVFs become obvious later, occurring throughout the affected limb, particularly near the joints.
- Assess leg length.
- Muscles and joints are not usually involved in fast flow anomalies.
- MR angiography and MR venography are useful to detect arterial feeders.

Treatment:
- _Conservative:_
  ○ compression stockings;
  ○ shoe raise;
  ○ sclerosis of superficial veins.
- _Surgical:_
  ○ epiphyseal stapling for length discrepancy;
  ○ staged resection;
  ○ amputation.

Complex regional pain syndrome
See _Reflex sympathetic dystrophy_.

Composite grafts
- Composite grafts commonly contain skin, as well as other tissue such as fat or cartilage.
- Useful in _Nasal reconstruction_ and ear reconstruction.

- In general, any composite graft >5 mm distant from a vascular bed is at risk for necrosis of skin and fat
- Initially, a graft is white then cyanotic from venous congestions with a change to a pink colour after 3–7 days.
- Improve take of a graft by maximizing the contact of the graft with vascularized tissue.
- Post-operative cooling initially may improve.

Congenital hand anomalies
Incidence:
- 1:600. Most isolated.

Embryology:
- Limb bud develops at 4 weeks.
- 33 days hand paddle.
- 50 days digital separation.
- 50 days full bony structure.
- Complete development at birth except for myelination which is complete by 2 years.

Classification: International Federation of Societies for Surgery of the Hand Classification of Congenital Hand Anomalies. Seven types.
- Failure of formation (developmental arrest).
- Failure of differentiation.
- Duplication.
- Overgrowth.
- Undergrowth.
- Congenital constriction syndrome.
- Generalized skeletal abnormalities.

Failure of formation:
- _Longitudinal arrest:_ pre-axial:
  ○ pre-axial deficiency, See _Radial club hand_;
  ○ central ray deficiency, See _Cleft hand_;
  ○ post-axial deficiency, See _Ulnar club hand_.
- _Transverse arrest:_
  ○ complete deficiencies;
  ○ intercalated deficiencies.

Failure of differentiation:
- _Soft tissues:_
  ○ _Syndactyly_;
  ○ _Camptodactyly_;
  ○ _Trigger thumb and finger_;
  ○ _Clasped thumb_.
- _Skeletal:_
  ○ _Clinodactyly_;
  ○ _Symphalangism_;
  ○ _Arthrgryposis_;
  ○ _Windblown hand_.

Duplication:
- *Ulnar polydactyly.*
- *Central polydactyly.*
- *Radial polydactyly.*
- *Ulnar dimelia.*

Undergrowth:
- Hypoplastic fingers (*Symbrachydactyly*).
- Brachydactyly.
- *Thumb hypoplasia.*

Overgrowth:
- *Macrodactyly.*

Constriction ring.
Generalized skeletal abnormalities.

Congenital naevus
- Any *Naevus* present at birth.
- A naevus refers to abnormal growth. Most are melanocytic naevi (CMN).
- Melanoblasts migrate early from the neural crest to differentiate into melanocytes. When this migration is disturbed, the result is an ectopic population of cells.
- Histologically congenital naevi differ from acquired in being deeper into the dermis with nests of melanocytes.

Size:
- *Small:* <1.5 cm diameter.
- *Medium:* >1.5 cm <20 cm diameter.
- *Giant:* (GHN) many definitions, >20 cm diameter, >100 cm^2, >5% surface area. <1:20,000 newborns.

Malignancy:
- There is an association between giant naevi and melanoma.
- The quoted risk is variable, ranging from 2 to 30%.
- A study by Quaba suggested an 8% risk of malignant change for a lesion >2% TBSA in the first 15 years of life.
- 50% of malignancies occur in the first 3 years.
- There is also a 4% incidence of extra-cutaneous melanomas, usually CNS or retroperitoneal.
- Melanomas in a GHN may have a worse prognosis.

Clinical features:
- Pale at birth, darken with age.
- Borders are well demarcated, but irregular.

- Most are raised with follicular, pebble stone surface.
- They develop hairs as the lesion matures.
- Giant (GCMN) may be associated with underdevelopment of underlying tissue. They are more common on the lower back or thighs, *Neurocutaneous melanosis*
- Head and neck naevi may be associated with epilepsy. Over the spine there may be underlying spinal defects.

Treatment:
- Controversial, ranging from observation, to treatments such as dermabrasion to complete excision and reconstruction.
- Dermabrasion, split skin graft and laser do not get rid of all of the naevus cells, though may be more effective early before the cells migrate deeper.
- Excision with tissue expansion and advancement flaps can treat very large lesions.

Consent
The situation in England:
- Adults are assumed to be competent unless demonstrated otherwise. The question to ask is 'can this patient understand and weigh up the information needed to make this decision?'
- Consent is not a one-off event, but a process. Patients can change their minds.
- Children. Over 16, individuals are presumed to have competence. Younger children can also give consent if they understand fully. If not, someone with parental responsibility can give consent on the child's behalf unless they can't be reached in an emergency. A parent cannot override a competent child who consents. If a competent child refuses, then legally a parent can consent, but such a situation would be rare.
- The person treating should consent, or someone who can also treat or who has been trained to do so.
- Information needs to be given otherwise the consent may be invalid.
- Consent must be given voluntarily.
- Consent can be written, oral or non-verbal.
- Competent adults may refuse treatment. The only exception is when the patient is detained under the Mental Health Act 1983.

A competent pregnant woman may refuse any treatment even if detrimental to the foetus.
- No-one can give consent on behalf of an incompetent adult. They can be treated if it is in their best interests.
- If an incompetent patient has clearly indicated in the past, while competent, that they would refuse treatment in certain circumstances and those circumstances arise, you must abide by that refusal.

Constricted ear
See _Lop ear._

Constriction ring syndrome
- Probably due to premature rupture of amnion causing strands of amniotic tissue, which create tight bands leading to ischaemia in limbs.
- Incidence 1:15 000.
- May get compromised vascularity and oedema.
- Sporadic.
- Assess urgency, assess circulation and neurology. Note intrinsic muscles.

Classification: Patterson described 4 types:
- _Group 1:_ simple, a groove in the skin.
- _Group 2:_ distal deformity +/– lymphoedema.
- _Group 3:_ distal fusion – _Acrosyndactyly_.
- _Group 4:_ amputations.

Treatment:
- Release early when oedema gross use circumferential Z-plasties.
- Amputation may be required.
- If thumb is shortened the structures proximally are normal. may need phalangization, metacarpal lengthening, toe-hand, digital transfer.

Converse flap
See _Scalping flap._

Copper
Needed for lysyl oxidase used for collagen metabolism.

Cormack and Lamberty: fasciocutaneous flaps
Classification of _Fasciocutaneous flaps_.
- _A:_ multiple perforators, direct and indirect, e.g. _Pontén_ flap.

- _B:_ single perforator, usually direct, which runs along the axis of the flap. E.g. _Scapular_ and parascapular.
- _C:_ segmental perforators – from same source vessel, e.g. _Radial forearm flap_, _Lateral arm flap_.

Coronal synostosis
Unilateral coronal synostosis:
- 8–10% of _Craniosynostosis_.
- Premature fusion of one of the coronal sutures results in plagiocephaly (a Greek term meaning oblique skull).
- 1 of 10 000 live births.
- Superior growth elongates the forehead.
- Inferior growth deforms the middle cranial fossa and bows the greater wing of the sphenoid causing proptosis and the _Harlequin_ sign.
- There is a bulge of the ipsilateral temporal bone.
- The fused suture is ridged.
- _Surgery:_ bifrontal craniotomy and supraorbital rim osteotomy with fronto-orbital advancement. The frontal bone is reshaped and fixed.

Bilateral coronal synostosis:
- 9–20% of synostosis, many are syndromic.
- Tower-shaped, but short, head – turribrachycephaly.
- The skull is wide and elongated vertically.
- _Surgery:_ total calvarial remodelling with barrel stave osteotomies to increase the capacity of the vault. The frontal bone is remodelled and advanced as above.

Cortical ring sign
- Seen in scapho-lunate advanced collapse (SLAC).
- Palmar tilting of the scaphoid results in a ring appearance on a PA.
- Also get _Terry Thomas sign_.
See Carpal _Instability_

Cosmetic camouflage
- _Counteract:_ with neutralizers or colour correctors. A yellow colour negates red (neutralizer) colour correctors act as a primer and are followed by foundation.

- *Cover:* camouflage cream. These cover any scars, pigmentation, etc., that foundation won't hide being thicker and more opaque.
- *Create:* using contour shadow. Correct the brows, eyes and lips.

Cottle sign

- To assess the internal nasal valve.
- If lateral cheek traction improves airway obstruction (positive Cottle sign), then spreader grafts may be of benefit.

Coup de sabre

Sharp depression in forehead with _Hemifacial atrophy_.

Cowden disease

- Keratoses of the palms and soles.
- Multiple _Tricholemmomas_.
- Mucosal papillomas and fibromas.
- Internal organ involvement including thyroid, GIT, ovaries, breasts.
- High incidence of breast cancer.

Crane principle

- Described by Millard in 1969 to provide a platform for complex soft tissue reconstructions.
- A flap is transposed to cover the defect.
- The flap is then split into two lamina with the skin and outer lamina being returned to the original site after a delay period.
- The soft tissue now adherent to the wound providing a stable platform for skin grafting.

Cranial bones

- *Five bones:* 2 frontal, 2 parietal and occipital.
- *Intramembranous ossification:* a centre of osteogenesis develops first into cancellous bone and then into compact bone. They grow until they touch adjacent bones at the sutures. Once they contact, they only grow at the sutures. The metopic suture ossifies in the second year, but the rest ossify in the 30s. After the age of 8 the single plates of bone become two plates of compact bone separated by cancellous bone.
- *Endochondral ossification:* the method of bone formation in the cranial base. Cartilage models are replaced by bone and they articulate with cartilage – synchondrosis.

Craniofacial clefts

- A soft tissue and a bony disruption in the normal growth pattern of the face.
- Sporadic incidence and occurs 1:25 000 births.
- Formation of face between 4th and 8th.
- If the correct cells are not in the correct place then malformations may occur.
- Probably multifactorial.
- A lot occur in developing countries.
- Viruses, toxoplasmosis, teratogens such as anticonvulsants and steroids, and metabolic disorders have been implicated.
- Some overlap between clefts and other hypoplastic syndromes. Treacher Collins is hypoplastic and also Tessier 6, 7, 8 cleft.
- Clefts can affect any layer of the face.

Classification: _Tessier_.

Pathogenesis: key theories.

- *Failure of fusion:* this theory suggests that the face is the site of union of the free ends of the facial processes. After contact penetration by the mesoderm completes the fusion. Disruption leads to a cleft.
- *Mesodermal migration and penetration:* suggests that there are no free ends, but instead the face is a continuous sheet, demarcated by epithelial seams. Mesenchyme migrates into this. The craniofacial skeleton is derived from neuroectoderm. If the neuroectoderm fails to penetrate then the epithelium breaks down. Partial penetration will lead to a partial cleft.
- *Amniotic bands:* with intrauterine compression.

Craniofacial genetics
Orofacial clefts:

- Over 200 syndromes, but most clefts are isolated events.
- CL with or without CP is distinct from isolated CP.
- There may be two forms of CP. An autosomal dominant type and a non-familial, which is caused by environmental factors.

Orofacial cleft syndromes:

- _DiGeorge sequence/Velocardiofacial syndrome:_ diagnosis has been aided by molecular genetic techniques, especially fluorescently tag DNA probes, which shows only one signal as opposed to two when the deletion is present.

- *Stickler syndrome:*
- *Robin sequence:*
- *Van der Woude Syndrome.*

Craniosynostosis:
- Premature fusion can occur alone or with other anomalies.
- Most *Apert's* are sporadic with a few cases of autosomal dominance.
- Two-thirds of *Crouzon's* are familial.
- Both result from mutations of fibroblast growth factor receptor 2 (FGFR2) localized on chromosome 10.
- Most syndromic cases are confined to the coronal suture.

External ears and face:
- *Mandibulofacial dysostosis* (*Treacher Collins Syndrome*): the genetic defect is localized to the long arm of chromosome 5 (5q32-q33.1). The gene has been labelled *TCOF1*, which codes a protein called treacle. This protein probably has a role in early human facial development.
- *Hemifacial microsomia*/*Goldenhar syndrome*: most are sporadic.

Craniofacial surgery
Craniofacial surgery can be classified as:
- *Clefts*.
- *Synostosis*.
- Hypoplastic conditions: *Hemifacial microsomia*, *Treacher Collins*, *Hemifacial atrophy*.
- Hyperplastic and neoplastic conditions: *Fibrous dysplasia*.

Craniopagus
- Rare anomaly seen in 1:600 twin births and 1:60 000 live births.
- It consists of identical twins joined at the skull, brain and/or scalp.
- It may be partial or total.
- Problems with separation include the complex sharing of brain and particularly venous drainage. Skin separation has been facilitated by tissue expansion.

See *Scalp reconstruction*.

Craniosynostosis
- First described by Hippocrates in 100BC.
- Virchow described the condition in 1851.

- Premature fusion of one or more cranial suture *in utero* or shortly after birth. Growth perpendicular to the suture is restricted and parallel to it is increased. Purely deformational conditions do not have a compensatory bulge.
- 1:2200 live births.
- Apert's syndrome occurs 1:150 000 live births.
- Most are sporadic.
- 50% involve the sagittal suture.
- Syndromes often associated with malformations of limbs, ears, and heart.
- Rarely non-syndromic craniosynostosis are hereditary.

Anatomy: See *Cranial bones.*
Pathogenesis:
- The stimulus for growth is the expanding brain. It is 50% of the adult volume at 6 months of age.
- The primary problem is probably in the cranial suture.
- The cranial base may be the site of the primary problem.
- The causes may be multifactorial – in non-syndromic metabolic, such as vitamin D deficiency or brain malformations, in syndromic chromosomal abnormalities.
- The biomechanical model suggests that there are fibre tracts running through dura from cranial base to suture. Abnormalities in the cranial base result in transmission of abnormal stresses to the vault resulting in premature fusion.
- The model may be more biochemical, but the dura seems to be important.
- Lots of molecules have been shown to be important in this process such as FGF and TGF-β.
- TGF-β1, 2 and 3 appear to play different roles with perhaps TGF-β2 inducing fusion and TGF-β3 aiding suture patency.
- At least 5 genes have been identified which, when mutated lead to craniosynostosis – MSX2, FGFR1-3, TWIST.

Radiology:
- *CT*: requires GA so only if a procedure is planned.

- Plain XR look for primary and secondary signs:

Primary signs:
  - partial or total suture absence;
  - indistinct zones along the suture;
  - perisutural sclerosis.

Secondary signs:
  - calvarial shape;
  - *Harlequins sign*: ipsilateral elevation of the lesser wing of sphenoid causing an abnormally shaped orbit;
  - hypotelorism with metopic suture.

Clinical progression:
- *Raised intracranial pressure:* up to 60% of Crouzon's, which present later. Note papilloedema and *Thumb-printing/copper beaten* XR sign.
- Eye signs:
  - exorbitism with corneal exposure;
  - papilloedema and optic atrophy;
  - ocular motility problems and strabismus.
- *Hydrocephalus:* particularly with Apert's syndrome. It may be due to increased venous pressure in the sagittal sinus secondary to obstruction of the venous outflow.
- *Harlequin deformity*.
- *Torticollis*.
- *Airway obstruction:* due to choanal atresia leading to obstructive sleep apnoea.

Classification:
Characteristic skull shape depending on which suture is involved.
- *Metopic:* triangular – trigonocephaly.
- *Sagittal:* elongated keel shape – scaphocephaly.
- *Unilateral coronal:* twisted anteriorly – frontal plagiocephaly.
- *Unilateral lambdoid:* twisted posteriorly – occipital plagiocephaly.
- *Bilateral coronal:* frontal brachycephaly.
- *Bilateral lambdoid:* occipital brachycephly.
- *Sagittal and bilateral coronal:* oxycephaly.
- *Multiple:* clover leaf – Kleeblattschädel.

Non-syndromic craniosynostosis:
- 94% of craniosynostosis.
- *Sagittal suture synostosis*: the commonest.
- *Metopic synostosis*: midline forehead ridge and hypotelorism.
- *Coronal synostosis*.

- *Lambdoid synostosis:* must be differentiated from deformational plagiocephaly. True lambdoid synostosis is very rare.
- *Deformation plagiocephaly:* results from extrinsic forces. These can be intrauterine or post-natal positioning. The ear moves forward with deformational plagiocephaly and back with lambdoid synostosis. More common due to the back to sleep campaign.

Syndromic craniosynostosis:
- More complex as many sutures including the base of skull and face are involved.
- The problems are not easily correctable and require multiple procedures.
- Get specific mutations.
- Need to perform:
  - fronto-orbital advancement, at 9–12 months;
  - posterior release, at 12–24 months;
  - midface advancement.
- Syndromic craniosynostosis include:
  - *Apert's*.
  - *Saethre-Chotzen*.
  - *Carpenter's*.
  - *Pfeiffer's*.
  - *Crouzon's*.
  - Jackson-Weiss.

Treatment:
- Aim to correct functional problems and improve appearance.
- *Ocular:* topical protection, tarsorraphy, fronto-orbital advancement.
- *ICP:* shunts, treat airway obstruction, vault expansion.
- The treatment of the cranium range include strip craniectomies, fronto-orbital advancement and total calvarial remodelling.
- Midface hypoplasia can be addressed with Le Fort 3 osteotomies and advancement with bone grafts or distraction osteogenesis. A monobloc advancement advances the fronto-orbital and Le Fort 3 segments as one block.

Complications:
  - hypovolaemia;
  - sagittal sinus injury;
  - SIADH;
  - air embolism;
  - infection.

Cranium reconstruction
- *Split cranial bone graft*.
- *Rib graft*.
- Alloplastic materials such as *Methylmethacrylate*, infection is a problem. Contraindicated when there is exposure to sinuses or nasal cavity.

See Scalp reconstruction.

Creep
- Refers to the permanent stretching seen in *Tissue expansion*.
- Collagen is convoluted and allows stretching up to a certain point after, which there is sudden resistance. Recoil is due to elastin fibres.
- Prolonged loading causes irreversible extension.
- During creep there is a change in collagen fibre bonding and collagen fibre realignment.
- Creep may also be due to displacement of water from the ground substance.

CREST
- Calcinosis.
- Raynaud's.
- Esophageal problems.
- *Sclerodactyly*.
- Telangiectasis.

Two out of the 5 are needed for a diagnosis of CREST.

Critical ischaemia time
- The maximum period of ischaemia that tissues can withstand and remain viable.
- It is temperature and tissue dependent.
- Skin grafts can survive 3 weeks at 3–4°C.
- Digits can last over 24 hours when hypothermic.
- Normothermic skin flaps have a CIT_{50} (time when 50% of flaps would necrose) of 9 hours.
- Muscle has a higher metabolic requirement and is more sensitive, as is bowel.

Cross-finger flap
- Vascularized pedicle flap from dorsum of one finger to volar aspect of the adjacent finger. Pedicle is divided after 2 weeks.
- A de-epithelialized flap can be used to cover the dorsum, and can be used to preserve length with volar defects.

- Side cross-finger flap is useful for thumb tip injuries. A proximally based flap is raised from the side of the donor digit and rotated 90° to inset it. The donor site can be on the ulnar side.

Technique:
- Draw a pattern of the defect on the dorsum of the middle or proximal phalanx.
- The flap is based laterally along the midlateral line and elevated above the level of paratenon.
- Preserve veins near the base.
- Cleland's ligaments need to be divided to mobilize the flap.
- Suture the flap in place and immobilize the finger by suturing together.
- Graft the defect and divide the flap 3 weeks after the surgery.

See Fingertip injuries.

Crouzon's syndrome
Bicoronal synostosis, midfacial hypoplasia with exorbitism and normal hands.
- A syndromic craniosynostosis.
- Coronal, but also sagittal and lambdoid cranisynostosis.
- Midface hypoplasia.
- Shallow orbits, and ocular proptosis (defining feature) may get exposure keratitis, poor vision and blindness.
- Development is normal in 95% of patients.
- Usually present after 2–3 years.
- Conductive hearing loss in over 50% of cases.
- Incidence is 1:25 000 with variable expression.
- Two-thirds are familial, the rest are sporadic.
- Mutation in fibroblast growth factor receptor 2 (FGFR2).
- Similar to *Apert's* syndrome, but without the hand anomalies.

See Craniofacial genetics. See Craniosynostosis.

Cryptotia
- Congenital anomaly of the ear where the upper pole of ear is buried beneath the scalp.
- More common in Japanese.
- Non-surgical treatment is with splints.
- Surgical treatment is used to create sulcus with SSG or flaps.

See Ear reconstruction.

CSAG cleft lip and palate

- *CSAG:* clinical standards advisory group established 1996.
- Study into the quality of the UK cleft service was triggered by Eurocleft results where UK had the worst results.
- Survey of UK centres performing cleft repairs auditing 5- and 12-year-old unilateral cleft lip and palate.
- *Results:*
  - ○ 700 new cleft babies per year;
  - ○ 57 units 77 surgeons with poor organization and results;
  - ○ 21 centres could not even provide basic data;
  - ○ only 4 units had more than 30 cleft referrals a year;
  - ○ 6 units were well organized.
- *Recommendations:* 8–15 units with 80–100 cases and 2 surgeons.

CT scan

- Computerized tomography.
- Differentiate from MRI as the bone is white.
- Scout films show the levels and spacing of the cuts.
- Bone weighted scans are darker and demonstrate bone architecture.
- Lymph nodes are significant if >1 cm. Malignant nodes have a radiolucent core and a radio-opaque periphery.
- Spiral CT is fast. Five separate scanners move along the body. A chest can be scanned in 10–15 seconds.
- *Positive points:* good for bones, quick, cheap, easily accessible, better for ill patients.
- *Negative:* artefacts from bones, patients receive dose of radiation.

Cubital tunnel syndrome

- *Ulnar nerve compression* at the elbow.
- Second commonest compression in the upper limb.
- Distinguish from compression in Guyon's canal by assessing sensation on the dorsum of the little finger as the dorsal branch of the ulnar nerve commences proximally to Guyon's canal.

Anatomy:
- Fibro-osseous tunnel beginning at the humeral condyle with the medial epicondyle anteriorly.

- Lateral border and floor is the medial collateral ligament and elbow joint.
- Medial border is head of FCU.
- The roof is a fibrous aponeurotic band – Osborne's ligament.

Compression points:
- Arcade of Struthers (fascial band above the elbow).
- Compression of overlying muscles (medial head of triceps).
- Arcuate ligament (fascial arcade of FCU).
- Local mass effect (osteophytes, tumour).
- Osborne's ligament (roof of cubital tunnel).
- Cubitus valgus.

Treatment:
- Cubital tunnel release.
- Medial epicondylectomy.
- Anterior transposition of the nerve:
  - ○ subcutaneous;
  - ○ submuscular deep to flexors;
  - ○ intramuscular.
- Approach nerve by marking a line from the medial epicondyle to the olecranon. Draw a line from the midpoint of this. Find the nerve proximally before it enters under Osborne's ligament.

Cup ear
See Lop ear.

Cup size: bra

- Measure in centimetres or inches.
- First measure under the breasts at the level of the inframammary fold – the underband.
- Next measure around the breast at the most prominent point (some suggest the owner lifts her breasts up to the desired level) – the overbust.
- Round up to the nearest unit.
- The back size is the underband add 4 inches if even and 5 inches if an odd number.
- For the cup size compare overbust to back size. If equal it is an A, then for every inch over the cup size increases. If less it is an AA.
- Most women requesting BBR wear the wrong cup size.

Curreri formula

- Used for assessing nutritional requirements in burns patients.

- The adult daily caloric requirement is 25 Kcal/kg + 40 Kcal/% burn.
- For children, the formula is 60 Kcal/kg + 35 kcal/% burn.
- This formula appears to be accurate in assessing moderate-sized burns in young healthy patients.
- Caloric requirements are overestimated with this formula in large burns or in the elderly.

See Burns.

Cutaneous horn

- Arise from underlying epidermal lesions, usually *Actinic keratosis*.
- Up to 10% may have an underlying *SCC*.
- It may also be associated with keratoacanthoma, sebaceous adenoma or Kaposi's sarcoma.
- Excise for histology.

Cutis hyperelastica

See Ehlers–Danlos syndrome.

Cutis laxa

- Degeneration of elastic fibres in the dermis.
- Associated with COAD, pulmonary infections, cor pulmonale, diverticuli.
- Due to a deficiency of lysyl oxidase.
- May benefit from facial rejuvenation.
- The patient has coarse drooping skin.

Cutis marmorata telangiectatica congenita
(Van Lohuizen syndrome)

- Get dilated dermal capillaries and veins.
- Usually localized on trunk and extremity.
- May get ulceration.
- The condition improves over the first year of life, but the cutaneous atrophy, vascular staining and venous ectasia persist.

See Telangiectasis.

Cutler–Beard bridge flap

- Upper *Eyelid reconstruction* with a pedicled flap from the lower lid.
- Two-stage reconstruction for large full-thickness defects of the upper lid.
- Create the defect then pull edges together to judge the width.
- Draw horizontal line 5 mm inferior to lash line on lower lid.

- Draw vertical lines to orbital rim. Incise full thickness (including conjunctiva) and lift up flap under lower lid. Suture in 3 layers place, leave for 6 weeks, then divide.

Cyanoacrylates

- The cyanoacrylates are quick-setting, biodegradable, polymeric tissue adhesives.
- Useful tissue-bonding agents and haemostatic.
- They work well on a moist surface.
- Histoacryl is butyl-2-cyanoacrylate.
- Degradation of the cyanoacrylates yields the tissue toxic metabolites, alkyl cyanoacetate and formaldehyde.
- The longer alkyl chain compounds, such as histoacryl degrade more slowly than the methyl and ethyl cyanoacrylates, and therefore cause less tissue toxicity.

See Alloplasts.

Cyclic loading

A method of intra-operative *Tissue expansion* with 3–5 minutes of stretch followed by 2 minutes rest.

Cylindroma: turban tumour

- Solitary or multiple, pink nodules up to several centimetres occurs.
- Predominantly on the scalp or forehead.
- Slow-growing in adulthood.
- Autosomal dominant form associated with trichoepitheliomas covers the scalp like a turban.
- Treatment – excision.

Cytokines and growth factors
Summary:

- Cytokines and growth factors are essential for wound healing and host defence.
- They are polypeptide regulatory molecules crucial in initiating, sustaining and regulating the post-injury response.
- They are also implicated in impaired wound healing and abnormal scarring.
- The term cytokine is used for polypeptides essential for host defence and growth factors are primarily concerned with cell maturation, but these activities are often very similar.

Pro-inflammatory cytokines:
- *TNF-α:* initiates immune cascade, anti-TNF in sepsis.
- IL-1-like TNF, but stays longer.
- IL-2 T-cell activation.
- IL-6 fibrosis, marker for severity.
- IL-8 chemotaxis.
- INFγ wound remodelling.

Anti-inflammatory cytokines:
- IL-4.
- IL-10 – both regulate pro-inflammatory cytokines.

Growth factors:
- *PDGF:* initiates and maintains healing rPDGF improves healing.
- *TGF-β:* effects includes fibroblast migration, important in fibrosis.
- *FGF:* mediator of angiogenesis and epithelialization.
- *KGF:* one of FGF – important for keratinocyte proliferation.
- *EGF:* directs epithelialization, important for wound remodelling.
- *VEGF:* angiogenic.
- *IGF:* stimulates fibroblasts, keratinocytes and collagen synthesis.

Treatment: PDGF licensed. Anti-TNF for sepsis, anti-TGF for scarring.

Pro-inflammatory cytokines:
Tumour necrosis factor-α (TNF-α):
- Released by macrophage-monocyte.
- Initiates immune cascade in response to injury or bacteria.
- Involved in maturation of cellular component of inflammation.
- Excess TNF-α is associated with multisystem organ failure.
- High levels of TNF-α have been found in non-healing chronic venous ulcers.

Interleukin-1:
- Similar to TNF-α.
- Also promotes other cells to secrete pro-inflammatory cytokines.
- May be responsible for long-term host defence.

Interleukin-2:
- Produced by T lymphocytes.
- Involved in T-cell activation.

Interleukin-6:
- Wide variety of effects.
- B and T-cell activation.
- Found early after injury and stays around for over a week.
- Stimulates fibroblast proliferation.
- Less in foetus that may contribute to scarless healing.
- May be used as a marker for severity of wound.

Interleukin-8:
- Secreted by macrophages and fibroblasts.
- Increase neutrophil and monocyte chemotaxis.
- Elevated in psoriasis and reduced in foetus.

Interferon-γ:
- Important in tissue remodelling.
- Reduces wound contraction.

Anti-inflammatory cytokines
Interleukin-4:
- Inhibition of pro-inflammatory cytokines.
- Increased in scleroderma where it may be implicated in fibrosis.

Interleukin-10:
- Inhibits synthesis of major pro-inflammatory cytokines.
- Found in high concentrations in chronic venous ulcers.

Growth factors
Platelet-derived growth factor (PDGF):
- Essential in initiating and sustaining wound-healing response.
- PDGF is released from platelets early.
- Causes activation of immune cells and fibroblasts.
- PDGF is then secreted by macrophages and stimulates collagen synthesis.
- Found to be decreased in non-healing wounds.
- Recombinant PDGF improves healing in acute and chronic wounds. Approved for use in diabetic neuropathic ulcers.

Transforming growth factor-β (TGF-β):
- Released by platelets, macrophages and fibroblasts.
- Central for wound healing.
- Effects include fibroblast migration, maturation and extra-cellular matrix synthesis.

- Elevated levels are found in fibroprolifera- tive states, such as keloid scars.
- TGF-β appears to play an important role in tissue fibrosis.
- Three iso-forms. Type 1 and 2 promote wound healing and scarring. Type 3 decreases wound healing and scarring.
- Not present in foetal wounds.

Fibroblast growth factor (FGF):
- Important mediator of angiogenesis and epithelialization.
- Ten members of the family isolated.

Keratinocyte growth factor (KGF):
- Member of the FGF family.
- Important regulators of keratinocyte proliferation.

Epidermal growth factor (EGF):
- Secreted by keratinocytes and directs epithelialization.
- Important in wound remodelling.

Vascular endothelial growth factor (VEGF):
- Released by keratinocytes.
- Levels rise steadily.
- Potent angiogenic factor.
- It is elevated in ischaemia.

Insulin-like growth factor (IGF):
- Produced primarily in the liver, but also found in wounds.
- Stimulates fibroblasts and keratinocyte pro- duction, and collagen synthesis.

 D Daniel/Taylor to Dystopia

Daniel/Taylor

1973: performed the first free flap in a human using a groin flap.

Darrach procedure: resection distal end of ulna
For _DRUJ instability_.

Operative procedure:
- Incise proximally over ulna head, preserve dorsal cutaneous branch ulna nerve. Find ECU and mark out a flap with the base radi- ally and the distal end running along ECU. The flap should be big enough to split prox- imal half for use as a sling and distal half to take under tendons to cover ulna bone after head excision.
- Incise extensor retinaculum on ulna border to enter 6th compartment (ECU). Enter 5th compartment and preserve EDM. Reflect and preserve joint capsule, perform synovec- tomy. Place Howorth and Mitchell trimmer around head of ulna and resect with oscillat- ing saw. Avoid ulna nerve and artery deep to head. Take only head, resect approximately 1 cm of ulna. Perform synovectomy.

- Close capsule over ulna head. While doing this, flex elbow and supinate to bring ulna in volar direction. Ask assistant to apply gentle pressure to ulna. Split extensor retinaculum into two. Pass one half under ECU and suture to capsule to hold head down. Pass other half around ECU and suture retinacu- lum to itself to bring ECU dorsally over ulna to assist in holding ulna down. Insert size 8 drain. Close skin. Apply above elbow back- slab with volar slab at wrist in supination.

Modifications: Swanson caps ulna, flap of ulna capsule sutured to dorsal ulna stump. Ulna stump can be tethered with distally based strip of ECU.
See _Ulna, Distal – arthritis_

DCIA flap
See _Iliac crest_

Debridement
- Usually refers to the surgical removal of dead tissue and foreign material from a wound, but can also be:
  - _autolytic:_ using digestive enzymes;

○ *chemical:* enzymes such as streptokinase and collagenase; also lava therapy;

○ *other mechanical:* such as pulsatile jet lavage and saline gauze.

Deep palmar arch

• Formed at the level of metacarpal bases by the anastomosis of radial artery and deep branch of ulnar artery.

• It gives off metacarpal branches to 2nd–4th intermetacarpal spaces and dorsal perforating branches to join the dorsal metacarpal arteries.

See Superficial palmar arch.

Degloving injuries

See Arnez and Tyler classification. See Ring avulsion injuries.

Delaire technique

• Regime for treatment of *Cleft lip and palate*.

• The lip and soft palate are repaired between 6 and 9 months of age.

• The remainder of the palate is repaired between 12 and 18 months of age.

• The rationale is an attempt to improve facial growth by delaying hard palate repair.

Delay phenomenom

• The delay procedure is where a portion of the vascular supply to a flap is divided before the definitive elevation and transfer of the flap.

• This extends the longitudinal reach of the flap's vascular pedicle as there is an extended random component.

• *Tagliacozzi* used delay with his nasal reconstruction.

• Milton experimented on pigs to find that a bipedicled incision was the most effective.

• The flap is usually raised 10–14 days after.

Mechanism of action:

• Multifactorial.

• *Sympathectomy:* an alteration of sympathetic tone producing vasodilatation.

• Reorientation of the blood supply along the length of the flap.

• Dilation of choke vessels.

• Tolerance to ischaemia: cells become conditioned to a hypoxic state after the initial delay procedure. Less tissue necrosis occurs after the second operation.

• *Hyperadrenergic state:* which results in vasoconstriction. This would not be as severe in a delayed flap.

Current applications of delay include TRAM flap reconstruction in high risk patients.

Deltopectoral flap

• Described by Bakamjiam in 1965.

• Outlined along the inferior border of the clavicle, beginning at the sternum extending lateral to acromion process. Returning at the level of 5th rib.

• *Blood supply:* sternal border to deltopectoral groove supplied by first 4 perforating branches of the internal mammary artery, particularly the 2nd and 3rd. At the upper portion of the groove, the thoracoacromial artery supplies the upper mid portion. The area of flap overlying deltoid is supplied by perforating vessels. This portion of the flap is, therefore, a random pattern supply. This may require delay to improve reliability.

• Elevation beneath the level of the pectoralis muscle fascia, lateral to medial.

• Provides only skin, subcutaneous tissue and fascia.

Dental

See Teeth.

De Quervain's disease

• Stenosing tenosynovitis of first dorsal compartment, involving APL and EPB sheaths at the radial styloid.

• Inflammation, oedema, adhesions and fibrosis restrict tendon glide.

• Get local tenderness and moderate swelling of the extensor retinaculum over first dorsal compartment and positive *Finklestein's test*.

• May occur through repetitive use of the wrist and hand.

• Most common in women between 30 and 50 years.

• Get crepitus: the *Wet leather sign*.

• APL and EPB pass through a tight canal 1 cm long. There are a lot of variations in the number of tendons in the sheath.

• *Differential diagnosis:* CMC OA, scaphoid fracture, *Intersection syndrome*, *Wartenberg's syndrome*

Treatment:
- *Conservative:* rest, immobilize, steroid, NSAID. Often fails.
- *Operative:* release of the first dorsal compartment. Make a 2 cm transverse incision 0.5 cm proximal to the tip of the radial styloid. The sheath can incised or excised or leave a radially based flap attached to the radius, incise dorsal ligament over EPB. This may help prevent subluxation on wrist flexion.

Complications:
- Neuroma, radial artery injury, tendon subluxation, scar tenderness, CRPS, failure to release all subcompartments.
See Tenosynovitis.

Dercums disease
- The literature describes two conditions.
- Multiple lipomata, which are sometimes painful.
- It is more commonly used to describe a condition where the predominant symptom is debilitating pain also called adipose dolorosa.
- This latter condition is far more common in women (20:1) and is usually associated with obesity. The pain exists within the fatty layer mainly in the knees, trunk, forearms and thighs. It is autosomal dominant.

Dermabrasion
- An abrasive process to remove epidermis and superficial dermis to smooth contours.
- Good for peri-oral rhytids.
- It has less bleaching and the contrast between treated and untreated skin is less than for *Chemical peels*.
- Not as effective as phenol for rhytids but more effective for acne scarring.
- Patients usually require 2–3 sessions.

Technique:
- Acyclovir is given if there is a history of herpes simplex. Topical treatment with tretinoin may hasten re-epithelialization.
- Dermabrasion is usually performed with a motor-driven instrument attached to either wire brushes, cylinders of sandpaper or steel burrs. When driven at relatively low speeds, a superficial- to medium-depth plane

is produced. The correct level is determined by the multiple fine bleeding points.
- After abrasion the area is irrigated with saline and a moist gauze placed on top. The appearance during healing is similar to *Phenol peels*.

Dermagraft
Human neonatal dermal fibroblasts seeded onto a synthetic mesh.
See Biological skin substitutes.

Dermal angiomyoma
See Vascular leiomyoma.

Dermatochalasis
- Horizontal redundancy of skin of the eyelids caused by aging.
- Herniation of intra-orbital fat.
- Common bilateral conditions.
- Male = female.
See Blepharoplasty.

Dermatofibroma
- Also called nodular subepidermal fibrosis, fibroma simplex, sclerosing haemangioma, noduli cutanei, fibroma durum and histiocytoma.
- Papule or nodule, usually in the extremities.
- Usually solitary, but 20% of patients have more than one.
- Slow growing, attached to the skin. Vary from 1 to 2 cm.
- Histologically composed of proliferating fibrocytes, collagen, vessels and monocytes.
- Either no treatment or excise.
See Mesodermal tumours.

Dermatofibrosarcoma protuberans
- Considered a malignant form of fibrohistiocytic tumour, though metastasis is virtually unknown. Tendency to local recurrence.
- Usually arises in the dermis of the trunk and proximal extremities.
- More common in men. Peak incidence in the 30s.
- Presents as a firm plaque-like bluish-red nodule with a keloid-like appearance.
- May remain unchanged for years and then develop a rapid growth phase to form a multinodular mass.

- Histologically, there is a characteristic 'cart-wheel' pattern of fibrous bundles in a non-encapsulated tumour that extend finger-like processes into adjacent subcutis and fascia. Mitotic figures may be numerous.

Treatment requires wide and deep local excision with a margin up to 5 cm.

See *Mesodermal tumours*. See *Sarcoma*.

Dermatosis papulosa nigra

- *Seborrhoeic keratosis* in dark skinned individuals.
- Occur most frequently on the upper cheeks, and are small, pedunculated and heavily pigmented with minimal keratosis.

Dermoid cyst

Two types, congenital inclusion dermoid and acquired implantation dermoid.

Inclusion dermoid:

- Subcutaneous cysts present at birth.
- Situated along embryonic lines of fusion, where ectodermal tissue becomes sequestered.
- Contain well-defined epidermoid structures.
- Also see inclusion dermoids.

Scalp:

- Assess carefully for relation to cranial sutures as they may extend intracranially, particularly if over a fontanelle or lambdoid suture.

Lateral brow:

- Commonest site.
- Asymptomatic, slow growing, usually superficial.
- May be fixed deeply, particularly in the area of the frontozygomatic suture.
- CT scan is not usually necessary unless it feels fixed.
- Excise through an upper lateral lid incision or lateral brow incision.

Frontonasal:

- Usually have a cranial origin.
- Situated from glabellar to nasal tip.
- Due to incomplete obliteration of a tract from the foramen caecum to nasal tip or foramen caecum through the frontonasal suture.
- Any failure of obliteration will leave both ectodermal and glial tissue.

- A CT scan is essential.
- A midline dermoid may have a pit possibly with hair and a wide nasal dorsum.
- The child may present with a brain abscess.
- Simple cysts can be approached through a dorsal nasal incision.
- If there is an intracranial extension, approach through a small frontal bone flap.

See *Epithelial cysts*.

Dermolytic bullous dermatitis

The most severe subtype of *Dystrophic epidermolysis bullosa*, which results in hand fibrosis and syndactyly.

Desmoid tumour

- Unencapsulated accumulation of fibrous tissue arising from the musculo-aponeurotic layers to the torso.
- Usually females in 30–50s, often after pregnancy.
- They are histologically benign, but locally invasive.
- Treat by full thickness abdominal wall resection.
- Even after aggressive surgery, local recurrence occurs in up to 40% of patients.
- Adjuvant RT may reduce recurrence.

See *Abdominal wall reconstruction*.

Dexon

- Synthetic suture composed of polyglycolic acid.
- It is degraded by hydrolization.
- It loses its strength by 3 weeks and is absorbed by 3 months.

See *Absorbable polymers*.

Dextran

- A low molecular weight polysaccharide available as 40 000 and 70 000.
- It is a product of the fermentation of sucrose.
- It has anti-platelet and anti-fibrin functions. The exact mechanism is unknown.
- It may work by the formation of a negative charge on the platelet surface or inactivation of von Willebrand's factor.
- It also is a plasma expander.
- Need to give a test dose of Dextran-40.
- Give 15–25 ml/hour for 3 days.

- Generally used in microsurgery if there has been a complication.
- There is a lack of evidence supporting its routine use.
- There are some significant complications associated with its use including anaphylaxis and ARDS.

See _Microsurgery_.

Diabetes

Wound healing:
- _Wound healing_ is significantly impaired in diabetes.
- Diabetic rats have diminished wound tensile strength which correlates with hydroxyproline content.
- Glycosylated collagen is less stable.
- Get impaired epithelialization and neo vascularization.
- Leucocyte function is impaired, which will diminish inflammatory response and higher infection rates.
- Capillary basement membrane thickens in all organs causing hypoperfusion.

Lower limb:
20% of diabetic admissions are with foot problems, 50% of non-trauma amputations are in diabetics.

Pathophysiology: multifactorial.
- _Neuropathy:_ get segmental demyelination. Compression neuropathies are increased. Compression and double crush may account for some symptoms. Get motor, sensory and autonomic which leads to arch collapse and a dry insensate foot.
- _Vascular disease:_ diabetics develop peripheral vascular disease which may start earlier and be more distal. Get pedal sparing.
- _Haemorheology:_ blood flow is reduced and viscosity increased with increased platelet aggregation.
- _Immunology:_ PMNs and T cells have reduced functions. Raised glucose encourages bacterial growth. Fissures provide an entry for infection.

Biomechanics:
- _Charcot foot:_ joint collapse from trauma caused by insensitivity to pain. Collapse of the arches, gait disturbance, ulceration and infection.
- _Achilles tendon:_ may be tight with reduced ankle movement which contributes to Charcot's joint. Lengthening may be required.

Assessment:
- Radiology to assess bones and presence of osteomyelitis.
- MRI is the most useful investigation. Vascular studies.

Management:
- Limb salvage.
- After amputation patients may not mobilize and those that do have much higher energy expenditure.
- 30–40% of amputees will require contralateral amputation.

DiGeorge sequence
- Associated conditions are _Velocardiofacial syndrome_, 22q11.2 deletion syndromes.
- Generally sporadic.
- 90% have a specific deletion of 22q11.2.
- Composed of:
  ○ aortic coarctation;
  ○ thymicaplasia;
  ○ parathyroid abnormalities with low calcium.

See _Craniofacial clefts_.

Disability
According to the WHO:
- Dysfunction inside the person is impairment.
- Dysfunction of the person affecting activities is disability.
- Dysfunction outside the person affecting the role in life is handicap.
- Disablement is the negative impact of the injury-healing process. This is a dynamic process.

Discoid lupus erythematosus (DLE)
- A chronic dermatitis that results in extensive atrophic scarring.
- The lesions may occur on the scalp, face, arms and trunk.
- They are often induced by exposure to sunlight.
- Treatment is with topical steroids and antimalarial drugs.

- Persistent scarring and deformity of the nose and face may occur.
- The lesions are usually discrete, and can be excised and reconstructed with skin grafts.
- Previously radiotherapy was used to treat DLE leading to a high incidence of SCC. Chronically active DLE lesions should be excised.
- Sun protection is important.

DISI/VISI
- Dorsal and volar intercalated segmental instability.
- Refer to the static posture of the lunate on a true lateral XR.
- *DISI:* lunate dorsal, scapholunate ligament degeneration. This is the most common carpal instability pattern
- *VISI:* lunate volar, lunotriquetral rupture *See*n in association with rupture or degeneration of the scapholunate ligament.
See Carpal instability.

Dissecting cellulitis of the scalp
See Perifolliculitis capitis abscedens et suffodiens.

Distal interphalangeal joint
Anatomy:
- Similar to *PIPJ*.
- ROM from −20 to 80º.
- Angulation of each is slightly different.
- Ligamentous support is similar to PIPJ, but also the insertion of flexor and extensor increase stability. Dislocation is less common.

Dislocation:
- More common dorsally.
- Reduction may be prevented by FDP getting trapped behind a condyle or volar plate interposition.
- Treat with reduction and splint.
- If dislocated for more than 4 weeks surgery is required to reduce. Release volar aspects of collateral ligaments and a dorsal capsulotomy. Fix with K wire.

Arthritis:
- OA affects the DIP joint most commonly.
- It is rarely functionally disabling.
- They may be associated with a *Mucous cyst*.

- Osteophytes are termed *Heberden's node*.
- Pain, deformity and instability may require *Arthrodesis*.

Dog ear
- Forms at the end of a closed wound when either the ellipse is made too short or one side of the ellipse is shorter than the other.
- They may flatten but primary correction is best.
- Either the ellipse can be lengthened or the dog ears excised as two triangles.

Dorsal carpal arch
- Formed from radial and ulnar dorsal carpal arteries.
- Also a branch from the anterior interosseous artery.
- It gives off dorsal metacarpal branches to the 2nd–4th intermetacarpal spaces.
- The 1st dorsal metacarpal artery supplying the thumb and index finger usually arises from the radial artery before it passes between the two heads of the 1st dorsal interosseus muscle.

Dorsal infections: upper limb
- *Dorsal subcutaneous space:* overlies the dorsum of the hand and communicates with the palm through the web space.
- *Dorsal subaponeurotic space:* lies below extensor retinaculum.
- Drain by incisions over the 2nd metacarpal and between the 4th and 5th metacarpal.
See Infection.

Dorsalis pedis flap
- Not very frequently used because there is a high rate of donor site problems.
- The skin is thin and pliable, and supplied by the superficial peroneal nerve.
- It can be harvested with underlying metatarsal bone or MTP joint.
- Based on the dorsalis pedis artery (DPA), which is 2–3 mm in diameter, a continuation of the anterior tibial artery as it passes beneath the extensor retinaculum.
- The first dorsal metatarsal artery within the deep interosseous muscle supplies periosteal circulation to the second metatarsal and articular branches of the joint capsule.

Technique:
- Centre skin over DPA distal to extensor retinaculum and no further than the interdigital web space.
- Incise over extensor retinaculum, and isolate DPA, venae comitantes and deep peroneal nerve.
- Include extensor hallucis brevis with the flap as it lies between skin and the 1st dorsal metatarsal artery (DMTA). Include some interosseous muscle.

Double crush phenomenom
Compression at one point of a peripheral nerve lowers the threshold for compression neuropathy at another site.

Doughnut circumareolar mastopexy
See _Benelli_ mastopexy.

Down's syndrome
Defects:
- Epicanthus.
- Oblique lid axis.
- Strabismus.
- Hypoplastic nose.
- Hypoplastic jaw.
- Macroglossia.
- Lip ectropion.
- Microgenia.
- Submental fat collection.
- Protruding ears.

Dray and Eaton classification
For PIP joint _Hyperextension injuries_.
- _Type I:_ volar plate avulsion, usually distally. Finger unstable in extension.
- _Type II:_ dorsal dislocation of the middle phalanx with middle phalanx dorsal to proximal. Volar plate is disrupted and collateral ligaments split.
- _Type III:_ fracture dislocations where the volar plate is attached to the fragment. These are stable if <40% of articular surface because dorsal collateral ligament is intact and unstable if >40%.

Dressings
- The ideal dressing should:
  - provide a sterile moist environment;
  - be cheap;
  - remove necrotic material;
  - promote healing;
  - protect the wound.
- _Low adherent dressings:_ e.g. _Melolin_, _Inadine_, paraffin gauze-based dressing such as jelonet and _Bactigras_.
- _Semipermeable films:_ permeable to gas and vapour, but impermeable to liquids and bacteria, e.g. omniderm, opsite, tegaderm.
- _Hydrogels_.
- _Hydrocolloids_.
- _Alginates_.
- _Synthetic foams:_ usually used in concave wounds. They conform to the cavity, obliterating dead space. They are suitable for heavily exuding wounds. An example is lyofoam.
- _VAC_ dressing.

DRUJ
- Distal radioulnar joint consists of the articular surface of the radius sigmoid notch and the ulnar head.
- It is separated from the radiocarpal joint by the Triangular fibrocartilage (_TFCC_).
- Stability is due to TFCC, ECU sheath, interosseous membrane, pronator quadratus, and the shape of the bones.
- _Rotation:_ supination and pronation occur by rotation of radius around a fixed ulna.

Dislocation:
- Described by the position of the ulnar head relative to the distal radius.
- So in a dorsal dislocation the ulna head is dorsal to the radius.
- Dorsal dislocation occurs by forced pronation.
- Reduce by supinating the wrist.
- The reverse is true for palmar dislocation. A long arm cast is applied.
- Chronic dislocation may require ligament reconstruction.

See _Galeazzi_ fracture.

DRUJ instability
- Prevent with splinting, steroid and synovectomy.
- Treat with:
  - _Darrach procedure_.
  - _Sauvé-Kapandji procedure_.
  - Resection hemiarthoplasty.

Du Pan syndrome

Thumb hypoplasia with a constriction band at the base.

Duchenne's sign

- In *Ulnar nerve palsy*.
- Ring and little finger clawing due to loss of intrinsics and inability to flex at MPJ, and unapposed flexion at PIPJ.

Duckett procedure

- Preputial skin island flap to treat *Hypospadias* with a one-stage procedure.
- Use when meatus is too proximal for more distal procedures or when there is significant chordee.
- Uses a vascularized flap of prepuce on a pedicle which is tubularized.
- Either split the glans or tunnel.
- Urethral plate can be preserved and the flap sutured to it.
- Skin coverage is obtained using Byars flaps – dorsal preputial skin that is split in midline and redistributed.

Dufourmental flap

- Variation of rhomboid flap in which the angles differ from standard 60/120°.
- Usually use angles of 30/150°.
- Use for coverage of defect in shape of rhomboid rather than rhombus. A rhomboid has acute angles of varying degrees.
- Diagonals are not of equal length.
- Planning is more complex and it is often easier to convert the rhomboid into a rhombus.
- A line is drawn as a continuation of the short diagonal and another line is a continuation of one of the sides. This angle when bisected, is the side of the flap.
- The length of the edge is the same as the length of the side.
- The other edge of the flap is made with an incision parallel to the long axis.

See *Rhomboid flap*.

Dupuytren's contracture

- First described by Sir Astley Cooper then by Dupuytren in 1831.
- Proliferative fibroplasia of palmar and digital fascia leading to nodules, cords, and flexion contracture of MCP and PIP joints.

- Normal fascia is called a band, when abnormal it is a cord.
- Commonest in the little and ring finger.

Incidence:
- Affects 1–3% of the population in North Europe and USA.
- M:F 10:1. Incidence increases with age.
- 10–44% have a family history. Autosomal dominant with variable penetrance.

Anatomy: See *Retinacular system*.
- In the palm the fascia involved are pretendinous band and natatory ligament.
- Transverse fibres of the palmar aponeurosis are usually uninvolved.
- In the finger the involved fascia is the spiral band of Gosset, *Grayson's ligaments* and retrovascular tissue.
- MCP joint contracture is caused by the pretendinous cord.
- PIP joint contracture is caused by the central, spiral and lateral cords.
- The spiral cord combines the distal prolongation of the pretendinous cord through the spiral band, which comes dorsal to the NVB at the MPJ. It joins the lateral digital sheet and distally joins Grayson's ligament.
- DIP joint contracture is caused by the retrovascular cord, located dorsal to the neurovascular bundle, palmar to *Cleland's ligaments*. It arises from the periosteum of the proximal phalanx and attaches to the side of the distal phalanx.
- The NVB is displaced superficially and towards the midline by the spiral cord.

Association:
- Diabetes (more radial, probably due to microangiopathy).
- Alcoholism (often thickening of the palmar aponeurosis without significant contractures though can be severe).
- Liver disease.
- Epilepsy (probably due to barbiturates).
- Smoking.
- Chronic lung disease.
- HIV.
- *Occupation:* trombonists, jockeys, vibrating tools.

Diathesis:
Aggressive. Starts early, strong family history. Often with knuckle pads (Garrod's pads)

plantar disease (Ledderhose's disease) and penile (*Peyronies* disease).

Pathology:
- *Intrinsic theory:* begin with activity in the perivascular fibroblast within normal fascia. The cords form along normal fascial bands (except the central cord).
- *Extrinsic theory:* Hueston suggests that the fibrous tissue starts superficial to palmar fascia and the cords overlay the aponeurosis.
- *Synthesis theory:* suggests that nodules arise de novo and cords from normal fascia.
- *Murrell's hypothesis:* age, genetics and environment create microvessel stenosis, localized ischaemia and free radical generation. This causes fibroblast proliferation.
- The fibroblast changes to become the myofibroblast. The actively contracting fascia is seen in the proliferative phase and the dense network in the involutional phase, in the residual phase myofibroblasts are replaced by more dormant fibrocytes. Type 3 collagen predominates in the early phases of the disease. The proportion of type 1 collagen increases as the disease progresses.
- Microtrauma may be a cause for Dupuytren's. In genetically predisposed individuals, tension causes rupture of the collagen with healing by hypertrophic scarring.

Indications:
- *Hueston's tabletop test*: usual indication for surgery is joint contracture. MCP joint contracture is usually correctable. >30° becomes troublesome.
- PIP joint contracture is more difficult to correct fully and any degree of contracture is an indication for surgery.

Non-surgical treatment:
- Splints, vitamin E, radiotherapy, enzymes have been tried, but not very effective.
- Steroid injection can help reduce symptoms from early palmar nodules.
- TGF-β may be found to be effective.

Surgery:
- Nodules can be painful and may require limited excision.
- Limited or regional fasciectomy:
  - ○ subcutaneous fasciotomy can be used in patients unfit for more extensive surgery, can be performed percutaneously;

- *fasciectomy:* regional excises all diseased fascia retaining transverse fibres, a limited regional fasciectomy excises diseased fascia in a digit and a radical fasciectomy involves removal of all palmar fascia;
  - ○ dermofasciectomy for recurrent disease or Dupuytren's diathesis, arthroplasty or arthrodesis of the PIPJ, amputation;
  - ○ open palm (McCash) reduces haematoma, pain, oedema and CRPS.
- Joint release.
- Joint replacement or arthrodesis.
- Incisions – Brunner, Z-plasty, Y–V, McCash. Skoog – transverse palmar incision with extensions into the fingers.

Complications:
- *Intraoperative:* NVB division, ischaemia.
- *Early post-operative:* haematoma, flap necrosis, graft failure, infection.
- *Late post-operative:* decreased movement, extensor block, CRPS I, recurrence, scar related.

Durken's test
- Test for *Carpal tunnel syndrome*.
- With the forearm supinated the examiner presses his/her thumb into the median nerve.
- Numbness or tingling within 30 seconds is a positive result.

Dysaesthesia
Abnormal unpleasant sensation whether spontaneous or evoked.

Dysgeusia
Distortion or absence of sense of taste.

Dysplastic naevus
- Larger than ordinary naevi with more ill-defined borders.
- >5 mm diameter.
- Variegated, flat, but with palpable dermal component.
- Mainly trunk and extremities. Usually acquired in adolescence.
- May be familial or sporadic.
- Syndrome is described if >100 dysplastic naevi are present.
- Familial are at increased risk of developing melanoma.

- Sporadic has less risk.
- Patients should be examined regularly and excision recommended for changing naevi.

See Melanoma, Naevus.

Dystopia
See Orbital dystopia.

E   Eagle–Barrett syndrome to Eyelid tumours

Eagle–Barrett syndrome
See Prune belly syndrome.

Ear
Anatomy:
- Normal adult ear 5.5–6.5 cm. Width 55% of height. 85% of ear development occurs in 1st 3 years. Position is one ear length posterior to lateral orbital rim, lateral protrusion of helix is 1.5–2.0 cm. Inclination of the ear is 20°.
- *Blood supply:*
  - *superficial temporal artery:* lateral surface;
  - *posterior auricular artery:* main blood supply to posterior surface and lobe;
  - *amputation:* anastomose posterior auricular artery and posterior auricular vein;
  - *occipital artery:* minor contribution;
  - venous flow is to the posterior auricular, superficial temporal and retromandibular veins.
- *Nerve supply:*
  - great auricular nerve;
  - auriculotemporal nerve;
  - lesser occipital nerve;
  - Arnold's nerve (auricular branch of vagus).

Ear replantation:
- Practised in 17th century following punitive amputation. Prynne, a lawyer had his ears amputated (for publishing an offensive book). When brought before a tribunal a second time the judge was surprised to see two normal-looking ears.
- Small segments can be placed as composite grafts. Larger pieces are unlikely to survive.
- Partial avulsion on a narrow pedicle may succeed due to the good blood supply.
- Cartilage can be banked, but tends to flatten.
- Posterior skin can be excised and lifted later, and cartilage can be fenestrated.

Prominent ear correction:
- 5% of Caucasians, 2/3 having a family history.
- The commonest deformity is absence of anti-helical fold and conchal hypertrophy. Also may have lobular hypertrophy.

Non-surgical treatment: Splinting (such as ear buddies) can be performed in the neonatal period and for up to 3 months. Maternal oestrogens circulate from 3 days to 3 weeks after birth. Long-term outcome is not known (Matsuo 1984).

Surgery:
- *Alter concha* by:
  - *Furnas setback:* suturing concha to mastoid fascia;
  - conchal excision;
  - anterior scoring.
- *Alter anti-helical fold* by:
  - Mustardè stitch;
  - grooving the posterior surface of the cartilage;
  - Gibson's 'release of interlocked stresses' anteriorly – Chongchet scores the anterior surface and Stenstrom used a rasp;
  - through-incision of cartilage or tubing method; a single through-incision permits folding creating an anti-helix fold (Luckett procedure); this gives a sharp fold so two incisions can be made.
- *Alteration of the upper pole:*
  - suture auricular cartilage (triangular fossa or scaphoid fossa) to temporal fascia;
  - scoring of the anterior cartilage
- *Alteration of soft tissues:*
  - *earlobe:* the fibrofatty core can be sutured to the concha or skin can be excised posteriorly;

○ *excision of auricularis posterior muscle and soft tissues:* this provides a space for the concha to sit in for the Furnas setback.

Complications:

- *Early:* haemorrhage, haematoma, infection, pressure necrosis.
- *Late:* under- or over-correction, irregular anti-helix, telephone ear, shallow sulcus, keloid.

See also *Constricted ear, Stahl's ear, Cryptotia.*

Ear reconstruction:

Classification of congenital ear anomalies: Tanzer.

Indications:

- *Cancer:* 9:1 ratio M:F. SCC equals BCC. SCCs have high recurrence rate and metastatic potential, higher than any other site.
- *Microtia:* incidence – 1:7000. M:F = 2:1. A component of first and second branchial arch syndrome (*Hemifacial microsomia*). Possibly linked with viruses, drugs, and inheritance.

Surgery:

- *Reconstruction for microtia.*
- *Composite graft.*
- *Helical rim defects:* helical rim advancement. Free entire helix from scapha through sulcus incision, not including posterior skin. Free up entire helix and advance – V–Y of helical root.
- *Upper third defects:*
  ○ helical rim advancement;
  ○ *Banner* flap;
  ○ *Bilobed* flap;
  ○ contralateral conchal cartilage;
  ○ *Concha* rotated as chondocutaneous composite flap.
- *Middle third defects:*
  ○ helical advancement;
  ○ wedge resection with accessory triangles;
  ○ tunnel procedure;
  ○ advancement flap.
- *Lower third – earlobe:*
  ○ use soft tissue flap from behind or below the ear;
  ○ *split earlobe:* from traumatic avulsion of ear ring – either close the defect completely or use the lining of the cleft to create a tunnel for future ear ring use.

Planning for total ear reconstruction: Trace normal ear on XR film and reverse. Tape template in position to find correct place.

First stage: This involves making and inserting the cartilage framework. This is most reliably obtained from rib though alloplastic and prosthetic frames have been used.

- Rib is taken from contralateral rib. Remove through an oblique incision just above the costal margin.
- Helical rim is fashioned separately. Ribs 6 and 7 provide enough cartilage for the main block.
- Aim to fabricate a framework with an exaggerated rim and distinct details of the antihelical complex. It is achieved with scalpel blades and a rounded wood-carving chisel.
- Create the pocket with an anterior incision.
- Cartilage remnant is excised. Used suction to prevent haematoma and oppose the skin to the cartilage. Infection can be treated with an antibiotic drip irrigation into the pocket.

Second stage:

- the posterior auricular groove is developed and the ear is kept in position with a posterior cartilage block. Temporoparietal fascia is used to cover the posterior ear, covered with a SSG. If it had already been used in the first stage then deep parietal fascia can be used.

Subsequent stages:

- *Rotation of the lobule:* performed more accurately as a separate procedure. This is accomplished by Z-plasty transposition of a narrow inferiorly based triangular flap.
- *Tragal construction and conchal definition:* this can be performed in a single operation. A crescent-shape conchal cartilage graft is harvested as a composite graft and placed as a shelf to recreate tragus.
- *Detaching the posterior auricular cartilage:* separate the ear from the head and apply a thick split skin graft.
- *Managing the hairline:* this may need to be removed from the ear at a later stage by electrolysis.

Eaton–Glickel classification: CMC OA

Grades the XR changes.

- *Stage 1:* widening of joint space, <1/3 subluxation.

- *Stage 2:* more than 1/3 subluxation, small bone deposits.
- *Stage 3:* larger fragments with narrowed joint space.
- *Stage 4:* advanced changes, major subluxation, cystic and sclerotic changes, lipping and OA formation.

See CMC joint arthritis.

Eccrine acrospiroma

Clear cell hidradenoma or nodular hidradenoma.

- May occur anywhere on the body, usually as a single, solid or cystic nodular lesion.
- Flesh-coloured or reddish and most often 1–2 cm in diameter.
- A few are tender on pressure, and a few show drainage or ulceration.
- Treated by simple excision.
- Rarely malignant variants have been reported. Eccrine glands.

See Sweat glands.

Eccrine hidrocystoma

- May resemble Syringoma in distribution, but the lesions are translucent.
- Situated on the face of older women.
- They are exacerbated by the heat and reduce in a cool environment.
- The lesions are obstructed sweat ducts.
- Treatment involves a cool environment and puncturing of the lesions.

Eccrine poroma

- Usually occurs on plantar or palmar skin.
- Firm red nodular tumour.
- Can be confused with pyogenic granuloma, amelanotic melanoma or Kaposi's sarcoma.
- Treatment is excision for histology.

Eccrine spiradenoma

- Can be tender.
- Severe pain may lead to confusion with glomus tumour.
- Usually solitary lesions on the upper body.

Eccrine tumours

See
- Syringomas.
- Eccrine hidrocystoma.
- Eccrine acrospiroma.
- Eccrine poroma.
- Eccrine spiradenoma.

- Cylindroma.

Ectopia cordis

- Very rare anomaly, may be seen prenatally, with varying degrees of abdominal involvement. The heart is located in an abnormal position.
- Thoracoabdominal defect, if any pressure on a dressing will get a tamponade.
- Usually lethal.
- Cover heart with biobrane, custom-made expanders and a silicon cage.

Ectropion

Eversion of the lid margin producing scleral show. May lead to significant exposure keratinization.

Causes: Paralytic, involutional, cicatricial, mechanical.

Surgery:
- *Cicatricial:* release tethered structures and reconstruct with flap or graft.
- *Involutional:* caused by laxity of eyelid. The best method for reconstruction depends on the site of laxity and stability of canthal tendons. If medial laxity and the medial canthus stable then perform a medial wedge excision. If lateral laxity and the lateral canthus is stable, perform Kuhnt–Szymanowski procedure. If lateral and lateral canthus unstable then perform a lateral canthal sling procedure.

See Eyelid reconstruction.

Ehlers–Danlos syndrome

- Group of connective tissue disorders with hypermobile joints, hyperextensible skin and fragile connective tissues.
- Genetically transmitted.
- They have defects in cross-linkage of collagen.
- This leads to decreased wound strength and delayed healing.
- May be associated with bleeding.
- Caused by inadequate production of the enzyme lysyl oxidase.
- These patients are at great risk of complications from surgery.

Elective lymph node dissection (ELND)

- Refers to lymphadenectomy of the primary lymphatic basin when clinically negative.

- The presumed advantage is clearing disease *if* it has spread to the lymph nodes.
- The disadvantage is the morbidity. 80% of intermediate thickness *Melanoma* (1–4 mm) will be node negative.
- The rationale has been to perform ELND on intermediate thickness melanomas as thinner have very few positive nodes and thicker are more likely to have haematogenous spread.
- Trials looking at survival have been conflicting. Overall there was no difference in survival but the subgroup of 1.5–4 mm thickness did have improved survival.
- Retrospective studies showed a survival advantage for ELD in intermediate group.
- WHO trial – no difference in survival.
- Large retrospective review by Sydney melanoma group – no difference.
- United States Cooperative reported by Balch (Intergroup Melanoma Trial) studied ELND for intermediate thickness elective lymph node dissection for intermediate-thickness melanomas. For patients with tumour thickness of 1.1–2.0 mm who were 60 years old or younger, a 96% 5-year survival was demonstrated for those who had elective node dissection, compared with 84% for those who did not.
- With head and neck melanomas it was noted that involved LNs were always in adjacent nodes.

Head and neck cancer:
- Use ELND to stage disease or if there is a >20% incidence of occult LN metastasis. If occult it should be selective.
- High-risk primaries can be judged by:
  ○ *site:* tongue, floor of mouth;
  ○ *thickness:* >4 mm have high incidence of metastasis;
  ○ character of tumour histologically.
- Also, particularly in America non-compliant patients, or patients who cannot attend follow-up or have thick necks are considered for ELND.

Embolization and sclerotherapy
- Used in the treatment of *Vascular malformations*, usually just prior to surgical excision to reduce blood loss and the morbidity of surgery.

- Superselective catheterization of 1 mm vessels is possible. The flexibility of the catheters is improving. The success depends on the number of loops of the vessel as with each loop, friction increases. Materials used are either solid or liquid.
- *Solids:* particles of polyvinyl alcohol foam (PVA) are irregular and adhere to the vessel wall. 30% ethanol can be added which increases occlusion but also necrosis. Occlusion is not permanent so this is used preoperatively. Coils made of platinum can be used for permanent occlusion. Their thrombogenicity is increased by attaching fibres to the coils.
- *Liquids:* silicone can be made radiopaque by adding tantalum, bismuth or tungsten powder. It solidifies after injection. Tissue necrosis is greater. Hydroxy-ethylmethacrylic glue solidifies after contact with blood so it can be used for occluding A–V fistulae. Pure ethanol is a good sclerotherapy agent when used in slow flow lesions. There is a risk of tissue necrosis. Use with venous angiomas. Do not inject intra-arterially.

Embryology
Branchial apparatus:

First branchial arch: gives rise to
- Maxillary and mandibular prominences.
- The maxilla, zygoma and squamous portion of temporal bone form by intramembranous ossification.
- The trigeminal nerve supplying the muscles of mastication, anterior belly of digastric, mylohyoid and tensor veli palatine.

Second branchial arch:
- Facial nerve comes from 2nd branchial arch.
- The muscles are the muscles of facial expression, posterior digastric, stapedius, stylohyoid.

General:
- Branchial arches are paired swellings, which lie along the developing neck. There are six paired swellings. The first and second are the most important in facial development. The grooves are branchial clefts, their inner surface is called pharyngeal pouch. The branchial cleft between the first and second arch becomes the external auditory meatus.

- The paired branchial arches decrease in size from cranial to caudal, with each pair merging midventrally to form 'collars' in the cervical region.
- Each branchial arch contains four essential tissue components:
  o *cartilage;*
  o *aortic arch artery:* these arteries course through the pharynx, joining the heart, which is ventrally located, to the aorta, which is dorsally located;
  o *nerve:* these comprise both sensory and motor fibres from the respective cranial nerves;
  o muscle.
- The embryological origin of muscles can be determined by their nerve supply and, although they may be intimately associated, two muscles may migrate from different origins, e.g. tensor veli palatini supplied by trigeminal nerve and levator veli palatini by vagus. Also muscle development and innervation are closely linked as seen in <u>*Möbius' syndrome*</u>.
- The branchial arches are separated by a series of clefts, which are termed 'branchial grooves'. All are obliterated except the dorsal end of the first branchial groove which deepens to form the external acoustic meatus.
- When the second, third or fourth branchial grooves are not completely obliterated, this can result in a branchial fistula, sinus or cyst,

Facial development:

- The frontonasal process is not a branchial arch derivative. Get paired placodes on the inferior border. Medial part forms medial nasal process, lateral part forms lateral nasal process and between the two is the nasal pit which becomes the nostril.
- Merging of the medial nasal prominences forms the philtrum and Cupid's bow region of the upper lip, the nasal tip, the premaxilla and primary palate, and the nasal septum. The lateral nasal prominences form the nasal alae.
- The frontonasal process merges with the paired maxillary and mandibular processes.
- Merging of the paired mandibular prominences produces the lower jaw.
- Failure of fusion of maxillary process and medial nasal process results in cleft lip.

- Failure of fusion of maxillary process and lateral nasal process results in a cleft along the alar margin – <u>*Tessier 3*</u> cleft.
- Failure of fusion of maxillary and mandibular process results in macrostomia, a Tessier 7 cleft.
- A median cleft lip is due to incomplete merging of the medial nasal prominences in the midline and is associated with midline furrowing of the nose, and a bifid nose – a number 0 Tessier cleft.
- Failure of the mandibular prominences to unite in the midline produces a central defect of the lower lip and chin, which is referred to as a number 30 cleft by the Tessier classification.

The palate:

- The palate represents both the frontonasal (median) and maxillary (lateral) prominences – the primary and secondary palates.
- All 3 elements are widely separated with the tongue in-between.
- At week 8 the lateral palate elements move from a vertical to a horizontal position.
- The jaw protrudes forward to give space to the descending palate and tongue.
- The medial edge of the palatal shelf undergoes apoptosis to enable fusion.
- The nasal septum also fuses with the palate.
- The median palatine process subsequently gives rise to the premaxillary portion of the maxilla and forms the primary palate; the lateral palatine processes give rise to the secondary palate.
- The primary palate and anterior secondary palate ossifies to become the hard palate and the posterior part of the secondary palate becomes the soft palate
- Cleft palate results from failure of the lateral palatine processes or the medial nasal prominences to meet and fuse with each other – resulting in a cleft of the primary or secondary palate.
- Delay in elevation of the palatal shelves from vertical to horizontal is part of the underlying mechanism of cleft palate formation.
- In Pierre Robin sequence with micrognathia, glossoptosis and cleft palate, the tongue fills the oropharynx because the mandible is small, so the shelves can't meet.
- *Epstein's pearls:* midline palatal microcysts occur along the median raphe of the hard

palate and at the junction of the hard and soft palates during the process of apoptosis due to cystic degeneration of the epithelial remnants. The external ear.

The ear:

- The auricle arises from the first and second branchial arches.
- Three anterior hillocks of the first branchial arch form the tragus, helical crus and superior helix.
- Three posterior hillocks of the second branchial arch form the anti-helix, anti-tragus and lobule.
- The external acoustic meatus develops from the dorsal aspect of the cleft between the first and second branchial arches, or the first branchial groove.
- Although the auricle and external acoustic meatus begin in the cervical region, they migrate cranially to reach their normal location.
- Patients with microtia or partial arrest in auricular development may have a caudally placed ear with respect to the contralateral normal ear.
- Spread of lymphatics follow embryology. Cancers of former origin drain to parotid nodes, the latter drain to mastoid nodes. Cancers of concha and meatus drain to both.

Chest wall and breast:

Skin from ventral portion of embryonic head fold. Ribs and muscles from ventral migration of dorsal mesoderm. The sternum is paired midline Mesodermal bars which fuse in the 7th week. Mammary ridges disappear from the 4th week. The breast bud is a downgrowth of epidermis into the mesenchyme.

Reproductive organs:

Internal organs:

Arise from:

- *Paramesonephric duct:* also known as Müllerian duct. In the female this develops into the fallopian tubes, uterus, cervix and upper part of vagina. In the male it degenerates to form the appendix testes.
- *Mesonephric duct:* also known as the Wolffian duct. It forms the majority of the internal sexual organs in the male. In the male the Sertoli cells within the gonad secrete a testosterone analogue, which acts as a Müllerian-

inhibiting factor. The Leydig cells secrete testosterone, which stimulates development of the mesonephric duct and genital tubercle. In the male the mesonephric duct gives rise to the epididymis, the ductus deferens, the seminal vesicles and the ejaculatory ducts.

- Mullerian Female → internal organs, Wolffian Male → internal organs.

External organs:

- *Indifferent stage:* mesenchyme cells migrate around cloacal membrane to form cloacal folds. These unite cranially to form the genital tubercle. Caudally they become urethral folds and anal folds. On either side of these, genital swellings become visible and become scrotum or labia majora.
- *Male:* genital tubercle elongates to form the phallus. It pulls the urethral fold forward to form the urethral groove. This does not reach the distal part of the glans. The groove forms the urethral plate. They close over to become penile urethra. The most distal part is formed in the 4th month from ectodermal cells of the tip which becomes the external urethral meatus:
  - *Timing:*
    - 3/52 – cloacal fold forms on cloacal membrane and the anterior part is the genital tubercle;
    - 6/52 – cloacal membrane → urogenital and anal membrane; cloacal fold → urethral fold and anal fold;
    - 6–11/52 – genital tubercle → phallus with urethral folds;
    - 12/52 – urethral folds form over groove to form urethra;
    - >13/52 – urethra canalized;
    - 7/12 – testes descend.
  - *Hypospadias* results from incomplete closure of the urethral folds during the 12th week of development.
  - *Epispadias:* urethral meatus is found on the dorsum of the penis. The genital tubercle seems to form in the region of the urogenital septum, so a portion of the cloacal membrane is found cranial to the genital tubercle and when this membrane ruptures the outlet of the urogenital sinus comes to lie on the cranial aspect of the penis
  - *Extrophy of bladder:* with epispadias. The abdominal wall is normally formed in

front of the bladder by primitive streak mesoderm, which migrates around the cloacal membrane. When this migration does not occur, rupture of the cloacal membrane extends cranially creating extrophy.

○ *Micropenis:* insufficient androgen stimulation.

○ Bifid or double penis occurs if the genital tubercle splits.

• *Female:* stimulated by oestrogen. Genital tubercle elongates slightly to form the clitoris. Urethral folds don't fuse but become the labia minora. Genital swellings become labia majora. Urogenital groove opens to form the vestibule.

Upper limb:

Embryogenesis is complete by the 8th week, but differential growth occurs until birth. Most congenital deformities occur between 3 and 8/40. Skeletal then muscle then nerve development.

Upper limb formation:

• *Proximal-distal sequence, apical ectodermal ridge (AER):* small buds of mesenchymal cells covered with ectoderm. Forms in response to signal from flank mesoderm. Initial bud formation is not cell proliferation, but decrease in cell proliferation. AER plays important role. *Progress zone* of undifferentiated mesenchyme at the end of the AER. Without the AER, mesoderm doesn't differentiate. AER controls limb-growth sequencing, but not the type of structure which is determined by mesenchyme. The time cells spend in the progress zone determines what they turn in to. So if they are in the PZ for short periods they will become more proximal structures.

• *Dorsal-ventral development (front to back):* controlled by ectodermal signals and interactions between ectoderm and the underlying mesenchyme. Dorsal structures are signaled by expression of Wnt-7a, which is found in limb dorsal ectoderm. When it is inhibited, a double ventral pattern is produced.

• *The anterior-posterior axis (head to tail):* controlled by signals from the *zone of polarizing activity* (ZPA). A region of mesenchymal cells on the posterior margin of the limb bud. Substances are produce which

in high concentrations produce posterior structures and in low concentrations produce anterior substances. Sonic hedgehog protein and BMPs may be responsible. Mirror hand results from duplication of the ZPA.

Hand and phalangeal formation:

• The AER becomes flattened distally.

• Portions of rim degenerate forming web spaces.

• Tissue beneath AER condenses to become digits.

• *Programmed cell death* (PCD) is important in development in modelling the digits. PCD clears the web spaces and prevents extra digits forming. Digits are seen by 8th week.

Genetic encoding and molecular response:

Several regulatory molecules are expressed by genes of the AER.

• *FGF:* important for initiation of limb growth. FGF appears to have a significant role in signalling between the AER and the mesenchyme. FGF-4 appears to maintain proliferation and polarizing activity. FGF-8 appears to be a key regulator of limb induction initiation and development.

• Signals from the AER control several regulatory proteins, e.g. *Msx-1 and Msx-2.* Changes in expressions of these genes can occur rapidly supporting the idea of a continuous interplay between AER and mesenchyme during growth.

• Signals from AER are necessary for the proper expression of *HOX* genes. The HOX are 38 genes, which encode proteins responsible for the establishment of cell identity along the AP axis. The position of gene on the chromosome correlates with the axial level of the limb bud, where they are expressed. They determine timing and extent of local growth rates.

• *Retinoic acid:* found in high concentration in undifferentiated buds. It plays a role in limb development though its role is not well understood.

• *Sonic hedgehog (Shh):* a segment polarity gene. Shh is the endogenous polarizing signal. It is expressed in the posterior mesenchyme of limb buds. It patterns the AP limb axis. It may maintain the progress zone of the AER, while acting as a positional signal along the AP axis.

Encephalocoele

Frontonasal encephalocoele:
- Present at birth and can become huge. They change in size with crying.
- Much of the dural sac is CSF filled. It may contain herniated frontal lobe.
- The herniation is through the open foramen caecum and patent frontonasal suture.
- They may also herniate caudally through defects in the sphenoids and ethmoids with presentation in the mouth, associated with a wide cleft palate and midline cleft lip.
- Imaging is required prior to surgery.

Enchondromas
- Most common benign hand *Tumour*.
- 50% found in hand.
- They may arise from misplaced islands of cartilage, which are shed into the medullary substance.
- Usually in the 20s to 30s.
- Well-defined lucent lesion in diaphysis or metaphysis with sclerotic rim. Cartilaginous. Often expansile. May have internal calcification.
- Extraosseous chondromas may occur in joints, tendon sheaths or bursa.
- Most common site is the proximal phalanx.
- Usually found incidentally.
- Occasionally present with pain or fracture. Treat fracture by curettage with bone grafting.
- Lesions in the hand often require treatment, whereas in other sites they often change from an active stage 2 to a latent stage 1 lesion at skeletal maturity. Risk of malignant change is minimal
- Syndromic enchondromas such as *Ollier's* disease and *Maffuci's syndrome* usually present earlier in life and have a more aggressive histology. There is a malignant transformation rate of 30–50% usually after 30 years of age.

Endoscopic plastic surgery
The rod-lens endoscope was introduced by Hopkins in 1953. Composed of rod glass lenses with intervening air spaces. It is still the main scope for most plastic surgical procedures. Computer chip video camera has enabled the image to be displayed on a monitor.

Benefits:
- Scar reduction and placement in hidden areas.
- Good illumination with magnification.

Applications:
- Correction recti diastasis if skin excess is not great and patients wish to avoid large scar. Combine it with liposuction.
- Endoscopic neck lift and brow lift can avoid a long scar.
- Endoscopic breast augmentation through an axillary or an umbilical port.
- Carpal tunnel release to avoid a palmar scar.

See Breast augmentation.

Enneking's system
- For staging tumours of muscoloskeletal system.
- Allows selection of treatment, assessment of prognosis and evaluation of results.
- Based on histology, anatomy and metastasis.

Benign:
- *Stage 1 inactive:* may heal spontaneously, indolent course. Well encapsulated, often incidental finding. Can be observed.
- *Stage 2 active:* progressive growth. Well encapsulated, but may deform the boundaries. Require resection to prevent bone destruction. More aggressive treatment, sometimes with a margin of normal tissue.
- *Stage 3 aggressive:* locally invasive. Extend beyond natural boundaries. Some such as chondroblastoma may metastasize.

Malignant: I–III. Each split into A and B if intra or extracompartmental. Staging is determined by grade (G), tumour site (T) and metastasis (M).
- *IA:* low-grade intracompartmental sarcoma.
- *IB:* low-grade extracompartmental.
- *IIA:* high-grade intracompartmental.
- *IIB:* high-grade extracompartmental.
- *III:* regional or distant metastasis.

See Sarcoma. See Bone tumours.

Enophthalmos
- Posterior displacement of the eye.
- It could also be due to loss of volume, but in the post-traumatic patient is principally due to an enlarged orbit.

Assessment: Check visual fields, extra-ocular range of motion, forced duction testing, and exophthalmometry. Image with CT and XR.

Surgery:
- Complete exposure of the zygomatic complex and orbital walls is important.
- If severe scarring of the peri-orbital tissue is present, it can be incised to allow anterior movement of the globe.
- For mild deformities, the volume of the orbital contents can be increased with autogenous rib cartilage.
- Soft tissue repositioning is important.
- The lateral canthal ligament needs to be repositioned in a slightly overcorrected position,

See *Orbital fractures*.

Entropion
Inward rotation of the lower eyelid towards the globe. Trauma to the globe from the lid margin and eyelashes results in pain and corneal scarring.

Causes:
Congenital, involutional, cicatricial (CIC).

Surgery:
- Cicatrical entropion is caused by vertical deficiency in the posterior lamellar. It is treated by releasing cicatricial bands and grafting the resultant defect.
- Can also use everting sutures, transverse fracture of the tarsal plate and everting wedge excisions.

Epiblepharon
Anomaly common in Asian children where the eyelashes are in contact with the cornea.

Epicanthal folds
- Prominent vertical skin folds over the medial canthus.
- They occur in Down's syndrome, *Blepharophimosis*, people of Asian descent.

- They may be released with a jumping man flap.

See *Eyelid reconstruction*.

Epidermal naevus
- Benign hamartoma, with hyperkeratosis, acanthosis and hypertrophy.
- 60% occur at birth. M = F.
- Lesions are hyperpigmented, linear or papillomatous.
- Naevus verrucous is a solitary lesion present at birth.
- Naevus unius lateralis are extensive forms of epidermal naevus, which can cover more than half the body.
- Ichythyosis hystrix are widespread epidermal lesions in irregular patterns.
- Inflammatory naevi can be misdiagnosed as psoriasis.
- Epidermal naevi with other anomalies is called *Epidermal naevus syndrome*.

See *Naevus*.

Epidermal naevus syndrome
- *Epidermal naevi* with other anomalies.
- Get skeletal anomalies, CNS abnormalities and ocular abnormalities.
- May uncommonly get malignant degeneration.
- Vitamin A analogues can be used to treat.

Epidermodysplasia verruciformis
- Wart-like lesions on the face, neck, hands, feet and trunk.
- Autosomal recessive cell-mediated immunity disorder.
- Several subtypes of human papillomavirus induce verrucous lesions with transformation to *SCCs*.

Epidermoid inclusion cyst
- Present as slowly growing palmar lesions due to implanted epidermal skin elements.
- The cyst is filled with white material.

Epidermolysis bullosa
- Epidermolysis bullosa (EB) is a group of inherited bullous disorders.
- Formation of blistering after minor trauma (Nikolksy sign), healing with scarring.

- Excessive epidermal collagenase activity, which breaks down papillary dermal collagen fibres, where blister formation begins.
- The digits become cocooned in atrophic scar.
- There are varying degrees of clinical expression.
- There is no effective treatment.
- Topical steroid therapy may reduce blistering and scar formation.
- The most severe subtype is dermolytic bullous dermatitis (DBD), which results in hand fibrosis and syndactyly.
- Correction of hand deformities is usually short-lived.

Epignathus
- An oropharyngeal teratoma composed of cells from ectodermal, mesodermal and endodermal layers.
- Epignathi arise from the palate or pharnyx and protrude through the mouth.
- They often cause airway obstruction.
- Failure of fusion may lead to a midline nasopharyngeal teratoma.

Epispadias
- 1 in 30 000. Male: female 4:1.
- Abnormal development of cloacal membrane with failure of rupture and abnormal growth.
- Leads to failure or blockage of normal development of the dorsal surface of penis, abdomen and anterior bladder wall. These defects are considered as part of the same disorder.
- _Exstrophy_ with epispadias most common.
- Penis is short, wide and stubby, with flat cleft glans and a dorsal chordee. There is divarication of the recti, wide symphysis. Females have a short vagina, wide separation of the labia and a bifid clitoris.
- Epispadias distal to bladder neck are continent.

Repair:
- The repair of the epispadias is similar to hypospadias (also need chordee release).
- If the epispadias encroaches on the bladder neck then a Young–Dees–Leadbetter bladder neck reconstruction is performed. Bladder is released from symphysis and wedges of bladder neck excised to elongate

urethra. Urethra is closed and sphincter muscle wrapped around. Ureters may need reimplanting and the bladder may need augmenting.

**Secondary surgery:** often required because of persisting chordee and inadequate penile length. W flap technique – exposes base of penis. Persistent bowing is usually due to inadequate urethral length. Divide distally. May need dermal graft to tunica albuginea. Urethral reconstruction with full thickness skin graft or flap.

Epithelial cysts
- Most epidermal (sebaceous) cysts arise from occluded pilosebaceous follicles. Get a small keratin-filled punctum. Asymptomatic.
- Histologically the cysts are lined with true epidermis that forms a granular layer and keratin. The keratin forms laminated layers within the cysts.
- Malignant degeneration can occur.
- _Pilar cysts:_ also called wens or _Tricholemmal cyst_ occur in the scalp derived from the outer root of a hair follicle. Clinically indistinguishable from an epidermal cyst.
- _Milia:_ or whiteheads tiny epidermal cysts occurring on the face. They may follow skin trauma or burns. Treatment is to incise the top and express the contents.
- _Steatocystoma multiplex:_ autosomal dominant, multiple intradermal nodules in upper trunk. They contain oily fluid and lanugo hairs.
- _Dermoid cysts._
- _Gardner's syndrome:_ multiple cysts.

Epstein's pearls
Midline palatal microcysts, which are commonly located along the median raphe of the hard palate, and at the junction of the hard and soft palates. See _Palate embryology._

Erb-Duchenne palsy
Obstetric brachial plexus palsy of C5–C6.

Erb's point
Point at which the spinal accessory nerve exits from behind SCM at its midpoint.
See _Neck dissection._

Erythema nodosum
- Painful, palpable, blue-red lesions on the calves and shins.
- Due to lymphocytic vasculitis.
- Usually women.
- Usually a tissue reaction to streptococcal infection, drug ingestion, sarcoidosis and other infections.

Erythroplasia of Queyrat
- _Bowen's disease_ of mucous membranes.
- Most often affects the glans penis.
- Seen in the 50s to 60s, mainly in uncircumcized men.
- Get solitary or multiple erythematous lesions.
- It is more likely than Bowen's disease to become invasive with tendency to metastasize.

Essex–Lopresti injury
Longitudinal radioulnar instability with:
- Displaced fracture of the radial head.
- Disruption of the interosseous membrane and distal radioulnar ligament.
- Proximal migration of the radius.

See Ulnocarpal impaction syndrome.

Estlander flap
- Useful for _Lip reconstruction_ with medium-sized lateral defects of the upper and lower lip, which include the commissure.
- It can be performed in one stage.
- Based on the superior labial artery for reconstructing lower lip defects involving commissure.
- Include ½ dimension of the defect.
- It is a laterally based switch flap.
- Get indistinct commissure, but acceptable oral competence.

Ethics
- _Ethics:_ the philosophical inquiry into the nature and ground of morality.
- _Normative ethics:_ the ethics involved in hand's-on reasoning.
- _Applied normative ethics:_ the ethics of medicine also called medical ethics.
- General theories of normative ethics are:
  - _teleological:_ assess right and wrong by consequence (utilitarianism);
  - _deontological:_ suggests that an act is inherently right or wrong regardless of consequences.
- _Teleology:_ utilitarianism states that moral rightness can be measured by the amount of good. Good is measured by terms such as wealth, health and pleasure. These are non-moral. So utility assesses morality by balancing the positive and negative non-moral good that the action achieves – 'the greatest good for the greatest number'. Utilitarians differ on which good should be sought. Action's morality is judged by outcome. The problem is that different outcomes may conflict in medicine, e.g. long life and wholeness. Also whose good is being considered? One may need to consider consequences for individual, family, community or mankind. The main criticism of utilitarianism is that there are no unchangeable rights and wrongs.
- _Deontology:_ actions are morally right or wrong. So a disabled child has moral worth. The grounds for deontological theories vary. Kant said that the capacity and freedom to act rationally are human in nature and we should respect other persons. Kant looked at actions and tried to determine whether they can apply universally. If so then they were moral. Different moral criteria have been defined. Again these can come into conflict. For example benifience and patient autonomy. The other problem is one of absolutes. If something is morally good is it an absolute rule, e.g. preserving life?

Moral problem-solving: Often the two methods and variations of them are merged when making decisions.

Code of ethics in medicine:
- _Self-regulation:_ code of medical ethics form part of the structure of self regulation. Principles that determine the doctor's duties to others are external norms. Working for the patients good is part of the code, but the problem comes in defining it. If a doctor imposes treatment this is paternalism, if the patient decides this is autonomy. Autonomy has become more important. Codes related to others in the profession are internal norms.

- *Conflicts with norms:* problems arise when an external norm conflicts with an internal norm or when two external norms conflict. Advertising is an example. This conflicts with internal norms by drawing patients away from other physicians, but gives patients more choice. It does, however, also conflict with medicine's altruism, putting commerce above all. The fee structure frequently causes conflict of interest.
- As the profession becomes more divided in itself, it is less able to self-regulate and external regulation is required. In plastic aesthetic surgery, the economic model becomes more prominent than the medical model. Patients are consumers, surgeons are businessmen.

Plastic surgery and medical ethics – applied ethics: Many of the areas of difficult ethical dilemmas don't affect the plastic surgeon such as life and death decisions. *Tagliacozzi* recognized the psychological elements and this aspect distinguishes the plastic surgeon from other doctors. Ward breaks down ethics of plastic surgery into:

- *Bedside ethics:* day-to-day matters of patient care.
- *Armchair ethics:* involves the aspects of running a business, providing a service, sharing resources, This area relies less on clinical proficiency. The physician acts as the patient's advocate.
- *Ethics of the technological imperative:* this states that what can be done technologically should be done.

See Bolan case, see Bolitho case.

Ewing's sarcoma

- Primitive malignant *Bone tumour* with small cells with round nuclei and without distinct cytoplasmic border.
- Probably of neuroectodermal origin.
- Occur in 20s to 30s.
- Found in the upper limb in 20% of patients, the humerus is the most common site.
- Present with pain, raised ESR, anaemia, raised white count and low grade fever. Mimic osteomyelitis.
- The tumour infiltrates the Haversian canals without diffuse cortical destruction.
- *XR:* mottled radiolucent lesion, poor boundaries, onion peel periosteal reaction.

- Most are stage IIB. Patients have chromosome 11-22 translocation.

Treatment.
Excision with wide margin with ray amputation with neochemotherapy and/or radiotherapy.

Exophthalmos

- Excess orbital contents in a normal bony orbit.
- The most common cause is Graves' disease.
- Also orbital tumours, invasive sinus mucocoeles, and post-traumatic haematomas.

Examination:

- Get extraocular muscle dysfunction, eyelid retraction, and peri-orbital and conjunctival oedema.
- The Hertel exophthalmometer is useful in measuring the distance from the lateral orbital rim to the corneal apex. The normal range is 16–18 mm.
- Computed tomographic scan imaging preoperatively demonstrates skeletal and peri-orbital tissue abnormalities.

Treatment:

- It is difficult to alter the globe position by removing peri-orbital fat.
- Therefore, with moderate to severe exophthalmos, a three-wall orbital expansion is the best treatment for surgical correction.

Exorbitism

- Normal orbital soft tissue in the presence of decreased bony orbital volume.
- There is a risk of corneal exposure and the development of keratitis, pain, infection, ulceration and blindness.
- If severe, urgent surgery is required.

Causes:

- Craniofacial dysostosis, such as Crouzon's, fibrous dysplasia, osteoma, meningioma, frontal sinus mucocoele and traumatic bony fragments.

Surgery:

- With congenital hypoplastic orbits and normal globes, e.g. Crouzon's, treat by fronto-orbital advancement followed by Le Fort III osteotomy or monobloc frontofacial advancement.

- For acquired exorbitism, make an osteotomy in the zygoma to rotate it outwards and increase space by a 'blow out' medially and inferiorly.

Extensor carpi radialis brevis

Origin: Lateral epicondyle. Passes between ECRL and EDC. Through 2nd extensor compartment.

Insertion: Base of 3rd metacarpal.

Nerve supply: Radial nerve.

Action: Wrist extensor. Doesn't produce any radial or ulnar deviation.
See *Muscles*.

Extensor carpi radialis longus

Origin: Distal 1/3 of lateral supracondylar ridge of humerus and lateral epicondyle. It passes radial to ECRB and through the 2nd extensor compartment radial to Lister's tubercle.

Insertion: Base of 2nd metacarpal. It may give a slip with ECRB.

Nerve supply: Radial nerve.

Action: Wrist extensor, radial deviator. Acts as a reciprocal antagonist with FCU.
See *Muscles*.

Extensor carpi ulnaris
See *Muscles*

Origin: Common extensor origin and dorsal aspect of ulna. A long muscle with short fibres. It enters the hand through the 6th extensor compartment. It passes through a groove dorsal to the ulnar styloid.

Insertion: Ulnar aspect of the base of the 5th metacarpal.

Nerve supply: Posterior interosseous nerve.

Action: Wrist extensor, ulnar deviator. Stabilizes the head of the ulna.

Extensor compartments of wrist
Radial to ulnar:
- APL, EPB on radial styloid
- ECRL, ECRB through floor of anatomical snuff box
- EPL separated from 2, by Lister's tubercle

- EDC, EIP
- EDM
- ECU, over head of ulna

Extensor digiti minimi

Origin: The common extensor origin and intermuscular septum.

Insertion: Little finger. It passes through the 5th extensor compartment. It is larger than EDC tendon and often has two or more slips. It passes ulnar to EDC and unites with it just proximal to MCPJ.

Nerve supply: Posterior interosseous nerve.
See *Muscles*.

Extensor digitorum communis
See *Muscles*. Most radial of the superficial group of tendons.

Origin: The lateral epicondyle.

Insertion: It divides into 4 slips in the distal third of the forearm. They enter the 4th dorsal wrist compartment. The tendons are interconnected on the hand by the *Juncturae tendinum*. The tendons insert into the dorsal hood of index to little finger. The tendon to little finger is variable and may only be a fine slip.

Nerve supply: posterior interosseous nerve

Action: extends the MCPJ and in conjunction with intrinsics it extends the PIPJ.

Extensor indicis proprius

Origin: Dorsum of distal 1/3 ulna and interosseus membrane.

Insertion: Passes with EDC in 4th extensor compartment. Passes on the ulnar side of the index finger with EDC into extensor hood. It may be absent and may give a slip to middle or ring finger.

Nerve supply: Posterior interosseous nerve.

Action: Independent index extension. Weak muscle.
See *Muscles*.

Extensor pollicis brevis

Origin: Dorsum of radius distally to APL and interosseous membrane. It runs obliquely distal then dorsal to APL. They pass superficial to ECRL/B and brachioradialis. It passes through the 1st extensor compartment.

Insertion: Base of proximal phalanx of thumb and extensor hood, and base of 1st metacarpal in 20%. It is often in its own compartment which should be released in *De Quervain's disease*.

Nerve supply: Posterior interosseous nerve. See *Muscles*.

Extensor pollicis longus

Origin: Dorsum of middle third of ulna and interosseous membrane. Passes through the 3rd extensor compartment. It curves around Lister's tubercle, crossing ECRL/B. It receives an insertion from APB and AP.

Insertion: Base of distal phalanx of thumb.

Nerve supply: Posterior interosseous nerve.

Action: Extends IP and MCPJ. Adducts and extends 1st CMC joint. It supinates the thumb MC. Radial deviates the wrist. It pulls the whole thumb towards the plane of the hand (retroposition). Test by placing palm on table and lifting up thumb. Only EPL performs this action.
See *Muscles*.

Extensor pollicis longus tenosynovitis

- Pain on moving the thumb, swelling, tenderness, crepitus just distal to Lister's tubercle.
- Symptoms should be treated urgently to prevent tendon rupture.
- Rupture is called Drummer's palsy.
See *Tenosynovitis*.

Extensor retinaculum

- Thickened distal portion of antebrachial fascia, 2–3 cm long and 4–6 cm wide.
- Radially it covers FCR and base of thenar muscles.
- Ulnarly it attaches to the pisiform and triquetrum.
- It has two layers. The deep layer forms the floor of the tendinous tunnel. It acts as a powerful pulley.

- It also stabilizes ECU tendon and *DRUJ*.
See *Extensor compartments of wrist*.

Extensor tendon zones

- Tendon divides at proximal half of proximal phalanx into 3 slips, one central and two lateral. Wing tendons form from interossei on the ulnar side and interossei and lumbricals on the radial side.

Zones:
- *Fingers:* I–IX. I, III, V over joints. VI over metacarpals, VII beneath retinaculum, VIII in distal forearm and IX over muscles.
- *Thumb:* 5 zones with V being over wrist.
- *Extensors:* most commonly injured over metacarpal – zone IV in thumb and VI in finger.
- *Zone VII injuries:* more like the flexor injuries as each tendon runs in its own sheath and repair has to be carefully performed to prevent triggering.
See *Sagittal band*, *Triangular ligament*.

Extravasation injuries

See *Chemical injuries*. Most occur during intravenous injections, mostly in upper limb. Get inflammation followed by sloughing and ulceration. Get demarcation within a week.

Agents:
- *Osmotically active agents*: hypertonic solutions, such as calcium and potassium cause osmotic imbalance and cell death.
- *Ischaemia inducing agents:* such as catecholamines, dopamines cause cell death by ischaemia.
- *Cellular toxicity agents:* such as chemotherapy (commonly doxirubicin, vincristine, mithramycin), digoxin, sodium bicarbonate.

Presentation: An inflammatory reaction, which may progress to necrosis, eschar and infection. The recall phenomenom is the extension of necrosis following recommencing administration of the toxic substance (mostly seen with doxorubicin).

Treatment: Varying advice.
- *Remove agent*, remove line (though may keep it in to aspirate and administer antidote).

- Apply *cold* to cause vasoconstriction (varying affect on chemicals, reducing toxicity of doxorubicin, but increasing vinca alkaloids).
- *Warm* may help to dissipate chemical and reduce toxicity.
- *Antidotes* phentolamine opposes vasopressors.
- *Saline flush:* after injecting hyaluronidase, make several stab incision and using a blunt cannula flush copious volumes of saline to dilute the chemical.
- *Excision:* a well-circumscribed injury may require excision, and graft or flap.

Outcome: Most isotonic extravasations don't require special management. Most osmotically active and vasoconstrictive agents need non-operative treatment, and a few only need surgery. *http://www.extravasation.org.uk/home.html* for reporting and further information.

Exstrophy/epispadias
See *Hypospadias*, *Epispadias*, *Embryology*. Get divergent rectus with exposed bladder plate, low umbilicus, widened symphysis pubis, anterior anus, short penis with dorsal meatus (epispadias), short urethra, short vagina, bifid clitoris. Extrophy results from failure of cloacal membrane to rupture which prevents development of the lower abdominal wall.

Surgery goals: Abdominal wall closure, bladder closure with good capacity, continence, preservation of renal function, cosmesis and functional considerations. More serious abnormality than epispadias. If untreated get infections, renal impairment and bladder ca. Most are reconstructable, 5% require urinary diversion.
Functional closure: Bilateral iliac osteotomies, free bladder and close. Close abdominal wall. Leave with suprapubic catheter. Females have better chance of continence.

Eyelid anatomy
Eyelid:
- Each eyelid bilamellar divided by orbital septum.
- Anterior lamellar of upper and lower lid – skin and orbicularis oculi.

- Posterior lamellar of upper and lower lid – tarsus, levator aponeurosis and Muller's muscle (upper), capsulopalpebral fascia (lower), conjunctiva.
- The orbital septum is a fascial membrane.

Orbicularis oculi

Tarsus: Form structural framework. Upper is 10 mm, lower is 4 mm. Dense fibrous tissue with meibomian glands.

Levator palpebrae superioris: The principal retractor of upper eyelid. Striated muscle supplied by the 3rd cranial nerve. Originates from the superior/posterior orbit, broadens into levator aponeurosis, which inserts into tarsal plate posteriorly and orbicularis oculi muscle and skin anteriorly. It is tented over Whitnall's ligament. The length is 55 mm of which 15 mm is tendon. In some Asian people the levator only attaches to tarsal plate so the lid doesn't have a fold.

Whitnall's ligament: The superior sheath of levator condenses to form the superior transverse ligament of Whitnall, a check ligament. This attaches medially to the pulley of superior oblique muscle and laterally to the lacrimal gland. It functions as a pulley to facilitate the change in direction of the levator action from horizontal to vertical.

Müller's muscle: Smooth muscle with sympathetic innervation. Situated in the posterior lamellar of the upper lid and attaches to levator and tarsus. Origin – posterior border of levator. Insertion – superior border of tarsus. It is 10–12 mm long and 15 mm wide. It is adherent to conjunctiva.

Lateral canthus: Composed of a number of structures. Lockwood's ligament (inferior suspensory ligament), lateral extension of levator aponeurosis, continuations of pretarsal and preseptal muscles and check ligament of lateral rectus. This attaches to the lateral orbital wall at Whitnall's tubercle.

Medial canthus: The tendon is a complex structure which attaches onto the medial part of the orbit in a tripartite manner. Closely associated with the lacrimal pump mechanism. The lacrimal sac lies between the anterior and posterior insertions of the medial canthal tendon.

Supratarsal fold: Corresponds to dermal attachments of the levator aponeurosis. Approximately 10 mm above the eyelid margin. In ptosis, a high-positioned supratarsal fold may suggest a levator defect.

Fascial framework: Supports the globe and allows coordinated movement of the orbit. Consists of Tenon's capsule, fascial layers of the extraocular muscles, check ligaments.

Palpebral fissure: Vertical height of 10–12 mm and width of 28–30 mm. Upper eyelid rests 2 mm below the upper corneoscleral limbus. The lower lip rests at the lower corneoscleral limbus.

Orbital septum: A thin sheet of fibrous tissue that lies deep to the preseptal portion of orbicularis. It is a protective barrier and restricts protrusion of orbital fat. It spreads from periosteum to tarsal borders. In the upper eyelid it fuses with levator aponeurosis 2–3 mm above the upper border of tarsus. They then insert into the lower anterior surface of tarsus. In the lower eyelid the orbital septum attaches directly to inferior border of tarsus.

Peri-orbital fat: Between orbicularis and periosteum over the lateral half of the orbital rim. Also preaponeurotic (post-septal) fat between levator and orbital septum of the upper eyelid. Two pockets are found in the upper eyelid – medial and central and 3 on the lower eyelid – medial, central and lateral. Preseptal fat lies between septum and orbicularis oculi – retro-orbicularis oculi fat (ROOF) in upper eyelid and sub (SOOF) in lower eyelid

Lower lid: Similar structure to upper lid. The retractor of the lower lid is known as the capsulopalpebral ligament and is continuous posteriorly with Lockwood's ligament.

Blood supply: Ophthalmic branch of internal carotid and facial branch of external carotid.

Nerve supply: Sensation to upper eyelid is through trigeminal nerve. The ophthalmic branch divides into lacrimal, frontal and

nasociliary. The frontal nerve gives supraorbital and supratrochlear. Lower eyelid is supplied by infra-orbital.

Eyelid reconstruction
Assessment:
- Separate the component portions of the defect into deficiencies of:
  - the anterior and posterior lamella;
  - upper and lower lid;
  - the support structures of the medial and lateral canthus.
- Posterior lamella defects may require reconstruction of the tarso-ligamentous sling with shared tarsoconjunctival flaps, mucoperichondrium or cartilage grafts.
- Anterior lamellar defects may require local flaps or grafts.

Pathology: Trauma, *Eyelid tumours*, *Coloboma*.

Direct closure: <25% or slightly >25% with lid laxity – close directly. Make parallel incision along lid margin.

> 25% – selective lateral cantholysis of the superior crus of the lateral canthal tendon.

Skin graft:
- The best site for lower lid is upper lid. Take equal amounts from both sides.
- *Post-auricular skin:* the sulcus should bisect the planned defect. Needs to be thinned. The graft can be extended laterally and medially to act as a sling.

Lower eyelid:
- For a full thickness defect first see whether the defect will close comfortably. If not, perform a lateral canthotomy and closure.
- Lining is not a problem as it rotates in with the lower lid. If this is tight then mobilize the cheek laterally.
- A back cut may be necessary possibly with a Z-plasty or a cheek advancement.

Upper eyelid:
- Treat in a similar way to lower lid with direct closure/lateral canthotomy/cheek mobilization/Z-plasty.
- An Abbé flap can be used.

Posterior lamellar reconstruction:
- *Sliding tarsoconjunctival flap:* isolated defects of the medial or lateral upper eyelid

can be reconstructed with a sliding tarso-conjunctival flap taken from the under-surface of the remaining upper lid. A transposition flap is created based on adjacent conjunctiva for blood supply and lining. Base flap 4 mm superior to the inferior edge of remaining tarsal plate. Extend incision laterally and angled superiorly to the border of the tarsal plate. Transpose laterally. The anterior lamella can be reconstructed with a flap or graft.

- *Free tarsoconjunctival graft:* shallow defects of lower lid can be reconstructed with a free tarsoconjunctival graft from the upper lid. The upper lid is everted and a graft is taken preserving 4 mm of inferior lid margin. Separate tarsal plate from the overlying Müllers muscle. The graft is sutured in place and a skin muscle flap advanced.

- *Ear cartilage:* provides support. The exposed surface becomes epithelialized by conjunctiva in a couple of weeks. It should be harvested from scaphoid fossa as concha is too curved. Through a posterior incision an incision is made into cartilage 5 mm from helical rim.

- *Hard palate mucosal graft:* useful as it has both support and mucosal lining. Good for large defects of the lower eyelid. Also for cicatricial ectropion. The keratinized mucosa transforms to non-keratinized mucosa in several weeks. Prior to this it may be irritating and cornea should be well lubricated. Too thick for upper lid. Take mucosa lateral to the midline. Leave periosteum intact. Beware the palatine artery.

- *Oral mucosa graft:* if thin mucosal lining is required it can be harvested from upper or lower lip or buccal mucosa. Use to line musculocutaneous flaps. Split thickness grafts can be used to reconstruct episclera. Avoid Stensen's duct in the buccal recess.

- *Septal chondromucosal grafts:* a graft 25 mm square can be harvested and indications include total upper and lower eyelid reconstruction. The septal is infiltrated and the graft outlined and an angled incision made parallel to the dorsum and caudal septum, preserving 10 mm of septum as an L strut. Contralateral cartilage is separated. The graft is removed. Any perforations should

be repaired. A lateral rhinotomy incision (full thickness incision in the alar groove) is usually required to gain adequate access to the septum.

Medial canthal reconstruction:

- Loss of the medial canthus leads to loss of medial support and, to correct this, the tarsoligamentous sling needs to be reattached to bone.
- If there is residual tendon, it can be directly reattached.
- The point of fixation should be posterior to the lacrimal sac.
- If there is no tendon, a nasal periosteal flap can be elevated. This is posteriorly based.
- If bone is also lost, a Y-shaped miniplate can be used and the tarsal plate is sutured to an empty hole in the plate or use Mitek bone anchor. Alternatively use transnasal wiring.

Lateral canthal reconstruction:

- Lateral canthotomy is achieved by an incision in the lateral palpebral fissure with subsequent detachment of the lower limb of the lateral canthal tendon, which allows relaxation of the lateral portion of the lower lid and adjacent cheek skin.
- For reconstruction use separate points of fixation for the anterior and posterior lamella to the lateral orbital rim.
- The lower lid is adynamic and fixation supports it. The upper lid is dynamic and fixation provides the fulcrum point.
- If tendon is resected, a lateral periosteal flap can reconstruct it. It is released from the junction of deep temporal fascia. Tarsal plate is sutured to this. If upper and lower limbs are missing, used crossed lateral periosteal flaps. If periosteum has been resected, use drill holes for fixation. Lower lid may require a fascial sling and fascia lata is the best option. This is passed along the margin of the lower lid and attached to periosteum.

Anterior lamellar reconstruction:

- *Tenzel flap.*
- *McGregor cheek flap.*
- *Mustardé flap.*
- *Subperiosteal cheek advancement:* the cheek lift is particularly useful in patients with midfacial aging and tissue laxity. The cheek

flap is anchored to the deep temporal fascia lateral to the orbital rim.

- *Hughe's flap*.
- *Hewe's tarsoconjunctival transposition flap*.
- *Cutler–Beard*.
- *Fricke flap*.
- *Mustardé lid switch*.
- *Tripier flap*.
- *Glabellar flap*.
- *Nasolabial flap*.
- *Forehead flap*.

Eyelid tumours

Benign: Seborrhoeic keratosis, benign pigmented naevus, dermoid cysts and hamartomas.

Malignant:
- *BCC*: most often on the lower eyelid and medial canthus. Most are nodular.

- *SCC*: <2% of all lid tumours. typically arising in sun-damaged skin, but also on the inner conjunctival surface. Those on the inner surface or arising after RT have a much higher metastatic potential.
- *Sebaceous cell carcinoma*: third most common eyelid tumour.
- *Melanoma:* lentigo maligna, or malignant melanoma *in situ*, accounts for about 1% of all lid lesions and is treated by excision with a 5-mm margin.

Benign	Malignant
SK	BCC
Pigmented naevi	SCC
Dermoid	Sebaceous ca
Hamartoma	MM

F Face lift to **Furlow technique**

Face lift
Anatomy:
- *SMAS*.
- Retaining ligaments:
  - osseocutaneous ligaments pass from bone to skin; occur over zygoma and anterior mandible;
  - musculocutaneous ligaments; between skin and muscle fascia; occur between parotid fascia, and skin and masseter and skin.
- Frontal branch of *Facial nerve*.
- *Greater auricular nerve*.

History: Ask about smoking, BP, medication, healing disorders, DM, RA.

Examination: Look at distribution of skin excess, wrinkling, skin type, facial movement, hair.

Surgery:
- *Skin-only:* subcutaneous undermining. Extend to nasolabial crease. Get early recurrence

- *Skin and SMAS lift:* skin is dissected and SMAS as a separate layer. Zygomatic and masseteric ligaments are released. SMAS is secured anterior to the ear. Excess SMAS can augment the zygomatic arch.
- *Deep plane face lift:* under SMAS and skin not dissected separately. The composite flap is tightened. Indicated in smokers as the flap is thicker.
- *Mid-face suspension:* deep tissues of mid-face are dissected through lower blepharoplasty incision. Suture passed from cheek to temple and sutured to the deep temporal fascia.
- *Non-endoscopic subperiosteal face lift:* soft tissues are dissected in the subperiosteal plan through a number of open incisions.
- *Endoscopic face lift:* face is dissected endoscopically at a subperiosteal level. Once freed it is elevated and secured. Usually for younger patients.
- *Neck:* get divarication of platysma. Appearance can be improved by submental defatting, plication of medial borders of

platysma, resection of platysmal bands. Also laser resurfacing.

Complications: Haematoma, skin necrosis, nerve injury, alopecia, hypertrophic scars, change in skin pigmentation.

Facial fractures

Classification:

- Closed or open, or by the anatomic region.
- Anatomic areas in the upper face consist of the frontal bone, frontal sinus and supra-orbital areas.
- The orbit is divided into the rim and the internal orbit. Rim fractures are classified in three sections: supra-orbital, zygomatic and naso-ethmoidal. The internal orbit is classified into four areas.
- The maxilla, the nose and the mandible are the other anatomic areas.
- Fractures tend to occur in patterns as the bone demonstrates weak areas that fracture first despite the source or location of the impact.

Management principles: Need accurate diagnosis, early single stage surgery, good exposure, rigid fixation, bone grafting where needed, soft tissue reconstruction.

Incisions:

- Through existing lacerations if present.
- Bicoronal incision.
- Lower eyelid:
  - trans-conjunctiva;
  - subciliary;
  - mid-lid;
  - junction of eyelid and cheek.
- Upper or lower buccal incision.
- Dingman's lateral brow incision.
- Risdon's retromandibular incision.
- Lynch's medial canthus incision.
- Gilles' incision in the temple hairline.

Radiology:

- Straight PA views.
- *Caldwell views (forehead on plate):* inclined PA views with 23° head extension.
- *Water's views (chin on plate):* inclined PA views with 37° head extension.
- *Towne's views:* AP views with XR tube rotated 30° in a caudal direction.

- *Reversed Towne's views:* as above with tube and film reversed.
- CT and 3D CT (but a lot of radiation).

Management of soft tissue injuries:

- *Skin:* good blood supply so debride minimally. Excise edges.
- *Facial nerve:* repair branches lateral to lateral canthus, but medial branches are too small to repair. Muscle will often reinnervate spontaneously.
- *Infra-orbital nerve:* numbness suggests fracture of the floor of the orbit or zygoma. If the zygoma fracture is impacted into the nerve canal then decompression is advised. A branch of the nerve travels to the maxilla and supplies the teeth so numbness here suggests partial injury.
- *Parotid duct:* (<u>Anatomy</u>) closely related to buccal branch. If in doubt place a probe in the opening. If divided, repair over a thin stent, otherwise get salivary collections, fistulae, duct stenosis and parotiditis.
- *Lacrimal apparatus:* injuries to canaliculi, lacrimal sac or duct should be repaired over a silastic stent, which should be inserted along the length of the lacrimal system and tied externally to each other.

Timing: Other major injuries take priority. Fracture fixation can be:

- *Early:* preferred if the patient is stable.
- *Delayed primary:* 10 days after injury once swelling has settled, indicated if multiple injuries
- *Secondary:* try to avoid late surgery as soft tissues contract making realignment difficult.

Immediate management of pan-facial fractures:

ABC:

Airway: Stabilize cervical spine, remove loose teeth, clean vomit and blood from airway. If the patient is not maintaining the airway, distract mandible forward. It may be improved by relocating maxilla upwards and forwards. Obstruction may be due to swelling. Unrelieved obstruction may require intubation, cricothyroidotomy or tracheostomy. Never attempt nasotracheal intubation with midface fractures as brainstem may be impaled. Place gastric tube orally.

Breathing: Look for chest injury, and adequate ventilation.

Circulation: Significant haemorrhage is usually associated with upper Le Fort or nasoethmoidal fractures. Insert large bore cannula, start infusion. Send bloods (including drug and alcohol screen). Reduce bleeding by reduction of fractures, nasal packing. If still profuse, give blood, correct coagulopathy, take the patient to theatre, reduce fractures and hold with K wires. Consider facial bandaging, by packing nose and mouth followed by circumferential bandages. If it continues consider external carotid artery ligation through an incision behind the ramus of the mandible or endoscopically through the maxillary sinus or embolization.

Other injuries: Once stabilized exclude other injuries. 10% of patients with facial fractures have cervical spine fractures, and 10% have eye injury – need opthalmological assessment.

Mandibular fractures.
Zygomatic fractures.
Maxillary fractures.
Orbital fractures.
Nasal fractures.
Nasoethmoidal fractures.
Frontal sinus fractures.

Facial nerve

CN VII. Arises from the 2nd brachial cleft arch and is the motor to muscle of facial expression. It leaves the stylomastoid foramen and passes through the parotid gland.

- Intratemporally the facial nerve has sensory, as well as motor fibres:
  - the superficial petrosal nerve supplies the lacrimal gland;
  - the chorda tympani provides sensation to the anterior 2/3 of the tongue; parasympathetic nerves of facial nerve travels with the trigeminal nerve;
  - tympanic nerve is a small sensory branch;
  - the nerve to stapedius – if not functioning get hyperacusia.
- As it leaves it gives off:
  - the posterior auricular nerve to the occipital muscles and sensation behind the ear lobe (sensory fibres travel with the auricular branch of vagus);

  - a muscular branch to the posterior belly of digastric and stylohyoid;
  - *five branches:* temporal (frontal) zygomatic, buccal, mandibular and cervical
- As it leaves the foramen, it passes anterior to posterior belly of digastric, lateral to styloid process and external carotid artery, and posterior to the facial vein. Find frontal branch on *Pitanguy's line.*
- The facial nerve runs quite superficial, but always below the SMAS. In the midface there are communications between branches.
- Identify nerve by mobilizing the tail of the parotid, bring anterior sternocleidomastoid muscle laterally to find posterior belly of digastric. Follow the muscle up, separate parotid from cartilage of external auditory canal. Facial nerve lies 1 cm deep to tragal pointer.

Temporal branch: Frontal branch is deep to SMAS, but lies superficially over the zygomatic arch, lying between periosteum and temporoparietal fascia (TPF). Superior to the zygomatic arch it lies within or under TPF, superficial to the deep temporal fascia. The nerve enters frontalis on its deep surface where orbicularis oculi intersects with the lateral aspect of frontalis 1.5 cm above the lateral point of the eyebrow.

Zygomatic branch: Supplies orbicularis oculi. Division results in inability to close the eye.

Buccal branch: Divides into multiple branches, which travel along the parotid duct. They supply buccinator muscle and the muscles of the upper lip. Division causes difficulty emptying the cheek.

Marginal mandibular: Runs below border of mandible deep to platysma and superficial to facial vein. Supplies lower lip. Division results in elevation of the corner of the mouth.

Cervical branch: Runs downwards into the neck to supply the platysma muscle. There is significant cross-over between buccal and zygomatic branches of the facial nerve. Injury to either is compensated for. There is little cross-over with frontal and marginal mandibular nerves, and there is little compensation if they are injured.

Muscles: Posterior belly of digastric, stapedius. Muscles of facial expression – the muscles levator anguli superioris, mentalis and buccinator lie deep, and therefore are innervated on the superficial surface. All other muscles lie superficial to the plane of the facial nerve and receive their innervation on the deep surface

Bell's palsy:

Facial danger zones: All the nerves are below SMAS apart from frontal branch within SMAS.
- *6.5 cm below external auditory canal:* great auricular nerve.
- *Pitanguy's line:* temporal branch.
- *Midmandible 2 cm posterior to oral commissure:* marginal mandibular.
- *Anterior to parotid and posterior to zygomaticus:* zygomatic and buccal.
- *Superior orbital rim:* supra-orbital and supratrochlear nerve.
- *1 cm below inferior orbital rim, mid-pupil:* infra-orbital nerve
- *Mid-mandibular below 2nd premolar:* mental nerve.

Facial re-animation

History: Particularly note for onset. A slow onset is indicative of tumour, acute with infection, trauma, medication or vascular. Also note changes in hearing, taste and dizziness.

Aetiology: Congenital or acquired.

Congenital: Facial musculature doesn't develop. This is usually not complete. Usually unilateral and more rarely bilateral. *See Möbius syndrome*.
- *Acquired:* most common is Bell's palsy, which usually has spontaneous complete recovery. Also trauma, neoplasm and post-infective, e.g. Ramsay–Hunt syndrome:
  - ○ *Intracranial:*
    - vascular abnormalities;
    - central nervous system; degenerative diseases;
    - tumours of the intracranial cavity;
    - trauma to the brain;
    - congenital abnormalities and agenesis.
  - ○ *Intratemporal:*
    - bacterial and viral infections;
    - cholesteatoma;
    - trauma;
    - longitudinal and horizontal fractures of the temporal bone;
    - gunshot wounds;
    - tumours invading the middle ear, mastoid, and facial nerve;
    - iatrogenic causes.
  - ○ *Extracranial:*
    - malignant tumours of the parotid gland;
    - trauma (lacerations and gunshot wounds);
    - iatrogenic causes;
    - primary tumours of the facial nerve;
    - malignant tumours of the ascending ramus of the mandible pterygoid region, and skin.

Grading: by House and Brackman
- *1:* some mimetic movement.
- *2:* no mimetic movement.
- *3:* only mass action of facial muscles.
- *4:* unable to move eyelids.
- *5:* face remains symmetrical despite complete facial paralysis.
- *6:* asymmetrical face, no movement.

Examination:
- Upper motor neuron lesion presents with ipsilateral lower face paralysis as the upper face is supplied by both sides from the cerebral cortex.
- Intratemporal lesions involve sensory, as well as motor fibres. Test for intratemporal lesions with:
  - ○ *Schirmer's* test (for tear production);
  - ○ the stapedius reflex test;
  - ○ the electrogustatory test for the tongue.
- Look for scars, movement of upper eyelid. Test strength of eyelid closure, perform lower eyelid snap test, assess nasal valving and examine temporalis muscle.

Investigations: Plain XRs, CT scans and nerve conduction studies to assess whether the muscles are partially or completely denervated.

Anatomy: 17 facial muscles. Three sphincters – eye, nose and mouth.

Treatment:
Non-operative:
- Protect eyes with eye drops, glasses, taping closed at night.
- Ectropion can be taped.

- *Botulinum* toxin into the normal side may equalize the face.

Static operations:

Indicated in older patients where more complex procedures are less likely to be successful.
- Around the eye include temporary or permanent *Tarsorrhaphy*.
- The *Kuhnt-Szymanowski* procedure for ectropion.
- Lateral canthopexy.
- Insertion of gold weights or springs, brow lift or forehead skin excision.
- Around the mouth include unilateral face lift procedures and static slings with fascia lata.

Dynamic operations:

If proximal stump is present, neurotize the muscles with nerve grafts, if distal stump present perform ipsilateral nerve transfer or contralateral facial nerve grafting (CFNG).
- *Nerve repair:* If nerve divided attempt immediate repair and before 3 weeks for good results. Beyond a line dropped from the lateral canthus, repair may not be required due to the numerous anastomoses.
- *Nerve graft:* Require a good bed for the tissues. Use cervical plexus from ipsilateral or contralateral side. Also sural nerve. Return of facial movement occurs between 6 and 24 months. First tone improves then movement in the middle third of the face. This extends to the mouth, cheek and orbit but rarely to the forehead and lower lip. There is a deficit of emotional expression.

Reconstruction:

- *CFNG* (Scaramella 1970): uses motor axons from the normal contralateral facial nerve via nerve grafts. It allows the potential for symmetrical self-expression. Usually done as a two-stage procedure to allow assessment of the grafted nerve histologically. The disadvantage of CFNG is the use of a normal facial nerve. Assess the nerve regeneration through the graft with a Tinel's test and with conduction velocities. After CFNG a splint is placed limiting mouth movement to protect co-aptation sites. Anti-emetics are used and talking limited. After 6 weeks the area is massaged.
- *Ipsilateral versus crossover:* Ipsilateral procedures use other nerves such as hypoglossal.

However, facial movement is not co-ordinated. They can, however, be used to send strong motor fibres quickly to denervated muscles to maintain bulk performing the first stage of the CFNG. Only 40% of the nerve is used. When the second stage is performed the ipsilateral nerve is preserved to maintain muscle bulk, while the CFNG gives co-ordinated movement. Nerves that are used are the hypoglossal, glossopharyngeal, accessory and phrenic.
- *Free muscle transfer:* Used when the denervation time is long and muscle has atrophied. Nerve conduction studies quantify the severity of the denervation. A donor muscle should have the same length of excursion, be expendable, the right shape and have a reliable pedicle. Gracilis and pectoralis minor are most frequently used. If ipsilateral facial nerve is present this is used and co-apted immediately to the transferred muscle. If not, a CFNG is used.
  - *Gracilis*: has a predictable neurovascular pedicle, can be contoured and has the correct excursion but it is bulky and too long and requires contouring; debulking may lead to end plate damage and muscle weakening; it only has one direction of pull;
  - *pectoralis minor*: very useful in developmental facial paralysis in young children where the dimensions are ideal; it has a minimal donor site morbidity, good size and shape and multidirectional pull, but harvesting is difficult as is debulking; the neurovascular pedicle is short and the lateral thoracic artery is normally the dominant supply, but is sometimes shared making transfer impossible; cannot be used in muscular adults.
- *Local muscle transfers:* masseter and temporalis can be used. They are easier to perform and gives a quicker return of function, but it is not co-ordinated with the contralateral side. Supplied by Vth cranial nerve. They provide some motion and improved symmetry. Also anterior belly of digastric has been used to augment lip depression and eversion of the lower lip. These transfers do not produce a natural smile and abnormal movements can occur during chewing. Temporalis can be detached from its origin

and reflected back with a fascial sling or detached intra-orally from insertion into coronoid process and fed intra-orally to the commissure with a fascial sling extension.

Eyelid: Determine whether the upper or lower lid needs correction. A lower lid ectropion needs support using a tendon, such as palmaris longus. For the upper lid use a gold weight or an eyespring, which gives a better result but is more troublesome to fit. Local and free muscle transfer with CFNG can be used.

Lower lip: If mandibular nerve cannot be co-apted, use direct co-aptation of hypoglossal nerve or use a muscle transfer with platysma or digastric. Platysma is preferred as it gives co-ordinated movement being supplied by facial nerve, but if also paralysed digastric muscle with CFNG can be used.

Falconer's test

- Test for *Thoracic outlet syndrome*. Costo-clavicular compression.
- Perform with patient standing. Military brace position with shoulders pushed back, arms behind the back and shoulders depressed. (Like a diving falcon.)
- Feel both radial pulses and apply downward traction.

Fanconi's anaemia

See Radial club hand.
- Autosomal recessive aplastic anaemia presenting end of first decade.
- Associated with abnormal repair of damaged DNA.
- The carrier frequency is 1:300.
- Death is by bone marrow failure, leukaemia and solid tumours.
- The average life expectancy is 30 years.
- Associated with altered skin pigmentation, thumb and radial anomalies, abnormal male gonads, microcephaly, developmental delay.
- The thumb is usually present with this form of radial club hand.

Fasanella–Servat operation

- For correction of moderate eyelid *Ptosis*.
- Upper eyelid is everted. Conjunctiva and lower end of Müllers muscle is held in a clip.

A row of sutures is placed above the clip. Tissue held by clip is excised.

Fascia

See Retinacular system

Fascia lata graft

Useful in facial reconstructions when intrinsic support systems are absent or stretched. Used for lower lid ptosis, 7th nerve palsy, static sling.

Technique:
- Several transverse incisions are made over the middle 1/3 of the lateral thigh on a line between the greater trochanter and lateral condyle. Parallel incisions are made in the fascia lata and the fascia lata harvested directly or with a stripper.
- The thumb is usually present with this form of radial club hand.

Fasciocutaneous flap

- Any *Flap* that includes fascia to augment the blood supply.
- Fascia has subfascial, fascial and suprafascial network of vessels.
- The suprafascial network is the most significant and lifting fascia ensures this network is protected.
- Fascial perforators can be direct – going straight to skin – or indirect – ending in skin after supplying deeper structures.
- Fasciocutaneous perforators arise from septa and occur mainly in extremities.

Classification:
- *Cormack and Lamberty* (CandL).
- *Nahai-Mathes* (NandM).
- To summarize: CandL are multiple, solitary or segmental NandM are direct, septocutaneous or musculocutaneous.
- So CandL A have multiple perforators some being indirect are like NandM C CandL B with single perforator are like NandM A (e.g. groin flap), but would be like NandM B if it passes through septum.

To increase the length of pedicle of a flap:
- *CandL A:* dissect indirect perforators through muscle, e.g. periumbilical flap includes the deep inferior epigastric, but not muscle.

- *CandL B:* follow the perforator through septum to origin, e.g. circumflex scapular artery leads to the subscapular artery.
- *CandLC:* include entire source vessel, such as the radial forearm flap.
- The least reliable flaps are those based on indirect perforators.

Axis of flap: Determined by the predominant direction of flow – longitudinal in the extremities and oblique in the torso.
See *Neurocutaneous flaps*. See *Pontén flap*.

Fat anatomy
Fat cells arise from mesodermal adipoblasts. In children accumulation of fat is by increase in number of adipose cells (hyperplasia) for the first 5 years and again during adolescence. After adolescence, no new adipocytes are formed. After puberty the number is constant but the size of the cells enlarge (hypertrophy). Subcutaneous fat forms an insulating layer. In many regions there are deep and superficial compartments. The superficial compartment has dense tightly packed fibrous stroma, whereas the deep layer is more loosely arranged. With weight gain there is a disproportionate enlargement of the deep fat. Men deposit more fat intrabdominally than women.

Abdomen: The waist is the narrowest portion of the torso and is usually 2.5 cm above the umbilicus. With age the waist definition softens due to skeletal compaction, loss of muscle tone and increase in fat.

Thigh hip and buttock: Women have a double curve with fullness at the level of the iliac crest and also the trochanteric area separated by the gluteal crease.
See *Liposuction*.

Fat graft
- Used since 1893.
- Success is dependent on the injected volume and vascularity of the donor sites. A large injected volume has a peripheral area of viable adipocytes, an intermediate zone of inflammation and a central zone of necrosis.
- With a large graft up to 50% volume is lost.
- Fat alone or fat and dermis can be taken.

- To treat furrows. Incise at one end and free up the skin. Insert a strip of fat along the furrow. Over-correction is not necessary as with small grafts, take is 100%. The rate of absorption is variable.

Technique: Outline an ellipse of skin over the inguinal fold. Angle a blade just beneath the epithelial surface. Remove epithelium and then excise entire dermis leaving just a few fat cells. Cut into strips for transfer.

Fat injection
- Used since 1911.
- It has been used to eliminate facial lines secondary to age related ptosis and loss of volume.
- Opinions differ regarding effectiveness.
- Use lower quarter of abdomen and aspirate fate through a 17-gauge blunt tipped epidural needle or by liposuction.
- Transfer fat from one syringe to another with saline until there is no tinge of blood. This will also reduce the amount of free fat. Mark furrows clearly. Use a 19-gauge needle and release fibrous bands. Inject the fat. Over-correct. A disadvantage is the unpredictability. It also does not eliminate muscle function.

Felon
- Infection in the distal phalanx which is inhibited from side-to-side spread by the tight network of vertical fibres attaching to the skin of the distal phalanx.
- Spread occurs by erosion of the walls one by one. Progression can lead to osteomyelitis.

Femoral nerve: anatomy
- L2,3,4. Lies behind fascia iliacus, lateral to femoral artery.
- Terminates 4 cm below inguinal ligament. Divides into anterior and posterior branch. Supplies muscles of anterior compartment.
- Anterior division has 2 cutaneous branches (medial cutaneous nerve of the thigh and the intermediate cutaneous nerve of the thigh), and 2 muscle branches (sartorious and pectineus).
- Posterior division has 1 cutaneous (saphenous nerve to ball of big toe).

- Muscles of anterior compartment are sartorious, iliacus, psoas, pectineus, and quadraceps femorus (rectus femorus, vastus lateralis, astus medialis and vastus intermedias).

Femoral triangle

Boundaries: Inguinal ligament, medial border of Sartorius laterally, medial border of adductor longus medially, and the apex is where the two converge (some take the boundary as the lateral border of adductor longus). The floor consists of iliopsoas, pectineus and adductor longus.

Contents: The femoral artery and vein lie anterior to the fascia. Femoral and lateral cutaneous nerve lie deep to fascia.
See Groin lymph node dissection.

Ferguson–Smith syndrome
Condition linked to a single gene mutation in West of Scotland 200 years ago. Autosomal dominant. Multiple self-healing epitheliomas, which look like KAs.

Fibrillation potentials
- An action potential of a single muscle fibre.
- Arises from a spontaneously contracting muscle and is recorded with a needle electrode.
- Usually suggestive of denervation though they can be seen in healthy muscles. Fibrillations may indicate a lower motor neuron lesion such as arising from the anterior horn cell, nerve root, or peripheral nerve. Also in muscular dystrophy or polymyositis.
- After nerve injury it usually takes 14 days before fibrillation potentials are seen due to the delayed onset of denervation hypersentivity.
See Nerve conduction studies.

Fibrin glue
Prepared by a mixture of cryoprecipitate, calcium and thrombin. It has been shown to decrease subgraft haematoma rate and increase wound healing.

Fibroblast growth factor receptor
A family of tyrosine kinase receptors sharing a common protein structure. Binding of FGF to the receptor results in activation of the tyrosine kinase signalling pathways for cell replication and differentiation.

Fibroma of tendon sheath
Fibromas of tendon sheaths are difficult to distinguish from cysts. They are treated by excision with a small amount of sheath.
- *Juvenile aponeurotic fibroma:* a rapidly growing firm irregular mass on the sole of foot or palm of hand in children. They require conservative excisional surgery. Histologically, there may be infiltration into surrounding muscle, but no mitotic activity. Initial frequent recurrences become less frequent with age.
- *Recurring digital fibrous tumour of childhood:* occurs as multiple smooth masses on the dorsum of the fingers and toes of infants and children. They may appear simultaneously on several digits. Intracytoplasmic inclusion bodies are seen suggesting a viral origin. Treatment is conservative unless there is interference with function. Local recurrence occurs in >50% of cases.

Fibrous dysplasia (FD)
- A benign disease of bone representing 2.5% of all bone tumours.
- Normal bone matrix is replaced with fibroblastic proliferation, which contains irregular trabeculae of partially calcified osteoid.
- Its aetiology remains unclear, but it appears to be a congenital anomaly, which produces dysplastic growth of bone with incomplete maturation of mesenchymal tissue.
- It may be monostotic (one site) or polyostotic. Monostotic are more common and tend to involve ribs, femur, tibia and craniofacial.
- A subset have Albright's syndrome. Also Cherubism.
- Presents with pain from fracture, microfracture or skeletal insufficiency. 10s–30s.

XR:
- *Variable:* central metaphyseal or diaphyseal lesion with mild cortical expansion. Ground glass appearance.
- *3 types:*
  - I: pagetoid;
  - II: sclerotic;
  - III: cystic.

Histology: Immature trabeculae giving a Chinese letters appearance.

Craniofacial fibrous dysplasia:
- Ranges from a painless local swelling to a gross deformity. May get proptosis, optic atrophy and vision loss.
- May be confused with ossifying fibroma, Paget's and meningioma..
- *Malignancy:* rare. Risk greatest in males with polyostotic disease. The most common malignancy is osteosarcoma. Never use RT for FD.
- *Treatment:* curettage and cortical strut grafting. Options are observe, contouring or radical resection.
- FD divided by location into:
  - ○ *Zone 1:* around the orbit; may get displacement of the globe and this causes the greatest cosmetic problem; may require radical resection; perform en-bloc excision of all involved bone; reconstruct with cranial grafts (inner cortex), rib grafts or iliac bone.
  - ○ *Zone 2:* hair-bearing cranium; can be hidden.
  - ○ *Zone 3:* cranial base; resection hazardous and, therefore, conservative treatment if asymptomatic.
  - ○ *Zone 4:* teeth-bearing areas of maxilla or mandible; resection would require dentures.

See Bone tumours.

Fibrous tumours
- *Dermatofibroma.*
- *Pseudosarcomatous lesions.*
- *Dermatofibrosarcoma protuberans.*
- *Angiofibroma.*

Fibula flap
Free fibular flap can achieve a length of 26 cm, has a thick cortex, gives good structural strength, and minimal donor morbidity. It has a short pedicle and peroneal artery must be harvested. The periosteal blood supply is segmental and the endosteal blood supply is usually preserved so that multiple osteotomies are possible. Skin can be harvested, but much of the blood supply comes through septocutaneous and musculocutaneous perforators, which are

variable so reliability can be improved by taking some soleus with the flap.

Technique:
- Bend the knee. Plan to leave 10 cm of bone proximally and distally. Create osteotomies and apply fixation while the pedicle is still attached.
- If bone only is to be taken, make a mid lateral incision. If a skin paddle will be taken 6 cm width can be closed. Doppler perforators and include in flap. They are usually present in the distal and proximal 2/3.
- Elevate the skin island and find the perforators emerging through the intermuscular septum. The common peroneal nerve is protected.
- Peroneus longus and brevis and extensor hallucis are dissected off the fibula and a small cuff of muscle remains.
- Once the lateral half of bone is exposed an osteotomy is performed distally. Divide intermuscular septum and find the distal peroneal vessels. Divide attachments of FHL, TP and soleus. Preserve deep peroneal nerve. Perform a proximal osteotomy. Dissect the vascular pedicle. Apply a splint with crutches for 1/52.

See Mandibular reconstruction.

Fillet flap
Uses skin and vascular supply to an otherwise destroyed digit for reconstruction.

Finasteride
- Finasteride is a competitive inhibitor of 5-alpha reductase, which converts testosterone to dihydrotestosterone.
- It is licensed for treatment of androgenic alopecia in men.
- It is contraindicated in women of childbearing age due to the impaired androgenization of the male foetus.
- It has been used for *Hydradenitis suppuritiva.*

Fingertip injuries
- Distal pulp is divided by radial fibrous septa, which create a multipyramidal structure of fibroadipose tissue compartments.
- Digital nerve trifurcates at the level of the DIP joint.

- Determine the level and angle of tissue loss and what is left. Small defects can be left to heal.

Non-operative:
- If no exposed bone and <1 cm diameter, leave to heal by secondary intention. Healing occurs in 3–6 weeks. It may lead to loss of pulp volume and pulp sensitivity but gives good sensory return.

Operative:
- *Primary closure:* limited bone shortening may be required. If there is significant loss of terminal phalanx, germinal matrix should be excised.
- *Skin graft:* SSG or FTSG. Return of sensation is better with thicker graft. Sharply amputated tissue can be replaced as a graft.
- *Kutler lateral V-Y flaps:*
- *Atasoy volar V-Y flap:*
- *Moberg volar neurovascular flap:*
- *Cross finger flap:*
- *Thenar flexion crease flap:*
- *Littler neurovascular island flap.*
- *Venkataswami flap.*
- *Homodigital island flap.*

Finklestein's test
To confirm *de Quervain's* disease. The patient grasps own thumb within ipsilateral palm. Pain elicited when patient's wrist moves from radial to extreme ulnar deviation.

Finochietto–Bunnell Test
For contractures of interosseous. With MCP joint in extension, PIP joint flexion is prevented due to a contracted interosseous. Flexion of MCP joint releases PIP joint.

Fitzpatrick skin types
Six different skin types based on colour and reaction to sun exposure:
- *Very white or freckled:* always burn.
- *White:* usually burn.
- *White to olive:* sometimes burn.
- *Brown:* rarely burn.
- *Dark brown:* very rarely burn.
- *Black:* never burn.

Five-flap Z-plasty
See *Jumping man flap.*

Flag flap
Axial flap using skin from the dorsal index or middle fingers at the proximal phalanx based upon the dorsal metacarpal artery. It can be used to resurface skin loss over the base of the index or middle finger See *Foucher flap.*

Flap
- Tissue that remains attached to the donor blood supply or is revascularized to recipient vessels.
- *Pedicle:* base of the flap containing its blood supply and maybe other tissue.
- *Composite flap:* contains more than one tissue layer.
- *Blood supply of skin:* arises from either fasciocutaneous vessels, musculocutaneous perforators or direct cutaneous arteries. These supply a deep plexus at the junction of deep dermis and subcutaneous tissue and a superficial layer at the junction of papillary and reticular dermis.
- *Regulation of blood flow:* extrinsic and intrinsic factors affect flow and can either be due to the vessel, the blood or a combination.

Classification: 5 Cs, circulation, composition, contiguity, contour, conditioning.
- Circulation: *Random*, *Axial*.
- Composition: cutaneous, fasciocutaneous, fascial, musculocutaneous, muscle, osseocutaneous, osseous.
- Contiguity: local, regional, distant (pedicled and free).
- Contour: the method in which they are transferred into the defect. *Advance flaps*, *Transposition*, *Rotation*, *Interpolation*, *Crane principle*.
- Conditioning: by *Delay*.

Flaps: upper limb
- *Foucher flap.*
- *Flag flap.*
- *Maruyama flap.*
- *Posterior interosseous artery flap.*
- *Ulnar artery flap.*
- *Radial artery flap.*
- *Distant flaps:* with the development of free flaps there are less indication for pedicle flaps, but they are occasionally indicated – thoracoepigastric, anterior abdominal, groin

or contralateral extremity flap. They are easily dissected and reliable. The disadvantage is immobilization for 2–3 weeks.

• *Pedicle groin flap*.

Fleur-de-Lys abdominoplasty

• *Abdominoplasty* technique when lateral, as well as vertical skin excision is required usually after significant weight loss.
• The operation takes its name from the pattern generated when the first key stitch is placed to bring the skin flaps together.

Flexor carpi radialis

Origin: Medial epicondyle and common flexor pronator origin lateral to PT. Tendinous in mid-forearm. It crosses the wrist under the crest of trapezium.

Insertion: Volar aspect of base of 2nd MC. Sometimes it inserts into flexor retinaculum if there is no PL.

Nerve supply: Median nerve.

Action: Wrist flexor, weak elbow flexor and radial deviator. See *Muscles*.

Flexor carpi radialis tendonitis

Usually get pain and tenderness over FCR just proximal to the scaphoid tubercle and trapezoid crest. Worsened by resisted flexion.

Treatment: Rest, NSAIDs and steroids. Surgical release is performed by opening the fibroosseous tunnel from 3 cm proximal to wrist to the insertion of FCR.
See *Tenosynovitis*.

Flexor carpi ulnaris

Origin: Humeral head arising from the common tendon attached to the medial epicondyle of the humerus and an ulnar head from the medial aspect of the olecranon process of the ulna and the posterior border of the ulna. The two heads are united by a tendinous arch – Osborne's ligament. Long fleshy muscle with short fibres running into tendon almost to the insertion.

Insertion: Into the pisiform bone and by two ligaments, the pisohamate and pisometacarpal

ligaments into the hook of hamate and base of 5th metacarpal. Some fibres form a roof for ulnar artery and nerve.

Nerve supply: Ulnar nerve.

Action: Powerful flexor and wrist ulnar deviator. Stabilizes the wrist. Can be used in radial nerve palsy to restore wrist extension. See *Muscles*.

Flexor carpi ulnaris tenosynovitis

Volar wrist pain worsened by flexion and ulnar deviation.

Differential diagnosis: Pisiform fracture, *Pisotriquetral arthritis*, ulnar neuritis. See *Tenosynovitis*.

Flexor digitorum profundus (FDP)

Origin: Volar and ulnar aspect of proximal 2/3 ulnar, septum that separates profundus from FCU and ulnar half of interosseus membrane, occasionally from the radius. Independence decreases from the radial to ulnar with the index finger being the most independent. It lies beneath FDS. Lumbricals arise from the radial side in the palm.

Insertion: Distal phalanx.

Nerve supply: Radial half anterior interosseous nerve from the median nerve, ulnar half ulnar nerve.

Blood supply: Muscle belly by ulnar anterior interosseous and common interosseous arteries. Tendons at the wrist by branches of the superficial palmar arch. In the sheaths the digital arteries supply the tendons. The only tendon to flex the DIPJ. To test, immobilize the PIPJ in extension and for maximal effect with wrist and MPJ also in extension. Any flexion is caused by FDP.
See *Muscles*.

Flexor digitorum profundus avulsion

• Forced avulsion from the insertion is the next common tendon injury after laceration.
• FDS can be avulsed, but is rare.
• Most occur in the ring finger. A common muscle belly may make it more susceptible

to hyperextension. Also the insertion is weaker and the ring finger is longer in flexion.

Classification: _Leddy and Packer_.

Treatment:
- Repair is easier with early diagnosis and treatment.
- Ultrasound can locate the tendon.
- It should be retrieved and passed through the tunnel and inserted into the distal phalanx.
- Raise a periosteal flap and suture through drill holes to a button tied over the nail. A bony fragment should be fixed.

Flexor digitorum superficialis

Origin: Three heads – humeral from medial epicondyle, ulnar from coronoid process and radial from oblique muscular line of the radius. An aponeurotic arch connects radial to ulnar head and passes over median nerve and ulnar artery. The muscle divides into 4 distinct bundles. Four tendons, superficial are ring and middle, deep are index and little. Pass under TCL.

Insertion: FDS inserts into the volar aspect of the middle phalanx and flexes the PIPJ. FDP also flexes the PIPJ so FDP needs to be blocked to test FDS. FDP has a common muscle belly so holding the other fingers in extension will prevent contraction of FDP on the finger to be tested. As the PIPJ flexes due to FDS action the DIPJ remains extended as the FPD can't function. This may not occur in the index finger as the FDP may function separately. FDS to little finger may not appear to function because 15% are absent, 15% are not functional and some are adherent to the FDS ring thus blocking flexion if the ring is in extension.

Nerve supply: Median nerve.

Blood supply: Muscle is supplied by branches of the ulnar artery, as well as contributions of radial artery. Tendons at the wrist are supplied by branches of the superficial palmar arch. Digital arteries supply tendons in the sheath. To test FDS to index finger ask patient to squeeze a piece of paper between the index and thumb. If the FDS is functional the finger is

held in the pseudo-boutonniere. If absent the finger is held in the pseudomallet position.
See _Muscles_.

Flexor digitorum superficialis tenodesis

See _Proximal interphalangeal joint_. For chronic hyperextension injury. Take radial slip of FDS and fix to bone with interosseous wire or mitek.

Flexor pollicis brevis

Origin: Two heads. Superficial from anterior TCL, FCR tendon sheath and crest of trapezium. Deep originates from anterior surface of trapezoid and capitate. They unite, forming an arch for the passage of FPL. They insert into the lateral sesamoid and lateral tubercle of the base of the proximal phalanx.

Nerve supply: Mainly median nerve, but deep fibres have dual innervation.
See _Muscles_.

Flexor pollicis longus

Origin: Middle 1/3 of radius. An accessory belly may originate from the coronoid process – the accessory muscle of Gantzer. It passes through the carpal tunnel on the radial side of median nerve, bends around trapezium, runs between two heads of FPB, between the two sesamoids. May have an attachment to FDP – _Linburg's syndrome_.

Insertion: Distal phalanx of thumb.

Nerve supply: Median nerve.

Blood supply: Muscular perforators from the radial artery. It is usually supplied by two distinct vincula in the tendon sheath of the thumb.
See _Muscles_.

Flexor sheaths

The flexor sheath of the thumb and little finger are contiguous with the radial and ulnar bursa. That of the index, middle and ring finger originate at the metacarpal neck. Double-walled fibro-osseous tunnel sealed at both ends. Inner visceral and outer parietal layer. Floor is composed of periosteum and volar plate. The system of annular and cruciate _Pulleys_ holds the tendon close to the bone. The sheath forms a closed cavity.

Flexor sheath infection
See _Tenosynovitis_.

Flexor tendons
Anatomic relationship:
- In arm FDP deep to FDS with median nerve in-between.
- _FDS:_ middle and ring finger volar to index and little. In the palm they lie in the same plane. At the distal palmar crease each FDS splits to wrap around FDP. The two slips merge deep to FDP then insert along middle phalanx. The decussation distal to where the FDP tendon pierces the two slips is called Camper's chiasm.

Pulleys: A2 and A4 most important for function.

Flexion: Starts at PIPJ. FDP is the prime flexor. MCP joint flexion is resisted by the extensors. Flexion of PIP joint increases intrinsic tension which causes MCP joint flexion. Flexion of DIP joint is limited by ORL tightness. Flexion of PIP joint relaxes ORL allowing for DIP flexion.

Blood supply: From 3 sources.
- Point of bony insertion.
- The _Vincular_ and vessels in the palm.
- In the palm they are surrounded by paratenon containing vessels from the palmar arch.

Nutrition:
- Vascular perfusion (vincula).
- Diffusion of nutrients from synovial fluid (predominant system). Diffusion is probably more important within the tendon sheath than vascular perfusion.

Healing:
- Via fibroblastic response of the sheath through adhesions.
- Via nutrients supplied through synovial fluid.
- _Histology:_ three overlapping phases of inflammation, proliferation and remodelling. Invasion of white cells with granulation

tissue (inflammation). Fibroblasts produce matrix (proliferation). Endontenocytes and epitenocytes migrate into gap. After 6 weeks remodelling occurs with maturation of tissue and realignment of cells.

Incisions: Bruner incisions or midlateral incisions.

Flexor tendon repair:
Retrieval:
- Retrieve through the sheath in the least traumatic manner usually through funnel-shaped incisions in the cruciate pulleys proximal and distal to A4 pulley.
- Core sutures can be placed in each tendon through the closest window to assist retrieval.
- Milk tendon or blind retrieval.
- If it can't be retrieved, incise in the palm for fingers or wrist for FPL. A feeding tube can be used to feed tendon through pulleys.

Suture repair:
- Two types of suture, the core suture and the epitendinous suture.
- The strength of repair is proportional to the number of strands.
- The epitendinous suture increase strength and resists gapping.
- The core suture is usually a modified Kessler repair with the know internally. Place core sutures in the volar half of the tendon to preserve vascular supply.
- Repairing the sheath does not give a proven advantage.

Post-operative therapy: Tensile strength decreases for 7–10 days. A number of regimes used, but the Belfast regime is one of the commonest.

Partial tendon laceration: <60% mobilize without tenorrhaphy.

Outcomes:
- Different outcome measures.
- Distance from pulp to palm, extension deficit, composite joint flexion, flexion minus extensor lag at each joint. Strickland excludes MCP joint function, which is more dependent on intrinsics and measures flexion at DIP joint and PIP joint minus extension loss.

Late reconstruction:
Indications:
- Immediate repair or tendon graft may not be possible if there is significant trauma, infection, delay or failure of previous operation. Pulleys may have been lost.
- New sheath formation by the insertion of a silicone rod, developed by Hunter seems the most effective reconstruction.
- The ring and little finger require full flexion for strong grasp.
- The radial fingers require less flexion as they are used more for pinch.
- The thumb requires a stable post so full flexion is less important.

Tendon grafting: One-stage grafting is indicated for acute trauma with segmental loss, otherwise perform in two stages.

Operation:
- *Choice of motor unit:* contracture of the motor unit which is being replaced may prevent it from being used. A minimum of 2–3 cm amplitude is required. FDS is independent and should be used over FDP if available. FDP needs to be tensioned correctly to prevent the quadriga effect.
- *Donor tendon selection:* PL and *Plantaris*, or toe extensors (*EDL*).

First stage:.
- Expose the pulleys in the finger from A1–A5 with Bruner incisions. Remove FDP. Pulley reconstruction may be required. Make a wrist incision and pass a 4-mm Hunter silicone rod through the carpal tunnel then through the pulleys. Suture to periosteum. Suture to FDP in the wrist to help at the second stage. Perform the second stage in 3–4 months.

Pulley reconstruction: Use fascia lata, PL or extensor retinaculum. Use a single, double or triple loop encircling the phalanx or attach to volar plate. Double loop will need 10 cm of graft.

Second stage: Harvest tendon and perform Pulvertaft weave to proximal end. Distal the tendon can be attached with a pullout suture or mitek. Alternatively, the tendon can be passed through the pulp, tensioned and suture to the nail.

Flexor tendon zones
Zones:
- *I:* insertion of FDS (middle middle phalanx) to FDP insertion.
- *II:* A1 (distal palmar crease) to FDS insertion (middle middle phalanx).
- *III:* distal to carpal tunnel to A1 (distal palmar crease).
- *IV:* carpal tunnel
- *V:* roximal to carpal tunnel.
Thumb also has 5 zones
- *I:* distal to IPJ.
- *II:* A1 to IPJ.
- *III:* thenar eminence.
- *IV and V:* as above.

Described by Verdan. Zone II was described as 'no man's land' by Bunnell reflecting the poor results of tendon repair at this site.

Flexor tenolysis
Indicated if lack of movement is due to excessive scar formation. Adhesions are released followed by intensive hand therapy.
- *Operation:* perform under LA. Expose the sheath, preserve pulleys. Make transverse incisions between pulleys. Release scars to improve ROM. Steroid injection gives a higher rate of rupture. Active mobilization post-operatively.
- *Complications:* tendon rupture. If pulleys significantly damaged then staged reconstruction may be better. CRPS will compromise function obtained.

Flip-flap urethroplasty
Described by Mathieu for distal *Hypospadias*.
- Use if no chordee and meatal opening is adequate and if urethral plate flat and narrow and can't be tubularized.
- Use ventral shaft skin to make ventral wall by flipping over with closure over this by glans wings.
- Devine and Horton modified the flip-flap with triple glans flaps. If the native urethra is more proximal, FTSG is used to reconstruct the anterior urethra beyond the limits of the flip-flap.

Floor of mouth cancer
Present around 60 years. Related to smoking and alcohol. The area between tongue and

inner surface of mandible. Most are anterior. Tumours may involve Warton's duct causing submandibular gland enlargement. It begins as an inflamed ulcer.

Treatment:

- Small lesions can be treated with surgery or RT. Stenosis of Wharton's duct may lead to submandibular enlargement and confusion with lymphadenopathy.
- If they abut the mandible perform a rim mandibulectomy.
- Advanced lesions require a partial mandibulectomy.
- High incidence of neck disease so >T1 require neck dissection, surgery and RT.

Results:

- Stage I and II lesions have 70–90% 5-year cure rates with excision and interstitial radiotherapy. Large lesions have a much poorer prognosis, ranging from 30 to 60%.
- The overall 5-year survival rate has been reported as 65%.

See Head and neck cancer.

Foetal surgery

Prenatal diagnosis:

- By ultrasound, amniocentesis, umbilical blood sampling and chorionic villus sampling.
- Foetal cleft lip and palate can be diagnosed at 15–20 weeks of gestation.
- Foetal MRI is developing.
- A thorough assessment of all organs is required before a surgical intervention. A careful risk–benefit assessment is required for non-lethal conditions. Also accuracy must be 100%. Some conditions such as clefts are associated with undetectable syndromes.

Maternal risk:

- Particularly in having two GA operations in a short space of time.
- Tocolytics to prevent preterm labour have their risk.
- Pulmonary oedema can occur from magnesium sulphate.
- Hysterotomy can cause uterine rupture.
- There is a potential risk of infertility.

Foetal risk:

- All human subjects have delivered prematurely.
- Seven out of 33 foetuses had neurological injury.

Foetal surgical techniques:

- In experiments with monkeys, surgical procedures were performed through a hysterotomy in the upper segment of the uterus.
- *Open surgery:* US is used to localize placenta. Classic hysterotomy is used. Irrigate the foetus. Restore amniotic fluid with normal saline. Three layer closure to reduce amniotic leak.
- *Foetal endoscopy:* potentially less invasive. Require CO_2 insufflation as cautery doesn't work in amnion. The magnification allows earlier surgery. It may be useful for clefts, neural tube defects and amniotic bands.
- *Foetal surgical interventions:* performed for diaphragmatic hernia, obstructive uropathy, hydrocephalus.

Foetal indications in plastic surgery: there are presently **no** indications in plastic surgery.

- *Cleft lip and palate:* repair *in utero* may allow scarless healing. A rabbit model has shown good repair with normal midface growth. Endoscopic cleft repair has been performed on a lamb.
- *Craniosynostosis:* the pathology was created by performing a strip craniectomy and inserting demineralized bone matrix to cause fusion. Repair was then performed by excising the area, and the margins were wrapped with Gortex. All had open craniectomy sites.
- *Amniotic band syndrome:* constrictive bands. Lambs had limbs banded and 2 limbs were released, the other two left banded. The released limbs had normal development, whereas the unreleased limb showed gross changes.
- *Myelomeningocoele:* May be caused by failure of mesoderm migration with exposure and damage to the spinal cord. Lamb models have been performed with *lat dorsi* distally based flap. Though there was a high mortality, those that survived had near normal neurology.

Foetal wound healing

Scarless _Wound healing_ up to the early third trimester. Not all foetal tissues heal without scar. Doesn't follow adult pattern and normal tissue architecture restored by 5–7 days. There are many extrinsic and intrinsic differences.

- In adults the inflammatory process is orchestrated by the macrophage. In the foetus there are few inflammatory cells and the healing process is controlled by the foetal fibroblast and epidermis.
- Wound repair occurs by the rapid deposition of type III _Collagen_ with a ratio of 3:1, which remains unlike adult wounds where it is replaced with type I.
- The extracellular matrix also differs (ECM). Hyaluronic acid is elevated which aids fibroblast movement and favours scarless healing.
- Fibronectin is rapidly laid down providing a good scaffold for cells.
- Amniotic fluid plays a role, inhibiting foetal and adult fibroblast contraction.
- _Growth factors_ differ in foetal wounds. Some, such as TGF-β, PDGF, bFGF are reduced. They are expressed for only a short time.

Foot: anatomy

Four layers of muscles.

- Flexor digitorum brevis, abductor hallucis, abductor digiti quinti.
- Flexor hallucis longus, flexor accesorius, lumbricals.
- Flexor digiti quinti brevis, flexor hallucis brevis, adductor hallucis.
- Tibialis posterior, peroneus longus, interossei.

Foramen caecum

A blind opening formed between the frontal crest and the crista galli, which sometimes transmits a vein from the nasal cavity to the superior sagittal sinus.
See _Dermoid cyst_.

Fordyce's spots

See _Sebaceous hyperplasia_. Ectopic sebaceous glands on the vermilion border of the lips and oral mucosa.

Forehead flap

- Commonly used in _Nasal reconstruction_.
- Forehead is supplied by supra-orbital, supratrochlear, infratrochlear and dorsal, nasal and angular vessels.
- A vertically designed paramedian forehead flap is an axial flap. The distal flap can be thinned of frontalis and some subcutaneous tissue. The proximal flap is elevated over periosteum. The flap can be extended into the scalp with this area thinned and hair bulbs clipped.
- Pedicle can be divided at 3 weeks, but also it can be lifted as a bipedicled flap, attached at alars and still attached to forehead.
- Lateral forehead can be transferred on the unilateral superficial temporal artery.
- Forehead flaps can be expanded or delayed prior to raising.
See _Gullwing flap_.

Forehead rejuvenation

- _Botulinum toxin:_ ½ ml is injected into each corrugator. Ask the patient to frown. Palpate the muscle. Mark the injection site that is the medial end of the eyebrow at the supra-orbital rim. Inject at one site only. Paralysis usually lasts 4–6 months.
- _Fat graft:_
- _Transpalpebral corrugator resection:_ if there is no ptosis, but significant frown lines, corrugator resection can be performed through the upper eyelid. Corrugator is exposed cephalad to the orbital rim. Nerves are protected. Muscle is removed completely. Procerus is transected if active. Fat is placed in the space.
- _Brow lift_.

Forme fruste

Also called microform _Cleft lip_. Very mild or incomplete cleft lip. May have:
- A kink in the alar cartilage.
- A notch in the vermilion.
- A fibrous band across the lip.

Foucher flap

- A flap based on the radial side of the proximal dorsum of the index finger.
- The dominant branch of the radial artery travels in the base of the anatomic snuff box

before giving off terminal branches to the dorsal carpal arch and first dorsal metacarpal artery.

- The first dorsal metacarpal artery courses within the fascia and occasionally within the belly of first dorsal interosseous muscle adjacent to the second metacarpal bone.
- There is an anastomotic communication within the first web space with the palmar vessels.
- Veins run more superficially and venae comitantes run with the artery.
- It can also be raised with the vessel to resurface the thumb.
- Extend the incision proximally, and include superficial veins and fascia overlying first dorsal interosseous muscle.
- This tissue contains the first dorsal metacarpal artery and branches of the radial nerve.
- The flap can be tunnelled to the thumb defect.

See _Flag flap_. See _Maruyama flap_.

Four-flap Z-plasty
- Useful for correcting thumb-index web space and axillary contractures.
- Use 90° or 120° angle _Z-plasty_.
- Convert to four flaps by bisecting the angles.
- This produces greater lengthening (124%) with less tension on the flaps.
- Flaps ABCD becomes CADB (Cadbury).

Fractures: metacarpal and phalangeal

Instability: The primary problem leading to surgery. Leads to displacement. Get angulation, shortening or rotation. Rotation and lateral angulation are poorly tolerated. Shortening and dorsal angulation are better tolerated.

Pathology: An unstable fracture cannot be held in the functional position without fixation. Muscle balance causes dorsal angulation of metacarpal and volar angulation of phalangeal fractures.

Goals: Anatomic reduction, stability, early movement.

Free flap

Anticoagulation: The role has not been clearly defined. There is no definite indication in elective free tissue transfer. It may reduce the risk of anastomotic thrombosis, but will increase the risk of haematoma. Indicated following re-exploration. Aspirin, dextran and heparin used.

No-flow phenomenom: Failure to perfuse an ischaemic organ after re-establishing a blood supply. Related to endothelial injury, platelet aggregation, and leakage of intravascular fluid. Relates to ischaemic time.

Occlusion: If arterial the flap is pale with poor refill. If venous it will be bluish with a brisk refill.

Repair: Platelets are deposited on the injured intima. Pseudointima forms within 5 days. By 2 weeks new endothelium covers the anastomosis. Platelet deposition only leads to fibrin deposition and thrombosis if there is extensive intimal exposure.

Spasm: Topical lignocaine may relieve it. Papaverine dilates small vessels. Epidural and other regional blocks may block sympathetically mediated spasm.

Monitoring: Viability easier to assess with skin-bearing flaps. Assess colour, capillary refill, dermal bleeding. Also fluoroscein, surface Doppler, temperature probes, _Laser Doppler flowometry_, tissue pH, pulse oximetry and direct tissue oxygen measurements.

Free radicals
Atoms or molecules with unpaired electrons in the outer orbit.

French gauge
Measurement for catheters – diameter measured in millimetres.

Frey's syndrome
- Gustatory sweating.
- Post-ganglionic parasympathetic nervous system (PNS) secretomotor fibres destined for the parotid hitch-hiking in the auriculotemporal nerve – sensory nerve to the ear and temple.
- Trauma of parotidectomy divides PNS branches of the nerve which degenerate to the level of the cell bodies in the otic ganglion

and regenerate along the auriculotemporal nerve.
- These link up with sweat glands in the absence of parotid gland.
- Subsequent eating with activation of the salivation nerves induces sweating in the distribution of the auriculotemporal nerve.
- Incidence is 10–40%.
- Treat with antiperspirants, dermofat grafts, tympanic neurectomy.

Fricke flap
- Inferiorly based refers to a flap designed with the base at the lateral canthus and the limb extending above the eyebrow. It can be used for lower eyelid reconstruction.
- Superiorly based: also for eyelid reconstruction.

Froment's sign
- In *Ulnar nerve palsy*.
- Loss of pinch between index finger and thumb with IPJ flexing due to paralysis of first dorsal and second palmar interosseus and adductor pollicis muscles.

Frontal sinus fractures
- 'Le Fort IV' fractures.
- Often associated with other fractures as the force required to fracture the frontal bone is great.
- The frontal sinuses are small in children and really expand from age 7, therefore they are less likely to be involved in children.
- A blow associated with depression of the bone, CSF rhinorrhoea, supra-orbital anaesthesia, crepitus are all suggestive of frontal sinus involvement.
- Complications are due to obstruction of the nasofrontal duct and mucosal tears. Can get meningitis, sinusitis, osteomyelitis and cerebral abscesses.

Symptoms and signs:
- Bruising and swelling.
- Palpable bony step.
- CSF rhinorrhoea.
- Frontal lobe injury.
- Pneumocephalus and orbital emphysema.
- Visual loss.

Management:
- *Conservative:* if undisplaced, no CSF leak, intact posterior wall and unaffected drainage system.
- *ORIF anterior wall:* if displaced anterior wall, no CSF leak, intact posterior wall, unaffected drainage system.
- *ORIF anterior wall and obliteration of frontal sinus:* if displaced fracture, no CSF leak, intact posterior wall, damaged drainage system. Obliteration of frontal sinus is performed by complete removal of nasal lining, followed by spontaneous osteogenesis or bone graft.
- *Cranialization of frontal sinus:* if displaced fracture of anterior wall, CSF leak, minimally displaced fracture of posterior wall. Cranialization is achieved by complete removal of mucosal lining, plugging nasofrontal duct with bone graft, removing posterior wall, allowing brain and dura to expand into the resultant dead space.
- *Cranialization of frontal sinus with dural repair:* if displaced fracture, CSF leak, displaced fracture of posterior wall.

Frontalis

Origin: From epicranial aponeurosis at the anterior hairline.

Insertion: Into the dermis of the skin.

Nerve supply: Temporal branch of facial nerve.

Action: To elevate the eyebrow. See *Brow lift*.

Frostbite
- Three types of cold injury are tissue-freezing injury (frostbite), non-tissue freezing injury (trenchfoot, chilblain, pernio) and hypothermia.
- Frostbite occurs when the temperature falls to –2°C resulting in intracellular and extracellular ice crystals and microvascular occlusion.

Chilblain: High humidity and low temperature without freezing, particularly in mountaineers.

Trenchfoot: Extremities exposed to a damp environment at temperatures of 1–10°C. Heat is lost as it is wet and vascular flow is poor. Get numbness, tingling, pain and itching. Skin is red and oedematous then grey-blue. Symptoms resolve in 3–6 weeks, but get cold intolerance.

Cold uriticaria: Urticaria and angio-oedema due to exposure to cold temperatures, especially with aquatic activities. Anaphylaxis may occur. May be familial or acquired.

Aetiology: Temperature, wind, humidity, protection and mental state. Race affects susceptibility with blacks having a 2.5–6× greater risk of cold injury.

Pathophysiology: Tissue damage from direct cellular damage or vascular compromise. 3 phases.
- With reduced temperature get peripheral vasoconstriction but periodic cold induced vasodilatation to protect the periphery until the core temperature drops when the peripheral circulation shuts down by closing the AV shunts.
- Direct cellular trauma by freezing. Intra- and extracellular ice crystals. With rapid cooling get intracellular crystals, which are lethal to the cells unless they are small as in supercooling. With slow cooling get extracellular crystals, and an osmotic gradient with cell dehydration.
- With rewarming there is microvascular damage and a reperfusion injury. Endothelial cell damage leads to oedema and hypoxia. O_2-free radicals are released by neutrophils and thromboxane causes vasoconstriction.

Clinical: 4 degrees, 1 and 2 are superficial, 3 and 4 are deep. Get initial swelling and erythema followed by white waxy skin. With thawing there is vasodilatation with a purple colour, pain and blisters. Oedema in the region with deeper areas developing dry gangrene which demarcates over several weeks.

Treatment:
- Rapid rewarming. Immerse body in water at 40–42°C. Lower temperatures aren't as effective and higher will cause a burn. 15–30 minutes are required to restore core temperature.

- A number of treatments to improve the circulation have been tried with varying results;
  o dextran and heparin have been effective in some trials;
  o streptokinase was significantly beneficial;
  o recombinant tissue plasminogen activator (r-tPA) is fibrinolytic;
  o prostaglandin and thromboxane blockers may improve tissue survival.
- Give analgesia. Don't massage. Debride clear blisters, elevate, apply topical thromboxane inhibitor (aloe vera), systemic anti-prostaglandin, tetanus, whirlpool treatment.

Surgery: Not in acute management. Relieve constricting eschar. Amputation may be required, but wait until demarcation.

Other treatment: Alpha blocker to relieve spasm. Nifedipine for chilblains, heparin and streptokinase.

Late sequelae: Arthritis, cold sensitivity, hyperhydrosis.

Fungal hand infections
Most are treated by local or systemic antifungal agents. Surgery is generally not required though *Coccidiomycosis* may cause tenosynovitis, and blastomycosis and brucellosis may cause septic arthritis or osteomyelitis. _Aspergillosis_ is an exception, and surgery may be requested to rule out neoplasm.

Furlow technique
- Technique of _Cleft palate_ repair and treatment of _VPI_.
- Double-opposing Z-plasty technique.
- The technique lengthens the soft palate and attempts to place the muscle in a more posterior position.
- A Z-plasty of the oral layer includes the muscle on the posteriorly based flap.
- A Z-plasty of the nasal layer is performed in the opposite direction with the muscle again included on the posterior flap on the opposite side.
- The hard palate is closed with a vomer flap.
- Good for submucous cleft palate.

Galeazzi fracture

Fracture dislocation with fracture to the radius shaft and dislocation of the distal radioulnar joint.

See _DRUJ_.

Gamekeeper's thumb

Chronic attritional change to UCL noted in Scottish gamekeepers because of the technique of killing rabbits by twisting the head and neck. Often also applied to acute injuries.

Ganglion

The most common hand mass.

Pathogenesis:

- Herniation of fluid from a joint or tendon sheath. The cyst has a stalk which can be a one- or two-way valve.
- Ligament strain with mucinous degeneration.
- Embryological remnants of synovial tissue.

Site: around the wrist.

- Dorsal ganglia most frequently arise from the articulation of lunate and scaphoid.
- Volar ganglia may be adherent to radial artery and arise from radiocarpal or STT joint.
- Mucous cysts arise from the DIPJ in association with OA. They may arise from tendon sheath.

Presentation: 20s–40s. F:M 3:1.

Signs and symptoms: Many are asymptomatic or present with a dull ache.

Dorsal wrist ganglia:

- 60–70% of hand ganglia. They arise from the scapholunate ligament (SLL). The pedicle arising from SLL usually emerges between EPL and EDC. Occult SLL ganglia may cause pain by pressure on the SLL. Diagnose with USS.
- _Conservative treatment:_ 40% resolve spontaneously. Cysts can be aspirated and injected with sclerosants or steroids.
- _Surgery:_ dissect down to the SLL and excise ganglion off SLL. Recurrence rates of up to 40% are reported, so surgery is discouraged for asymptomatic ganglia.

Volar wrist ganglia:

- _20% of hand ganglia:_ originates from the scaphotrapezium-trapezoid joint (STT). They pass superficially radial to FCR. They may be attached to radial artery.
- _Treatment:_ excision is usually recommended. Aspiration may injure the radial artery.

Flexor sheath ganglia:

- Also called volar retinacular ganglia. 10% of hand ganglia. Occur at the proximal palmar sheath, arising from the A1 pulley. Most commonly in the middle finger.
- _Treatment:_ needle rupture and steroid injection can be tried prior to surgery. If resected this is done with a small portion of A1 pulley.

Mucous cyst:
Other:

- Capsular cysts also called daughter cysts may be a cause for recurrence.
- After resection some surgeons advise closure of the capsule.
- Arthroscopic excision has been described.
- Carpal ganglia are more difficult to treat and extensive resection may lead to capsular instability.
- Ganglion cysts may arise on the ulnar side of the wrist from the pisohamate joint or TFCC. They can stretch the dorsal branch of the ulna nerve giving pain.

See _Soft tissue tumours_.

Gantzer: accessory muscle of

An accessory belly of _Flexor pollicis longus_, which originates from the coronoid process.

Gardner's syndrome

- Multiple _Epithelial cysts_.
- Polyposis coli.
- Osteomas of the jaw.
- Intestinal desmoid tumours.

Garrod's pads
Knuckle pads associated with _Dupuytren's_ diathesis.

Gas gangrene
- Similar presentation as _Necrotizing fasciitis_.
- Patient presents very sick with surgical emphysema.
- Bloody blisters contain _Clostridium welchi_ (Gram ve bacilli).

Clostridial myonecrosis:
- Seen in _Abdominal_ infections as a post-operative complication.
- Get rapid progression of sepsis with crepitus. Patient is very toxic.
- Polymicrobial with _Clostridium_ usually _C. oedamatiens or C. septicum_. The most important exotoxin is lecinthinase.
- With myonecrosis get a small amount of gas and severe toxicity.

Gastric pull-up
- Used for _Pharynx_ reconstruction.
- Largely replaced by free jejunal transfer that has less morbidity and mortality.
- The only indications are for reconstruction of a pharyngolaryngeal defect when the inferior end extends into the superior mediastinum and when there are skip lesions.
- The viability of the stomach depends on the preservation of right gastric and right gastroepiploic arteries, as well as the entire gastroepiploic arcade.
- The spleen is left. The left gastric artery and branches are divided. The hiatus is enlarged and the lower oesophagus mobilized. Kocher manoeuvre and pyloromyotomy is performed. The oesophagus is removed by blunt dissection and the stomach passed up and anastamosed to the pharynx.

Gastrocnemius flap
- Proximally based flap of one head of gastrocnemius useful for soft tissue cover of the knee and upper tibia.
- Medial head has a longer reach than the lateral head, as it is longer at its insertion and lateral head has to pass around fibula.
- Fibres of the two may decussate in the midline.

- The sural nerve and lesser saphenous vein mark the midline.

Gastroschisis
- A full thickness defect of abdominal wall, which occurs lateral to the umbilical ring usually on the right side with cord in the normal position.
- The viscera are not covered by amnion. The bowel is not rotated and the midgut is short with a small peritoneal cavity. It lacks a covering sac and the intestines are usually matted and shortened.
- Mortality usually from sepsis, respiratory insufficiency and a prolonged ileus.
- 20–25% of patients with gastroschisis and omphalocoele have intestinal atresia, malrotation and volvulus.

Treatment: Primary closure if it doesn't produce too high intra-abdominal pressure. Otherwise slowly close on Teflon sheets.
See _Abdominal wall reconstruction_.

Genitalia reconstruction

Degloving: Either immediate skin grafting or bury shaft for delayed reconstruction.

Penile reconstruction: Radial forearm flaps are now the prime flap. Add a prosthesis but delay before inserting.

Vaginal reconstruction: Can use bowel (sigmoid colon), flaps, skin grafts or amnion.
See _Penis_, _Hypospadias_, _Extrophy/epispadias_.

Giant cell tumour of bone
- Found in long bones and 50% occur around the knee.
- In the upper limb, it is most commonly found in the distal radius. In the hand, they are mainly in the phalanges.
- 1/3 are aggressive stage 3 lesion with cortical breakthrough and a soft tissue component.
- 5% of patients develop lung metastasis.
- Excision frequently leads to local recurrence.

_XR:_ Expansile eccentric radiolucent lesion involving epiphysis and subchondral bone of distal radius. Cortex thinned with sclerotic margin. May get pathological fracture.

Histology: Numerous giant cells.

Differential diagnosis: Chondroblastoma, non-ossifying fibroma, brown tumour, fibrosarcoma, osteogenic sarcoma.

Treatment: Curettage with adjuvants such as polymethymethacrylate cement, liquid nitrogen or phenol, +/– bone grafting. Vascularized fibular graft.
See Bone tumours.

Giant cell tumour (PVNS)
Also call pigmented villonodular tenovaginosynovitis (PVNS).
- Benign soft tissue tumour seen over the palmar aspect of the fingers which slowly increase in size.
- Firm, nodular and maybe mobile.
- Treatment is excisional biopsy.
- Recurrence rate of 10–30%.
- Commonly occur in middle-aged women.
- They occur along tendon sheaths and other sites where synovial fluid is formed.
See Soft tissue tumours.

Giant condyloma acuminatum
- A fungating growth usually on the prepuce of an uncircumcized male.
- Locally destructive and may transform to a verrucous SCC.
- Frequently mistaken for condyloma (viral wart) and verrucous SCC.
- It probably has a viral origin.
- Recurrence is common following excision.

Gibson's principle
Of interlocking stress: Cartilage moves away from the scored surface.
See Prominent ear correction.

Gilles' fan flap
- Used for Lip reconstruction.
- Fan-shaped rotational advancement flap based on the superior labial artery, for defects over 50% of lower lip.
- Flap made around nasolabial fold with 1 cm back-cut.
- Extended version of the Estlander flap.

Gilles' lift
- Used in the treatment of Zygomatic fractures.
- For reduction of displaced fractures of the zygomatic arch.

- Make a radial incision above and anterior to the ear. Deepen through temporoparietal fascia (superficial temporal fascia). Incise the deep temporal fascia and insert a Gilles' elevator between it and temporalis muscle. This leads under the zygomatic arch. Elevate the fracture by lifting. Pivoting the elevator on temporal bone may result in a secondary fracture.

Gilula's lines
Lines on XR made by the proximal and distal carpal row.

Glasgow Coma Scale
- Best verbal response
  - *1:* none;
  - *2:* incomprehensible sound;
  - *3:* inappropriate words;
  - *4:* confused;
  - *5:* orientated.
- Eye opening
  - *6:* none;
  - *7:* to pain;
  - *8:* to speech;
  - *9:* spontaneously.
- Best motor response
  - *10:* none;
  - *11:* pain extension;
  - *13:* pain flexion;
  - *14:* pain withdrawal;
  - *15:* pain – localizes;
  - *16:* obeys command.
Highest score 15
Lowest score 3

Glioma
- Nasal gliomas are uncommon, smooth, non-compressible masses present at birth or early childhood. Either extra or intranasal.
- Lack of change in size with crying distinguishes it from an encephalocoele.
- If extranasal it may penetrate the bone in the frontonasal suture area and may have a broadened nasal root.
- Intranasal gliomas present with nasal airway obstruction.
- Need imaging prior to excision.

Glomus
A glomus is an arteriovenous anastomosis involved in thermoregulation.

Glomus tumour

- Benign vascular hamartomatous derivative of the glomus body – a normal intradermal arteriovenous anastomosis that arises from the normal neuromyoarterial glomus.
- Derived from smooth muscle cells and are usually solitary, occurring in nail bed and less commonly on the pulp. They can occur at other sites.
- They are tender blue-red 1–2 mm papules. They are very painful and sensitive to temperature change.
- The lesions may be single or multiple and most characteristically occur on the hands and feet, especially subungually. Glomus tumours have also been reported on the face.
- Treatment of symptomatic lesions requires complete excision, which dramatically relieves the severe episodes of pain. Subungual, highly sensitive lesions may be small and difficult to locate visibly.
- Usually present in adults.
- Multiple glomus tumours are inherited as autosomal dominant with incomplete penetrance. They develop 10–15 years earlier than solitary tumours, Pain is not as severe as in solitary glomus tumours. They can present as regional, disseminated or congenital plaque-like.
- _Haemangiopericytoma_ may resemble a painless glomus tumour
- Assess with _Love's sign_ and _Hildreth's sign_.

Treatment: Surgical excision.
See _Familial glomangiomatosis_.

Glossectomy

- Most commonly required for _Tongue carcinoma_.
- Tongue mobility is important for speech and food propulsion.
- With partial glossectomy the goal of reconstruction is to preserve mobility, restore shape and volume and sensation. Need adequate bulk and mobility.
- If >30% of the tongue remains, a thin pliable flap enables mobility and the radial forearm flap is used. It can also be made sensate. It is useful for tongue and floor of mouth as a sulcus can be created.
- If less tongue remains, a more bulky flap is used and the rectus abdominus flap is useful.

Sometimes there is too much bulk in which case skin and fat is excised leaving just muscle which can be grafted or left to re-epithelialize.
- Midline posterior tumours which require total glossectomy may be treated by brachytherapy to reduce the debilitating nature of the surgery.

Gluteal thigh flap

Blood supply: Descending branch of the inferior gluteal artery.

Surface marking: Midpoint between greater trochanter and ischial tuberosity. Distally, it can extend to the medial femoral condyle.
See _Pressure sores_.

Gluteus maximus

Origin: Lateral sacrum and posterior superior iliac crest.

Insertion: Greater trochanter of femur. Rotates and extends the hip.

Blood supply: Type III muscle with two dominant pedicles – superior and inferior gluteal arteries.

Nerve supply: Superior and inferior gluteal nerves. The inferior is more dominant.

Gluteus maximus flap
Gluteus maximus muscle flap:
- Upper half of muscle supplied by superior gluteal artery, lower half by inferior gluteal artery.
- Expose using a buttock rotation flap incision. detach insertion on femur and reflect as turn-over flap into sacral defect. Apply SSG.
Gluteus maximus rotation flap:
- As above, but raise in plane between gluteus maximus and medius.
- Divide origin from ilium to rotate into defect. If arc of rotation limited by superior gluteal vessels, these can be divided.
See _Reconstruction_. See _Pressure sores_.

Gold

Gold is resistant to corrosion, but has a low tensile strength. It is used primarily as an upper-eyelid weight to facilitate eye closing in *Facial palsy*. See *Alloplasts*.

Goldenhar syndrome

Hemifacial microsomia associated with epibulbar ocular dermoids and vertebral anomalies. Occurs in less than 5% of hemifacial microsomia.

Goldwyn

1963: Performed the first free flap (groin flap in a dog).

Gorlin syndrome

Also called basal cell nevus syndrome.

- The naevi are reddish brown and papular.
- Autosomal dominant though 20–30% are due to *de novo* mutations.
- Traced to a mutation in a suppressor gene located at 9q23.1–q31 – the Patched gene (PTCH).
- Get multiple basal cell naevi with malignant change to *Basal cell carcinoma* by puberty.
- Jaw cysts (adontogenic keratocysts).
- Pitting of the palm and soles.
- Calcification of the falx cerebri by 20 years of age.
- Also pseudohypertelorism, frontal bossing, syndactyly and spina bifida.

GOSLON index

- Developed by Michael Mars to assess cleft malocclusion in *Cleft palate* patients.
- Five models of malocclusion were made based on previous patients. These were graded 1–5. Cleft models are assessed by this yardstick and graded.
- Grades 4–5 are likely to require orthognathic surgery.

Gout

- M:F 8:1.
- High levels of uric acid with precipitation of sodium urate in the joint.

Aetiology:

- Primary hyperuricaemia – increased dietary intake (red wine and meat), enzyme abnormalities.
- Secondary hyperuricaemia is caused by diuretics and myeloproliferative disorders.

Acute gout:

- Painful synovitis.
- 90% of attacks are self-limiting.
- 60% are of 1st MTPJ. It can involve wrists and fingers.

Tophus: Deposits of sodium urate in joints and perarticular tissues. With chronic gout get extra-articular deposits.

Diagnosis:

- Identification of monosodium urate monohydrate crystals by polarized light microscopy.
- High uric acid levels are not diagnostic.
- Most patients with hyperuricaemia do not have gout.
- XR show punched-out erosions away from the joint margin.

Treatment:

- *Acute:* high-dose NSAIDs, colchicine.
- *Chronic:* low-purine diet, allopurinol (xanthine oxidase inhibitor), probenecid (uricosuric drug).

See *Pseudogout*.

Gracilis

Origin: Inferior margin of symphysis pubis, inferior ramus of pubis and adjacent ramus of ischium.

Insertion: Medial surface of tibial shaft, posterior to sartorious.

Action: Flexes knee, adducts thigh and medially rotates tibia on femur.

Nerve supply: Anterior division of obturator nerve.

Blood supply: Medial circumflex femoral artery from profunda femoris.

Gracilis flap

Thin strap-shaped muscle with consistent pedicle. Minimal morbidity. Donor site can be closed. Can be innervated by including the anterior branch of obturator nerve. Can be used for facial re-animation.

Blood supply:

- Dominant supply is the medial circumflex femoral artery from the profunda femoris.

- The pedicle runs from medial to lateral entering the undersurface of the muscle 10–12 cm inferior to the pubic tubercle.
- A 6-cm pedicle length can be achieved in adults.

Raising the flap:
- Dissect gracilis through a medial thigh incision. Gracilis lies posterior to adductor. Include fascial origin and divide tendon distally.
- For functioning muscle, before dividing, place muscle under maximum physiological stretch and mark every 5 cm with a suture.

Upper limb:
- Free muscle transfer is used with severe Volkmann's ischaemic contracture or where there is marked muscle loss.
- There must be an appropriate motor nerve to reinnervate the muscle, there should be skeletal stability and the hand should be sensate with intrinsics.
- For Volkmann's the preferred nerve is the anterior interosseous nerve, which is in a protected position and only rarely injured.
- FDP and FPL are woven into the distal muscle flap to provide independent movement of finger and thumb by splitting the gracilis, or they can be woven together.
- When joining, connect the donor nerve as close as possible to the muscle to reduce reinnervation time.
- Reinnervation begins in 3–4 months. Tenolysis is necessary in 1/3 of patients.
See *Pressure sores*.

Graft
Tissue that is separated completely from the donor bed. It depends on the ingrowth of vessels from the recipient bed for survival.
- *Autograft:* tissue transplanted within the same individual.
- *Isograft:* a graft exchanged between genetically identical individuals.
- *Allograft:* graft exchanged between genetically different individuals.
- *Xenograft:* interspecies graft.
- *Orthotopic* transplant is transferred into an anatomically similar site.
- *Heterotopic* transplant is transferred into a different site from its origin.

Granular cell myoblastoma
- Uncertain origin, but may come from Schwann cell sheath.
- Most common in 40–60 years in black skin.
- ⅓ are on the tongue, ½ are on the head and neck.
- Usually solitary.
- Treatment is excision.
See *Mesodermal tumours*.

Granulation tissue
The tissue underlying a healing wound consisting of inflammatory cells, capillary loops and fibroblasts.

Grayson's ligaments
- Present in the digits, these fibres pass transversely from the volar aspect of the flexor tendon to the skin.
- They lie in the same plane as the natatory ligament.
- They form the palmar wall of the compartment through which the neurovascular bundle passes and prevents them from bowstringing.
- They also stabilize the palmar skin in grasp.
- They form part of the spiral cord in *Dupuytren's contracture*.
See *Cleland's ligament*.

Greater auricular nerve
Branch of cervical plexus. Emerges from behind sternocleidomastoid 6.5 cm below tragus. It supplies sensation to the inner and outer aspect of lower half of ear.

Groin flap
- Type B (i.e. solitary perforator) *Cormack-Lamberty* fasciocutaneous flap.
- Fed medially by the superficial circumflex iliac artery and the superficial inferior epigastric artery and laterally from the deep circumflex iliac artery. Many variations in this configuration.
- The donor site is well hidden. Flaps up to 15 cm wide can be harvested. The flap is fairly thin and hairless. Good for the dorsum of the hand and thumb web space. However, the pedicle length is short.

Groin lymph node dissection

- Superficial lymph node dissection (LND) removes a block of tissue below the inguinal ligament in the femoral triangle.
- Radical groin LND involves division of the inguinal ligament with proximal dissection and possibly retroperitoneal dissection to the obturator-ilial, hypogastric and para-aortic nodes.
- *Operation:* make lazy S incision over NVB. Raise skin flaps – can include skin in specimen. Skeletonize femoral artery and vein. Saphenous vein is doubly ligated at saphenofemoral junction. Sartorius is transposed to cover NVB. Biopsy node of Cloquet separately. If positive, consider deep dissection. See *Femoral triangle*.

Growth factors

Polypeptides whose primary role is cell maturation. Involved with cytokines in wound healing and host defence.
See *Cytokines*.

Gullwing flap

- Design of *Forehead flap* for larger defects of the nasal tip, infratip and lobule designed by Millard.
- Transverse extensions are created on the standard paramedian flap. These can be used to cover extensive bilateral lobular defects.
- The donor site frequently can be closed primarily.
See *Nasal reconstruction*.

Gunshot wounds

- Degree of injury depends on mass and speed.
- Kinetic energy = mass × velocity^2/2G. Doubling the velocity squares the kinetic energy.
- Low-energy deposits travel at <1000 feet/ seconds and include hand guns.
- Shotgun pellets have a larger mass so are intermediate. They travel at 1200 feet/ seconds.

Gustilo-Andersen score

Scoring system for open lower limb fractures:
- *I:* skin opening <1 cm, minimal muscle contusion, simple fracture.

- *II:* laceration >1 cm, moderate soft tissue injury and stripping.
- *IIIA:* high energy, adequate soft tissue despite laceration or undermining.
- *IIIB:* extensive soft tissue injury and periosteal stripping with contamination, bone loss.
- *IIIC:* Gustilo IIIB with limb ischaemia.
See *Lower limb reconstruction*. See *Byrd* classification.

Guyon's canal

- The tunnel through which the *Ulnar nerve* and artery passes across the wrist.
- It begins at the level of the proximal edge of the wrist.
- Transverse carpal ligament and pisohamate ligament forms floor, the volar carpal ligament the roof and the pisiform and FCU the ulnar wall. The radial wall is formed by the hook of the hamate.
- The ulnar artery is radial to the nerve in the canal.
- To release the tunnel, use carpal tunnel incision. Incise more distally to find the superficial palmar arch. Follow the ulna branch, which will lead to ulnar nerve.

Gynaecomastia

- Excessive development of male breasts.
- No relationship with breast ca.
- *Idiopathic* occurs in of newborns (due to the transplacental passage of oestrogens), of pubertal boys, of men.
- Gynaecomastia may be unilateral, bilateral or asymmetrical. Usually asymptomatic.

Examination:
- *Breasts:* thickened breast tissue, if irregular mass suspect carcinoma.
- *Testes:* if small perform chromosome study, if asymmetric look for tumour.
- *Liver:* hepatomegaly, ascites.
- *Thyroid* enlargement, *nutritional status*.

Aetiology: Due to the increase in effective oestrogen-testosterone ratio.
- *Physiological:* newborn – 60%, puberty – 64% and old age –30%.
- *Pathology:* cirrhosis, malnutrition, hypogonadism, Klinefelter's, neoplasm (testicular, adrenal, pituitary, lung), renal, hyperthyoidism, hypothyroidism.

- *Pharmacological – mnemonic:* some (spironolactone) men (marijuana) can (cimetidine) develop (diazepam) rather (reserpine) excessive (oestrogens) thoracic (theophylline) diameters (digoxin).

Resolution: Gynaecomastia of puberty often regresses spontaneously within 2 years. Drug-related gynaecomastia may regress after cessation of drug.

Pseudo gynaecomastia: Increase breast size due to fat deposition.

Blood tests:

Medical treatment: Most effective during the active proliferative phase.
- Testosterone used for gynaecomastia secondary to testicular failure.
- Tamoxifen for middle-aged men.
- Danazol is a gonadotrophin inhibitor and reduces the pain and extent of gynaecomastia.

Indication for surgery: For adolescent males with enlargement for over 18 months, symptomatic patients fibrotic gynaecomastia, risk of carcinoma (e.g. Klinefelter's).

Classification: By _Simon_.

Surgical technique:
- *Grade 1-2:* excise breast tissue through semicircular areola incision (Webster) or transverse incision in axilla.
- *Grade 2-3:* skin resection is necessary with nipple transposition based on a superior pedicle. The nipple can be raised on a dermal bipedicled attachment and a horizontal extension either side to resect skin. Skin can be excised with a circumareolar incision or a LeJour vertical incision procedure can be performed.
- *Grade 3:* in massive gynaecomastia skin and breast tissue is excised and free nipple grafting performed. The graft is placed over the fifth rib.
- *Liposuction:* used in conjunction with surgery. Most successful with fatty breasts. Often leave a nubbin of firm breast tissue if used alone. Ultrasound assisted liposuction increases the scope for liposuction without open surgery.

Complications: Haematoma, seroma, nipple necrosis, nipples adherent to fascia if too much tissue resected.

 Haber's syndrome to **Hypothenar hammer syndrome**

Haber's syndrome
Familial variant of _Bowen's disease_ with rosacea-like eruption of the face and Bowen's lesions on the covered areas of the body.

Haemangioma
- This is a vascular tumour, which typically has rapid growth followed by involution.
- Most appear in the first couple of weeks of birth. 30% have a mark at birth.
- Congenital haemangioma is less common. 2% of newborns and 10% of 1-year-olds have a haemangioma. 23% of premature babies (<1 kg) have a haemangioma. Most appearing in adults were probably present previously, but not noted.

- 10% have multiple lesions.
- Female to male 3:1.
- Cells often have oestrogen receptors and grow with hormonal changes. Vascular lesions, such as spiders frequently develop in pregnancy.
- Haemangiomas are more commonly seen in the white population.

Pathology:
- Previously called capillary, cavernous or mixed.
- A lot of mast cells containing prostaglandins and leukotrienes are present.
- Each lesion is supplied by a single afferent arterial vessel. Outflow is by multiple veins.

- Regression occurs with thrombosis of the feeder vessels.
- The behaviour is variable, though when there is association with tissue, such as lymphohaemangiomas, they are less likely to resolve.

Natural history:
- Usually get rapid growth for 6 months, then remain static for 6 months then regress.
- Involution occurs between 5 and 12 years (50% by age 5, 70% by age 7 with no change after age 12). With normal skin being restored in 50%.
- 75–95% will not require intervention.
- 10% ulcerate – usually the very large ones in the expanding phase.

Differential diagnosis:
- Port-wine stain, AVM, *Pyogenic granulomas*, *Tufted angiomas*.
- A deep haemangioma can be confused with a lymphatic malformation and USS or MRI will differentiate.

Associated malformations: There are some rare associations.
- A large cervicofacial haemangioma may be accompanied by ocular abnormalities (microphthalmia, congenital cataract, optic nerve hypoplasia).
- Also other conditions such as sternal non-union, supraumbilical raphe.
- Cutaneo-visceral malformations: seen where there are multiple cutaneous haemangiomas, particularly intrahepatic. The baby may present with CCF, anaemia and hepatomegaly. Tumours may also occur in the GIT and CNS. Babies may also get CCF from a large solitary cutaneous or intrahepatic haemangioma.

Complications: 10% may require intervention. Conditions which may require treatment are:
- Airway obstruction.
- *Cardiovascular decompensation:* A–V shunting leading to high-output congestive heart failure. Also with multiple lesions. Symptoms usually develop within 2–8 weeks.
- *Ulceration or bleeding:* may result from platelet-trapping coagulopathy – *Kasabach–Merritt syndrome*.
- Infection.

- Thrombocytopaenia.
- Luminal obstruction.
- *Visual obstruction:* upper eyelid haemangioma can cause amblyopia and failure to develop binocular vision. Can also deform the cornea and produce astigmatism. This can occur with even a small haemangioma.
- Skeletal distortion.
- Pain.

Treatment: Most just require observation. Ulcerated lesions should be treated topically. See *Vascular malformations*. See *Salmon patch*.

Haemangiopericytoma
- May resemble a *Glomus* tumour.
- Rare and solitary; it may grow up to 10 cm in size.
- Rarely malignant.
- Women 30–50 years. 50% subungal.
- Pain, tenderness and cold intolerance.
- Treatment is excision.

Haines–Zancolli test
- Test for *Oblique retinacular ligament* tightness.
- Flexion of DIPJ is limited when PIPJ is in extension due to tension in ORL.

Hair
Three types:
- *Lanugo hair:* soft and fine, unpigmented and without a medulla. It is found on the foetus and is usually shed by the 8th month of gestation.
- *Vellus hair:* soft and unmedullated. Short, rarely exceeding 2 cm in length and may be pigmented. It replaces lanugo hair in the postnatal period and is spread over the entire body surface.
- *Terminal hair:* longer, coarser, pigmented and medullated. It replaces vellus hair at specific sites.
- Bald scalp has normal number of hair follicles though they are smaller and the hair is absent.
- The average scalp contains more than 1 million hair follicles with 100 000 terminal hairs. 90% are in anagen (growing) phase lasting 1000 days and 10% are in telogen (resting) phase lasting 100 days. Humans shed 50–100 hairs a day.

Hair follicle

- Each hair has a medulla, cortex and outer cuticle.
- The hair follicle consists of an inner root sheath derived from epidermis and an outer root sheath derived from dermis.
- Several sebaceous glands drain into each follicle. Discharge from these glands is aided by contraction of erector pili muscles.
- The living cells at the base of the hair follicle show active mitotic growth. A zone of keratinization forms above the dividing cells. The cells become dehydrated and are converted to a mass of keratin. The keratin filaments are cemented together by a matrix rich in cystine.

Hair restoration with flaps

Classification: *Juri.* Also Norwood classi fication.

Scalp reduction flaps:

- *Advancement flaps:* multiple procedures are necessary. Most create undesirable scars.
- *Bilateral occipitoparietal flaps (BOP):* useful for vertex balding. There is extensive undermining of the hair-bearing scalp. It will remove a width of bald scalp of 5–8 cm from the vertex. The superficial temporal artery should be Dopplered and protected as it will provide the majority of the blood supply. The whole scalp is mobilized to the nape of the neck and to the ear. It is advanced and the overlapping tissue is excised. Excessive tension may lead to necrosis. This is repeated several times often with hair transplantation. Some surgeons delay the flap by first ligating the occipital arteries.
- *Bitemporal flaps:* for midline alopecia but often performed 3 months after BOP flap to complete the excision.

Random flaps:

- *Temporoparietal short flap:* this is not delayed and narrower than the Juri flap and aims to create half of a frontal hairline. The larger delayed flap may give better results.
- *Nataf flap:* superiorly based to maintain natural hair direction and delayed. It rarely reached the midline.
- *Dardour flap:*

Temporoparieto-occipital flaps: *Juri flap:* 4 cm wide, based on the superficial temporal artery. It is long enough to extend across the entire width of the bald forehead. It uses 2 delays. The first cuts the superior and inferior border. After 1 week the distal quarter of flap is raised. The occipital vessels are divided. One week later the flap is transposed.

Scalp expansion: The advantage is to be able to move more tissue with tension free closures. It does, however, take more time with a cosmetic deformity for the duration of treatment.

Hair transplantation

- The most common cause for hair loss in both sexes is androgenic alopecia (AA) and progresses with age.
- Women tend to get thinning but the hairline is preserved.
- AA has multifactorial form of inheritance.
- Testosterone converts to dihydrotestosterone (DHT), which acts on the genetically predisposed hair follicle. The hair follicle becomes smaller and ends with fibrosis and hair loss.
- Hair transplantation is the most common cosmetic procedure performed on men for male pattern baldness (MPB) and is based on the principle of donor dominance. If a graft is taken from an area destined to be permanently hair-bearing, and is transplanted into an area of MPB or future MPB, it will continue to grow hair in its new site for as long as it would have in its original one. So the pattern of hair loss needs to be predicted.

Classification: See *Juri.*

Non-surgical treatment:

- Hairpieces, conditioners and permanents.
- Medical treatment include anti-androgens, *Minoxidil* and *Finasteride.* None are effective for the majority of patients.

Operations:

- *Grafts:*
  - *micrografts:* one or two hair grafts are sectioned from larger grafts or strip grafts and placed in holes created by 16–18-gauge needles;

o *minigrafts:* harvested using a trephine, scalpel or laser and sectioned into smaller grafts containing 3–6 hairs and can be round, linear or square; size is <2 mm;

o *standard grafts:* round or square containing 8–30 hairs, harvested with a trephine;

o *strip grafts:* more than 10 mm in length;

o *follicular unit grafts:* 1–5 hairs, each graft consists of a single hair follicle;

o *mixed grafts:* mini and standard grafts.

• *Planning:* design and placement are crucial. The hairline should not be placed too low as it will look unnatural in later years.

• *Recipient area:* with mini and micrografts, smaller spaces are left between grafts leaving a more natural result. However, increased density is sacrificed for decreased detectability. Mini-slits can be made and they should be at the correct angulation.

• *Graft preparation and insertion:* the graft is kept moist. The strip is sectioned with the blade parallel to the follicles. Glue helps to keep them in place.

<u>Scalp reduction:</u> This can be performed before or between hair transplantation procedures. This can be accompanied by prolonged acute tissue expansion where an expander is placed and inflated and deflated over 2 hours, thus allowing 200% more tissue removal.

Halo naevus
• Has a depigmented halo around the <u>Naevus</u>.
• A halo may be associated with melanoma.
• Halo naevi usually occur on the back of young adults and children and are exaggerated by a suntan.
• In time the pigmentation fades and becomes flesh-coloured.
• It is associated with vitiligo and thyroid disease.
• Excise if any doubt.

Hamartoma
• Congenital malformations consisting of normal tissue found in excessive amount or in abnormal relationship with surrounding structures. The cells usually retain normal histology and function. Malignant degeneration may occur.
• *Ectodermal hamartomas:* also called Naevi.

• *Neuroectodermal hamartomas:* arise from the neural crest. Two primary disorders – <u>Neurofibromatosis</u> and <u>Melanocytic naevi</u>.
• *Mesodermal hamartomas:* <u>Vascular malformations</u>.
• *Mixed origin hamartomas:* <u>Dermoid cyst</u>, <u>Nasal gliomas</u>, <u>Frontonasal encephalocoeles</u>.

Hamate fracture
Uncommon, 3 types.
• *Body:* Direct trauma. Also part of axial carpal instability injury.
• *Hook:* Direct injury in golf or racket sports, or avulsion by the TCL by falling on the outstretched hand. May get non-union that requires excision or bone grafting and fixation.
• Marginal fractures associated with fracture dislocation of ring and little metacarpals.

Hamate hook
Find hook by deep palpation over tip of hamular process in the palm by the examiner's thumb with dorsal/ulnar pressure with index and middle finger. Slide finger 2 cm distal from pisiform to locate hamular process. Running along the ulnar aspect of the base of the hook is the motor branch of the ulnar nerve. This can be injured in hook fractures. Usually the sensory portion is unaffected.

Harlequin deformity
The characteristic XR findings in unicoronal synostosis. Ipsilateral elevation of the lesser wing of sphenoid causes an abnormally shaped orbit. See <u>Craniosynostosis</u>.

Harris–Benedict equation
• Useful in predicting the basal energy expenditure (BEE) for a given patient.
• Calorie requirements in the burn patient can be predicted by doubling this BEE for a burn of greater than 30–40% TBSA.
• This method may well underestimate the caloric requirement for a given patient. Thus, averaging the figures obtained from the Harris–Benedict equation and the <u>Curreri</u> formula may allow a reasonable initial caloric target for nutritional supplementation.
• It is calculated based on gender, weight, height and age.
See <u>Burns</u>.

Harvey

1657: Described the heart as the centre of circulation.

Harvold classification

For _Hemifacial microsomia_.

- _Ia:_ classic type with unilateral facial underdevelopment.
- _Ib:_ Ia with microphthalmos.
- _Ic:_ bilateral asymmetrical type.
- _Id:_ complex type, which doesn't fit Ia–c.
- _II:_ limb deficiency type.
- _III:_ frontonasal type with hypertelorism.
- _IVa:_ unilateral Goldenhar with ocular dermoids +/– upper lid coloboma.
- _IVb:_ bilateral Goldenhar.

Hatchet flap

Also sickle flap.

- A variation of a local rotation flap with a Z-plasty in the tail to allow direct closure.
- Design flap adjacent to the defect with an arc two times the diameter of the defect. Place a backcut in the tail. Good for lower lid defects.
- The _Marchac dorsal nasal flap_ is a large version of the flap which can be rotated towards the tip of the nose.

Head and neck cancer

Incidence:

- 500 000 new cases with 270 000 deaths each year.
- ¾ are oral cavity and pharynx.
- Highest incidence in Melanesia (Papua), West Europe and south central Asia.

Aetiology:

- _6 Ss:_ smoking, spirits, spices, sharp teeth, sunlight, syphilis, smoking and alcohol account for ¾.
- _Smoking:_ stopping smoking reduces the risk to that of non-smokers after 15 years. Pipe smokers have a higher incidence of oral cavity ca. Users of smokeless tobacco develop cancers on the alveolar ridge or buccal mucosa.
- _Alcohol_ is associated with a sixfold increase in aerodigestive cancer compared with that in non-drinker. Carcinoma of the floor of the mouth is particularly associated with alcoholism. For oral cancer, this figure increases to 15 times when alcohol and tobacco are combined. Alcohol association is strongest for pharyngeal cancer. The synergistic effect between tobacco and alcohol is greatest between dark tobacco (pipe/cigar) and wine. Dark liquors, such as whisky, rum and cognac have higher incidences. Alcohol is not a known carcinogen, but may act as a solvent. It may also upregulate enzymes of cytochrome p-450 system required to convert procarcinogens to carcinogens.
- _Betel quid_ is mixed with tobacco giving rise to oral cancer.
- _Maté_ is a hot drink in South America associated with oral and oesophageal cancer.
- _Oral hygiene:_ loose-fitting dentures and mouthwashes may all be associated with oral cancer.
- _Wood dust:_ occupational exposure.
- _Human papillomavirus_ particularly with verrucous carcinomas. Most commonly found in tonsillar tumours. Also HIV, herpes simples and EB virus. Genetic factors such as Fanconis anaemia.

Diagnosis: Presentation depends on site.

- Nasopharynx ca may present with epistaxis or nasal obstruction, also cranial neuropathies and posterior cervical lymphadenopathy.
- Oral cancers may present with pain, ulcers or ill-fitting dentures.
- Oropharynx and hypopharynx cancers present late.
- Otalgia due to referred pain, may have hoarseness, dysphagia.
- 25% present with a neck mass.

Staging:

AJCC:

- _TX:_ primary tumour cannot be assessed.
- _T0:_ no evidence of primary tumour.
- _Tis:_ carcinoma _in situ_.
- _T1:_ tumour <2 cm in greatest dimension.
- _T2:_ tumour >2 cm, but <4 cm in greatest dimension.
- _T3:_ tumour >4 cm in greatest dimension.
- _T4:_ tumour invades adjacent structures (e.g. through cortical bone, into deep muscle of tongue maxillary sinus, skin).

- *NX:* regional lymph nodes cannot be assessed.
- *NO:* no regional lymph node metastasis.
- *Nl:* metastasis in a single ipsilateral lymph node, <3 cm in greatest dimension.
- *N2:* metastasis in a single ipsilateral lymph node >3 cm, but <6 cm in greatest dimension: in multiple ipsilateral lymph nodes, none >6 cm in greatest dimension; or in bilateral or contralateral lymph nodes, none >6 cm in greatest dimension.
- *N2a:* metastasis in a single ipsilateral node >3 cm, but <6 cm in greatest dimension.
- *N2b:* metastasis in multiple ipsilateral lymph nodes, none >6 cm in greatest dimension.
- *N2c:* metastasis in bilateral or contralateral lymph nodes, none >6 cm in greatest dimension.
- *N3:* metastasis in a lymph node >6 cm in greatest dimension.
- *MX:* distant metastasis cannot be assessed.
- *M0:* no distant metastasis.
- *M1:* distant metastasis.

Clinical staging:
- *Stage 0:* Tis.
- *Stage I:* T1.
- *Stage II:* T2.
- *Stage III:* T3N0 or T1–3 with N1.
- *Stage IVA:* T4 with or without N1 or any T with N2.
- *Stage IVB:* any T with N3.
- *Stage IVC:* any T or N with M1.

T classification for salivary gland tumours:
as for oral cavity except
- A signifies no local extension.
- B signifies local extension.

Prognosis:
- *Stage I:* >80% cure rate with dual modality treatment.
- *Stage II:* >60% cure rate. Second primaries are a greater problem than further trouble with the original primary.
- *Stage III/IV:* <30% cure.

Treatment: Usually combines surgery with radiotherapy. This improves local control but there is no improved survival.
- Stage I and II use single modality treatment, either RT or surgery. For oral pharynx this is usually surgery with a 1-cm margin. Get control rate of 60–90%. For hypopharynx RT is used rather than perform a laryngectomy.
- Stage III and IV require both with 30–60% control. Those unable to undergo surgery have palliative RT. SCCs are responsive to CT but no trials have shown improved survival. It is used for hypopharyngeal and laryngeal malignancy to allow organ preservation.

Access:
- Direct for anterior lesions, if access difficult, split the lip or perform a mandibular swing. If bone is involved, resect mandible. In the upper alveolus and palate, the underlying bone is frequently removed, the extent depending on the extent of involvement: It can range from removal of the alveolus to partial or total maxillectomy. In the latter cases a <u>Weber–Fergusson</u> incision may be necessary.

Nerve involvement:
- Symptoms of numbness, facial palsy and facial pain suggest nerve involvement.

	Oral cavity Oropharynx	Nasopharynx	Hypopharynx	Maxillary sinus
T1	Primary < 2 cm	One subsite	One subsite	Antral mucosa
T2	2–4 cm	>1 subsite	> 1 subsite, no-fixation	Bone below Ohngren's line
T3	>4 cm	Beyond nasal Cavity	Invades larynx	Bone above Ohngrens line
T4	Invading	Invades skull base or CN	Invades soft tissue	Adjacent structures

- Usually due to perineural lymphatic invasion.
- Involvement of the trigeminal ganglion is deemed irresectable.

Management of occult metastatic LN:

- *History:* general symptoms like wt loss, and local symptoms for primary.
- *Examination:* cachexia and secondaries. Intraoral examination.
- *Investigations:* biopsy – FNA or open. CXR, MRI, CT, panendoscopy with biopsy. On MRI, involved nodes are >1 cm, round not oval and have central necrosis.
- *Treatment:* neck dissection and RT to neck and likely primary sites.
- *Caucasians:* remove ipsilateral tonsil as this is a common site for the hidden primary.
- *Asians:* irradiate nasopharynx as there is a high incidence of nasopharyngeal ca.

Radiology: MRI, CT

Sites of head and neck cancer:

- *Nasopharynx:* common in China and Asia. Most present with nodal metastasis in the posterior neck. Lymphoepithelioma has a better prognosis than SCC. They are highly radiosensitive and RT is the treatment of choice.
- *Oral cavity:* the most common site of head and neck cancer. Bordered by lip vermilion, junction of hard and soft palate and anterior tonsillar pillar. Treatment depends on stage, age and functional result. Usually involves surgery.
- *Oropharynx:* bounded by the junction of hard and soft palate anteriorly to the hyoid bone, including soft palate, uvula, tonsil and pharyngeal wall. Often poorly differentiated and frequently has nodal metastasis.
- *Base of tongue:* posterior to the circumvallate papillae. Often occult. 75% present with nodal spread. Surgery is difficult and morbid. 5-year survival is 50% for stage I and 10% for stage IV.
- *Hypopharynx:* from hyoid to the lower border of cricoid cartilage split into larynx and hypopharynx. Most are seen in the piriform sinus. Occult until large and metastasized. 66% have LN, often bilateral. Require laryngopharyngectomy, bilateral neck dissection and RT.

- *Larynx:* most frequent site after oral cavity. Three anatomic areas. *Supraglottic larynx* is composed of epiglottis, aryepiglottic fold and false vocal cords. These are occult and present very large. They metastasize early. If present early treat with supraglottic laryngectomy or RT. If larger, need total laryngectomy, RT and neck dissection. *The glottis* comprises the true vocal cords. There are few lymphatics. Patients present early with hoarseness without neck metastasis. If early treat effectively with RT. T2 and T3 give CT and RT. *The subglottic larynx* is an infrequent site of laryngeal cancer. They are difficult to diagnose and present late. Treat with surgery and RT. Prognosis is poor.
- *Paranasal sinuses:* rare. Most commonly in the maxillary sinus, then the ethmoid sinus. Most are epidermoid, 10% are salivary, 10% are lymphomas, sarcomas or melanomas. T1 and T2 lesions treat with surgery or RT.
- *Alveolar ridge.*
- *Floor of mouth.*
- *Anterior tongue.*
- *Lip.*
- *Buccal mucosa:*
- *Retromolar trigone carcinoma.*
- *Palate.*
- *Tonsil.*

Neck dissection: Lymph node levels.

Complications:

- Salivary fistula may also occur and be difficult to deal with in the irradiated patient.
- The incidence of complications is increased when a simultaneous neck dissection is performed.
- If the carotid artery is exposed in the wound, especially if it is bathed in saliva and there has been previous irradiation, there is a considerable risk of catastrophic haemorrhage. Immediate cover with a muscle flap is advocated and may be performed prophylactically at the time of neck dissection.
- Chyle leak: may be repaired immediately if noticed, but usually become apparent once the patient is fed. Rarely require reoperation. Treat with fat free diet or TPN.
- Long-term complications include problems with the scar, shoulder pain and cosmesis.

- Because many patients have had a high alcohol intake, they must be observed post-operatively for delirium tremens. Parenteral vitamin B complex is administered when indicated. Operative mortality is low, but can be as high as 18% in elderly patients having extensive resection.

Radiotherapy: Consider if not cleared surgically or close, extracapsular extension, vascular invasion, multiple nodes. It can be given pre- or post-operatively, but the results are the same so there is no reason to give pre-operatively as the surgery is more difficult.

Heberden's node

Bony spurs on the dorsal aspect of the *DIPJ*. The most common clinical manifestation of OA. 10–20× more common in women. Rarely they may produce pain and require debridement.

Hemifacial atrophy

- Also called Romberg's disease and Parry–Romberg's disease.
- Usually unilateral. Sporadic. Unknown aetiology. Possibly viral or abnormality of sympathetic nervous system.

Clinical features: Get gradual wasting of one side of face and forehead. Usually starts between 5 and 20. It continues for several years before stopping. Get permanent soft tissue deficiency.
- *Skin:* localized atrophy.
- *Hair:* pigment changes.
- *Iris:* pigment changes.
- *Forehead:* sharp depression – coup de sabre.
- *Cheek:* soft tissue atrophy.
- *Skeleton:* hypoplasia.

Treatment: Generally none is performed when the condition is active and progressive. Reconstruction is performed once the condition is stable for at least 6 months. Options include:
- Fat and dermofat grafts.
- Temporoparietal fascia and temporalis muscle transfers.
- Free-tissue transfer – commonly scapular, parascapular, omentum.
- Osteotomies for skeletal abnormalities.

Hemifacial microsomia

Commonest of the *Craniofacial clefts*. Also called oculo-auriculovertebral spectrum and *Tessier* cleft no. 7
- 1:4000 births. 80% are unilateral. Bilateral are asymmetric.
- M:F 3:2.
- The second most common facial clefting condition after cleft lip and palate.
- Most are sporadic though autosomal dominant and recessive have been reported. Variable expression.
- May be caused by vascular disruption of the primitive stapedial artery (a temporary embryonic collateral of the hyoid artery)– on which the 1st and 2nd branchial arches are dependent.

Presentation:
- Affects the ears, eyes, mouth and mandible.
- A severe form has macrostomia, a furrow across the ear and *Microtia* of the ear.
- Cranial nerves V and VII may be involved.
- The zygoma, maxilla and temporal bone are hypoplastic, and the mandible may also be hypoplastic.
- Skin tags may be present between the first and second branchial arches.
- Ocular abnormalities include blepharoptosis, anophthalmia or microphthalmia. Epibulbar tumours are found in 1/3.
- Mandibular deformity:
- Muscles of mastication may be hypoplastic especially the lateral pterygoid muscle, which moves the mandible to the contralateral side.
- Cleft lip and palate may be present.
- Radial ray defects occur in 10%.
- Other abnormalities include lung, renal and congenital heart disease. *See Goldenhar syndrome*.

Classification:
- *Harvold* classification.
- *OMENS* classification.
- *Prozansky* classification.

Treatment:
- The surgical goals include normalizing the occlusal tilt and reconstructing the TMJ. Symmetry is important to prevent problems with the opposite TMJ. Auricular

reconstruction is planned and facial symmetry restored.

Operations:
- *Osseodistraction:* this is the commonest technique used for skeletal correction. There are many devices, including internal ones to prevent scarring. The timing is argued. Advance by 1 mm per day. Aim to overcorrect in the growing child. Get associated elongation of the soft tissues, particularly the inferior alveolar nerve. The biggest problem is that an absent TMJ is not restored and an absent zygoma is not addressed. It also does not correct the medial displacement, but only elongates an abnormally placed mandible.
- *Skeletal surgery:* those with mild involvement and an intact TMJ have a Le Fort I and a bilateral sagittal mandibular osteotomy.
- *Soft tissue:* dermal fat grafts for mild or moderate and free tissue transfer for severe defects.
- *Auricular reconstruction:* at age 6.
- *Facial clefts:* treatment of congenital macrostomia is performed early in life. Reconstitute the oral sphincter and the oral commissure. Closure is either as a straight line or Z-plasty. Noordhoff suggested a vermilion flap with a Z-plasty
- *Craniofacial microsomia:* if there is orbital dystopia and forehead involvement, start correction early. Use orbital wall grafts and 4-wall osteotomies. Advance the forehead.
- *Facial nerve paralysis:* most surgeons have not been treating it as there is often some residual function.

See Craniofacial genetics. See Tessier clefts.

Heparin
- Action is to inactivate thrombin in the clotting cascade by increasing the effect of antithrombin III.
- In *Microsurgery* in a multicentre trial into the use of heparin, dextran and aspirin in free flaps, only heparin given as DVT prophylaxis showed any difference to flap survival. Give a bolus intra-operatively if the anastomosis is redone or a clot develops.

Hereditary haemorrhagic telangiectasia
See Telangiectasis.

Hermaphrodites
Individuals with characteristics of both sexes. *See Ambiguous genitalia.*

Herpes
- Herpetic whitlow is a superficial viral infection of the fingertip.
- Medical and dental personnel are at the highest risk.
- Present with vesicles containing turbid fluid with local erythema and may also have fever and lymphangitis. Usually last 2/52.
- Don't perform IandD. Severe cases may require systemic acyclovir.

Hewe's tarsoconjunctival transposition flap
- Used for lower *Eyelid* reconstruction.
- For defects involving the lateral half of the lid margin.
- A laterally based tarsoconjunctival flap is moved from upper to lower lid to reconstruct the posterior lamellar.
- The skin muscle flap is advanced over this.

Hidalgo and Shaw: foot injuries
Classification of foot injuries into:
- *Type I:* soft tissue.
- *Type II:* major soft tissue, with or without distal amputation.
- *Type III:* soft tissue loss with fracture of ankle, calcaneous or bimalleolar.

See Lower limb reconstruction.

High-pressure injury
- Significant injuries, which may appear trivial initially.
- Often occur in the upper limb.
- The hand will rapidly swell in hours.
- Undetected or untreated it may lead to ischaemia and tissue necrosis.

Treatment:
- Is a surgical emergency. XRs may help establish the extent of injection. Give antibiotics, perform wide exposure with debridement

followed by serial debridement and aggressive hand therapy with early movement.
- There is a poor prognosis with delay, oil-based solvent, finger injection, high pressure or high volume.

Highet's scale for sensory testing
- *S0:* no sensation.
- *S1:* sensation to deep pain.
- *S1+:* sensation to superficial pain.
- *S2:* sensation to light touch.
- *S2+:* hyperpathia.
- *S3:* 2PD >15 mm.
- *S3+:* 2PD 7–15.
- *S4:* full.

Hildreth's sign
See *Glomus tumour*. Reduction of pain on exsanguination of the affected part.

Histiocytosis
- The benign reticuloendotheliosis are a group of diseases including eosinophilic granuloma, Hand-Schuller–Christian disease and Letterer–Siwe disease.
- Eosinophilic granuloma is the most common lesion.
- Get aggregates of xanthomatous histiocytes.
- Solitary lesions heal spontaneously.
See *Bone tumours*.

History of plastic surgery
Plastic is derived from the Greek word plastikos – to mould or give form. The word was first used by *Von Graefe* in 1818 in his Rhinoplastik. Goal of plastic surgery is the restoration of normal form and function and the enhancement of form.

Egypt: The Edwin Smith papyrus dated at 3000BC contains description of the management of facial trauma and fractures.

India: The first recorded scripts of actual plastic surgery were recorded in the Sanskrit texts 2600 years ago. This was required due to frequent acts of facial mutilation during conflict and for unfaithfulness. *Sushruta* wrote in the Samhita (encyclopaedia) about the forehead or cheek flap for nasal reconstruction. The Koomas caste of tile and brick makers may also have used full thickness skin grafts.

Roman: Celsus, the Roman medical writer included similar techniques to repair mutilated lips, ears and noses in his medical text. Oribasius, the 4th century Byrzantine physician devoted two chapters to the repair of facial defects including the use of flaps. He described bipedicle flaps and wound undermining.

Turkish: In the 15th century Serafeddin Sabuncuolu described treatment of gynaecomastia, eyelid surgery. He may be the first to describe a purely cosmetic procedure.

Italy: The nasal reconstruction was developed with a pedicle from the arm. It was performed by the Branca family in the 15th century and the technique kept a secret. This was learnt (not developed) by *Tagliacozzi* in the 16th century

Europe: The forehead flap was reported in the *Gentleman's Magazine* when a British bullock driver had his nose mutilated as punishment for transporting supplies for the British East Indian forces. His nose was reconstructed by a man from the brickmaker caste, observed by two British surgeons. The report was read and tried by *Carpue Von Graefe*.

Dieefenbach: Also described rhinoplasty, and was one of the first to use anaesthesia.

Cleft lip and palate history:

Skin graft history:

Microsurgery:

WW1: Great advances were made in reconstruction, particularly with the use of pedicled flaps. Gillies developed a unit in Sidcup, Kent.

WWII: At the start of WWII there were only 4 plastic surgeons in UK – Gillies, Kilner, Mowlem and McIndoe. With control of infection, early closure of facial wounds was advocated. Hand surgery developed during WWII led by Sterling Bunnell.

HIV
Post-exposure prophylaxis. Currently recommended regime is triple therapy with:
- Zidovudine 200 mg bid.
- Lamivudine 150 mg bid 3.
- Inidavir 800 mg tds.

Start as soon as possible and continue for 4 weeks. A negative test 6 months later suggests HIV infection is unlikely (*Annl R Coll Surg Eng* 2002;84:73).

Holoprosencephaly

- A disorder caused by the failure of the *prosencephalon* (the embryonic forebrain) to sufficiently divide into the double lobes of the cerebral hemispheres.
- This results in a single-lobed brain structure and severe skull and facial defects.
- Often the malformations are so severe that babies die before birth.
- In less severe cases, babies are born with normal or near-normal brain development and facial deformities that may affect the eyes, nose, and upper lip.

Classification:

- *Alobar:* in which the brain has not divided at all, is usually associated with severe facial deformities.
- *Semilobar:* in which the brain's hemispheres have partially divided, causes an intermediate form of the disorder.
- *Lobar:* in which there is considerable evidence of separate brain hemispheres, is the least severe form. In some cases of lobar holoprosencephaly the baby's brain may be nearly normal.
- *Premaxillary agenesis:* or median cleft lip is the least severe of the facial anomalies.
- *Cyclopia* is the most severe facial anomaly with a single eye located in the area normally occupied by the root of the nose, and a missing nose or a proboscis (a tubular-shaped nose) located above the eye.
- *Ethmocephaly* is the least common facial anomaly in which a proboscis separates closely set eyes.
- *Cebocephaly* is characterized by a small, flattened nose with a single nostril situated below incomplete or underdeveloped closely set eyes.

Holt–Oram syndrome

- The most common heart-hand syndrome.
- Autosomal dominant.
- Usually have an abnormal scaphoid with extra carpal bones.

- Thumb is abnormal.
- Get cardiac septal defects.

Horner

Described the Z-plasty in 1837.

Horner's syndrome

Consists of ptosis, meiosis, anhydrosis and enopthalmos. Due to the interruption of the sympathetic supply to the eye.

Horton's test

Artificial erection test. Tests for chordee. See *Hypospadias*.

HOX

- The HOX are 38 genes, which encode proteins responsible for the establishment of cell identity along the AP axis in limb development.
- The position of gene on the chromosome correlates with the axial level of the limb bud where they are expressed.

They determine timing and extent of local growth rates.

See *Embryology*.

Hueston's tabletop test

Test in patients with *Dupuytren's contracture*. Positive if the patient is unable to place fingers flat on the table. Usually surgery is indicated.

Hughe's flap

- Used for *Lower eyelid reconstruction*.
- A tarso-conjunctival flap taken from the upper lid.
- Cut out defect in lower lid. Evert upper lid and cut out proximally based flap of conjuctiva and tarsal plate 5 mm from lid margin to preserve inferior upper tarsus. Advance down to fill defect. Close anterior defect with FTSG or local flap.
- Divide pedicle after 3 weeks.

Human amniotic membrane

- composed of inner membrane (amnion) and outer membrane (chorion).
- Used as temporary dressings for ulcers, burns and donor sites.
- Can get freeze-dried gamma sterilized amniotic membrane.

- It may reduce bacterial count and pain.
- Neovascularization does not occur and it does not promote healing and get hypertrophic scarring.

See *Biological skin substitutes*.

Hutchinson's sign

Eponychial pigmentation in nail matrix melanoma.

Hyaluronic acid preparations

Preparations such as restylane and Perlane are composed of synthetically manufactured hyaluronic acid. 20–50% are absorbed by 6 months. They are typically injected superficially to treat wrinkles and increase lip definition.

See *Alloplasts*.

Hydradenitis suppuritiva (HS)

- Chronic disease with recurrent abscesses, sinus tracts and scarring occurring in areas of apocrine sweat glands.
- Incidence of 1:300. F:M 3:1, mainly 20s–30s. No racial difference.

Clinical features:

- Tender nodules usually start in puberty and in women flare premenstrually and may ease in pregnancy and after the menopause.
- It is related to obesity, acne and hirsutism.
- Deep abscesses develop which may resolve or discharge. Adjacent abscesses may become linked by scar tissue. Perianal HS may mimic Crohn's disease.
- Three conditions, which are similar and are called the follicular occlusion triad are acne conglobata, dissecting cellulitis of the scalp and HS.

Sites: In order of frequency – axillary, inguinal, perianal, mammary, buttock, chest, scalp, retroauricular, eyelid.

Pathology:

- Apocrine glands are compound sweat glands, which extend into the subcutaneous tissues. Each has a deep coiled secretory component, which drains via a straight excretory duct into a hair follicle. Secretion is malodorous due to surface bacteria.
- Though the condition only occurs where there are apocrine glands the primary event

seems to be follicular occlusion by keratinized stratified squamous epithelium. Apocrine glands which drain directly onto the skin are not affected.

- So it is a disorder of terminal follicular epithelium within apocrine gland-bearing skin. Follicular occlusion leads to rupture, spilling of contents including bacteria and keratin into the surrounding dermis. This leads to a vigorous chemotactic response, an abscess develops and this leads to destruction of the pilosebaceous unit. Epithelial strands generated from the ruptured follicular epithelium form sinus tracts.

Aetiology and bacteriology:

- There is no link to deodorants.
- Obesity exacerbates possibly by shear.
- There is an autosomal dominant inheritance. There is a strong influence of sex hormones.
- Incidence of smoking is higher in HS.
- Pus is usually initially sterile. Bacteria isolated are *Staph. aureus*, *Strep milleri*, *Peptostreptococcus* and *Chlamydia* (anogenital).

Medical treatment: is not very effective.

- *General:* weight loss, stop smoking, antiseptic soaps, tea tree oil, loose clothing.
- *Antibiotics:* e.g. oral clindamycin can be effective if used early.
- *Hormonal therapy:* the anti-androgen cyproterone acetate and ethinyloestradiol can be effective, but concerns are raised over the high doses required. *Finasteride* has been used to cause remission.
- *Retinoids:* isotretinoin has been useful for acne and has been considered for HS, but it has not been shown to be effective probably because it has the maximal effect on sebaceous gland activity. Acetretin 25 mg bd. does, however, appear to be effective and acts more on keratinization. Cimetidine has been tried.
- *Immunosuppression:* steroids may initially be effective, but relapse occurs when the dose is reduced. Intralesional triamcinolone can be effective.
- *Radiotherapy:* a recent German study had 38% complete relief of symptoms and 40% improved.

Surgical treatment:
- Most recurrence occurs due to a limited resection. The block of tissue need to be adequately excised in depth, as well as width as apocrine glands extend into the subcutaneous fat. Excise down to fascia or at least 5 mm of fat. The apocrine glands can be visualized by using the iodine/starch/oxytocin method.
- Reconstruct with direct closure, split skin grafts or local.
- Defects can be left to heal by secondary intention.
- VAC can be used on SSGs.
- CO_2 laser with healing by secondary intention appears effective. It can be used for mild to moderate disease without any need for hospitalization.

Complications: Fibrosis and scarring can lead to contractures. Fistulae can occur. SCC in anogenital HS has been described. *See Skin.*

Hydrocolloids
Hydrocolloid matrix backed with adhesive. It physically protects the wound, while absorbing fluid and maintaining a moist environment. Examples include granuflex and duoderm. *See Dressings.*

Hydrofluoric acid
- One of the most painful of chemical burns.
- Found in photography laboratory products, glass etching, rust removers and petrochemical refining.
- The fluoride ion rapidly extends through the epidermis into subcutaneous tissues and binds with calcium producing extreme pain. Acts more like an alkali than an acid.
- >2.5% TBSA will cause systemic hypocalcaemia and shock.

Treatment
- Irrigate with water and clip or remove involved finger nails.
- Neutralize using topical calcium gluconate 10% – crush calcium gluconate tablets into an aqueous gel.
- Apply until pain free.
- Subcutaneous injection is possible using calcium gluconate or magnesium sulphate in concentrations of 0.5 ml/cm^2.

- Biers block can be used with 10 ml of 10% calcium gluconate mixed with 40 ml of NS given over 20–30 minutes or arterial injection. *See Chemical burns.*

Hydrogels
Starch-polymer matrix, which swells to absorb moisture. They promote autolysis of necrotic material and are principally used to debride wounds. *See Dressings.*

Hydrogen cyanide
See Inhalation.
- Binds to and inhibits cytochrome oxidase.
- Rapidly fatal in concentrations of >20 ppm and serum concentration of >1 mg/L.
- Almond odour.
- Treat with amyl nitrite, which traps cyanide, also sodium thiosulphate and hydroxy-cobalamin.

Hydroquinone
Suppresses melanocytic activity and helps prevent hyperpigmentation.

Hydroxyapatite
- $Ca10(PO_4)6(OH)2$. Major inorganic component of bone.
- Coral of the genus *porites* has a calcium carbonate exoskeleton similar to bone. Exchange of carbonate for phosphate makes it identical to bone.
- This can bond to adjacent bone with no foreign body or inflammatory response.
- Comes as block and granules. Blocks are contoured and screwed.
- They are invaded by fibrovascular tissue with union in 2–3 months.
- HA implants are not resorbed. Blocks are brittle, but gain strength.
- Complication rates are 4–10% with low infection rate.
- BoneSource is a synthetic HA cement used for calvarial defects. HA can also be derived from bovine-deorganified bone.
See Alloplasts.

Hynes pharyngoplasty
- Used for the treatment of *Velopharyngeal incompetence (VPI).*

- Two superiorly based flaps are raised from either side of the pharyngeal wall.
- Each flap is 3–4 cm long and includes a portion of salpingopharyngeus muscle and overlying mucosa.
- The flaps are transposed medially and sutured to each other on the posterior pharyngeal wall.

Hyperaesthesia

Increased sensitivity to a stimulus such as light touch.
See RSD.

Hyperalgesia

Increased sensitivity to pain or enhanced intensity of pain sensation.

Hyperbaric oxygen

- Used for poor wound healing and radiation necrosis.
- In the normal wound a steep oxygen gradient exists between normal and damaged tissues.
- The mechanism by which hyperbaric oxygen can revascularize irradiated tissue is thought to occur through the creation of steep oxygen gradients naturally present in non-compromised wounds.
- These oxygen gradients allow the body to recognize irradiated tissue as being a true wound and the chemotactic and biochemical messenger response proceeds as in normal tissue angiogenesis.
- Clinically, HBO may or may not be effective in complicated wounds. See Radiation.

Hyperhidrosis

- Hyperhidrosis refers to excessive sweating on the palms of the hands, the soles of the feet, and the axillae.
- The situation may be improved in cool conditions though it often remains a problem.
- Medical sympathetic block or surgical sympathectomy has been effective in carefully selected patients.
- Axillary hyperhidrosis can be treated by wide excision of the axilla to include most of the eccrine sweat glands, which are concentrated in the axillary vault.

- Raising bipedicled flaps and excising dermis will also denervate the sweat glands and reduce sweating.
- Subcutaneous curettage can be performed to superficial and deep surface after undermining the area of hydradenitis.
- Botox injections are effective for several months.

Hyperkeratosis

See Skin. An increase in the thickness of the keratin layer.

Hyperpathia

Disagreeable or painful sensation in response to a normally innocuous stimulus (as touch).
See RSD.

Hypertelorism

- An increased interorbital distance.
- The interorbital distance (IOD) measures between the medial walls of the orbits at the junction of the frontal and lacrimal bones.
- The intercanthal distance is measured between the medial canthal tendons and an increase in this dimension with a normal IOD is called pseudo-orbital hypertelorism.
- In adults the average IOD in men is 28 mm and women 25 mm.

Classification.
- *Tessier*: based on IOD.
- *Munro*: according to shape.

Pathology:
- Hypertelorism is not a diagnosis in itself, but a description.
- All have nasal deformity with widening of the ethmoidal sinuses.
- The nose is usually short and wide. Get turbinate hypertrophy with airway obstruction.

Aetiology:
- Associated with many congenital malformations.
- Seen in midline clefts (see *Tessier*) craniofacial syndromes such as *Crouzon's* and *Apert's*, and sincipital encephalocoele. Also associated with dermoid cysts, teratomas.

Treatment:
- Usually after the age of 2. 3-D CT scans are useful.

- Combined intracranial and extracranial approach.
- Osteotomies are made in all walls of the orbit circumferentially.
- Structures within the interorbital space are resected. This may have an effect on facial growth. The cribiform plate should not be injured as olfactory function will be affected.
- Nasal reconstruction is usually required, with a bone graft to the nasal dorsum.
- 4-wall osteotomy.
- 3-wall osteotomy through an inverted U incision doesn't put the infra-orbital nerve at risk and is used in the primary or mixed dentition stages.
- *Medial wall osteotomy:* for mild hypertelorism or pseudohypertelorism. Lateral orbital wall may be in an adequate position. A triangular medial orbital wall osteotomy is performed. The ethmoid sinuses are completely removed. The orbits move by performing a medial canthopexy.
- Lamellar split orbital osteotomy: outer osseous table is separated from the inner table. It doesn't correct true hypertelorism but is useful in pseudohypertelorism. See *Orbital dystopia*.

Hypertrophic scar
- Excessive inflammatory response during healing.
- Remain within the borders of the scar, whereas *Keloid* scars extend beyond the borders.
- They may improve with time and may not recur if excised.
- Hypertrophic scars appear within 3/52, keloids after 3/12.
- M=F.
- Treat with intralesional *Steroids*, pressure, radiation, resection and other treatment.
- Good response rates, from 65 to 86%, have been reported in studies of topical silicone sheeting, although the mechanism by which the silicone produces its effect remains unclear.
- *Interferon* also of benefit. Laser, tamoxifen, calcium antagonists cryotherapy have been used.

In burns:
- All wounds contract, but the degree of contracture and hypertrophy is related to the time taken to heal as the longer the time the longer the wound is in the inflammatory phase.
- Excess inflammation increases the amount of the fibrogenic TGF ß1 and TGF ß2.
- Hypertrophy is also increased by shortage of tissue.

Hypospadias
- Congenital anomaly of penis and urethra. Get urethral meatus in ventral position with urethral plate distally to meatus.
- Associated with *Chordee*.
- Prepuce abnormal with dorsal hood.
- May get clefting of the glans and scrotal bipartition.
- Urinary stream affected and sexual function may be affected by chordee and small penis.

History:
- Paul of Aegina (7th century Greek physician) advocated glandular amputation to position the meatus at the tip of the penis.
- Mettauer (1830) described a two-stage procedure without a graft, the first stage being left to heal by secondary intention.
- Nové-Josserand (1897) first used a graft.
- Thiersche and Duplay – 2-stage procedure with first correction of chordee then tubularizing the urethra with lateral flaps.
- Cecil performed a 3-stage procedure with release of chordee followed by tubularizing ventral skin and burying in the scrotum. Later this skin is divided, but this means scrotal skin on the penis.

Incidence:
- Affects 1 in 300 males.
- 50% associated with inguinal hernias, 25% with other genitourinary anomalies. 15% have undescended testes. More proximal lesions more likely to have other anomalies.
- Father–son 8%, sibling 14%, not all identical twins.

Aetiology:
- Increase exogenous oestrogens.
- Decrease epidermal growth factor in penis during development.
- Androgen receptor deficiency.

Embryology:
Location:
- Anterior meatus (glanular subcoronal, distal penile shaft) 65%.
- Medial (midshaft) 15%.
- Posterior meatus (penoscrotal, perineal) 20%.

History: Ask parents about erections, penile curve, urinary stream.

Examination: Size of penis (testosterone cream may help), testicular descent (if not perform genetic analysis for intersex state), inguinal hernia (if present USS for upper urinary tract), watch urine flow and direction.

Techniques:
Aim to straighten, create normal calibre urethra, reposition meatus with good cosmesis and function.
- *One stage V two stage:* one stage has fewer operations, cheaper and less psychological trauma, but may shorten the urethra and the urethra, which is mobilized may be more mobile after. Two-stage is more versatile, easier, more reliable, more natural-looking.
- *Horton's erection test:* inject into corpus cavenosum.
- *MAGPI.*
- *BEAM.*
- *TIP:* tubularized incised plate urethroplasty (Snodgras).
- *Flip-flap urethroplasty.*
- *Preputial skin island flap* (Duckett):
- *Bracka repair.*
- *Van der Meulen.*

Complications:
- *Early:* bleeding, haematoma, infection, dehiscence, necrosis,
- *Late:* fistula, stricture, sacculation, residual chordee, spraying, urethral hair.
- *Fistula:* 90% detectable within 1 week of operation. In repairing, ensure that there is no distal obstruction. Wait for softening of tissues, close the hole and place a fascial flap over it. Test integrity of the repair.

See Penis.

Hypotelorism
Reduced interorbital distance seen in
- Binder's syndrome
- Down syndrome
- Trigonocephaly (metopic synostosis)
- Holoprosencephaly
- Arrhinocephaly.

Hypothenar hammer syndrome
- Thrombosis of the ulnar artery in Guyon's canal due to blunt trauma to the base of the hypothenar eminence.
- Get cold intolerance, pain and sometimes ulceration of the ring and little fingers.
- Treat by excision of thrombosed segment and vein graft.
- Allen's test positive.
- The localized sympathectomy caused by the resection may be important for recovery, allowing distal vascular dilatation or removal of a possible source of emboli
- The effectiveness of resection may be due to resection of sympathetic fibres.

See Vascular injuries.

Iliac crest: free flap to **Ito, naevus of**

Iliac crest: free flap
- A source of vascularized bone on a long pedicle.
- Curved and useful for mandibular reconstruction.
- Skin and muscle can be included with minimal morbidity.

- There is a limited amount of bone to transfer resulting in a marked contour deficiency and may get abdominal herniation.
- It can be raised on the superficial circumflex iliac artery, the deep circumflex iliac artery or the dorsal branch of the fourth lumbar artery.

Anatomy:
- The deep circumflex iliac artery (DCIA) arises from the external iliac artery and passes on deep surface of inguinal ligament. It continues along the inside of iliac crest. It supplies bone through muscle so muscle must be raised as well. Artery diameter is 2 mm.
- The vessels send branches to skin and the first branch supplies the internal oblique and transverses abdominus. A muscle flap can be isolated as a separate pedicle.

Mandible reconstruction: For mandible the crest forms the lower border of the mandible, the ASIS the angle and the AIIS the condyle. So, use ipsilateral crest. Difficult to shape for angle to angle defects. The skin paddle is good for facial skin, but not so good for oral lining. Use for lateral segment defects.

Operation:
- The skin ellipse is centred over the upper border of anterior iliac crest. The medial incision is along the inguinal ligament.
- Divide external oblique. The conjoined fibres of internal oblique and transverses are incised just inside the iliac crest.
- The DCIA can be palpated adjacent to the ilium. Dissect distally. The descending branch is divided 1 cm anterior and medial to the ASIS.
- Isolate the bone. Preserve ASIS. Remove the flap.
- Take at least a 1-cm cuff of iliacus fascia below the course of the DCIA. If the full crest is taken, the TFL and gluteal muscles are detached from the anterior lip. A 2–3 cm fringe of externally attached muscle along the crest is taken if a skin paddle is used. Close in layers anchoring the muscle to the remaining iliac crest through drill holes.

Ilizarov technique
- Distraction osteogenesis was introduced in 1951 when a patient reversed the compression rods of a ring fixator.
- New bone is regenerated by pinning fragments and performing a corticotomy.
- Preserve periosteum so open periosteum longitudinally and peel off cortex prior to osteotomy.

- Gradual distraction allows new bone to be generated at a rate of 1 mm/day.
- Too slow distraction results in union, too fast in non-union.
- Useful in craniofacial skeleton due to the rich blood supply and thin bony skeleton and for leg-lengthening procedures.

See Mandibular hypoplasia. See Bone.

Imiquimod
- An immune response modifier. Acts to stimulate immune pathways. Synthesis of cytokines, as well as induction of cells occurs.
- It has been used with success for Keloids following surgery with no systemic toxicity.
- It has also been used to treat molluscum contagiosum and BCC in children with xeroderma pigmentosa.

Implantation dermoid
See Epidermoid inclusion cyst.

Inadine
Rayon mesh impregnated with povodone-iodine.
See Dressings.

Incisional herniation
- Associated with infection, dehiscence, age, obesity, malnutrition, steroids.
- Transverse incisions have the lowest rate of herniation. Lateral traction on the recti increases the protrusion.

See Abdominal wall reconstruction.

Infection: upper limb
Infections caused by injury at home are most commonly *Staph. aureus.* Establish any underlying conditions such as diabetes.
See
- *Felon.*
- *Paronychia.*
- *Tenosynovitis.*
- *Collar-button abscess.*
- *Herpes.*
- *Mycobacteria.*
- *Osteomyelitis.*
- *Flexor sheath.*
- *Palm infections.*
- *Dorsal infections.*
- *Animal bite: Pasteurella multicida.*

- *Human bites: Eikenella corrodens.*
- *Sporothrix schenkii*: in nurseryman.
- *Aeromonas hydrophilia:* Gram-negative rod in freshwater lakes. Sensitive to tetracycline. Get rapid onset of cellulitis with abscess, myonecrosis and sepsis.

Infra-orbital nerve

- Travels in the floor of the orbit in a groove then in a canal.
- It exits 10 mm from the upper edge of orbital rim parallel to medial margin of cornea.
- V2 branch of trigeminal nerve emerges from the infra-orbital foramen and divides into 4 branches:
  - inferior palpebral;
  - external nasal;
  - internal nasal;
  - superior labial.
- They supply the lower eyelid, upper lip, lateral nose and ala, cheek, mucous membrane of cheek and lip.
- Block by palpating the infra-orbital foramen or notch which lies below the midline of the pupil with the eye looking straight.
- Inject into the cheek directly in through the upper buccal sulcus in the line of the canine.

Inheritance

Penetrance relates to frequency of manifestation and *Expression* relates to the extent.

Integra

- Integra is an artificial skin composed of a 2-layer composite of dermis and epidermis.
- The dermal template is a porous bovine tendon collagen and shark glycosaminoglycan – condroitin-6 phosphate fibrous matrix arranged in a 3D pattern.
- It provides a biodegradeable framework in which host fibroblasts migrate and lay down host collagen.
- The neodermis replaces artificial dermis and inherits a vasculature to become permanently incorporated as host.
- The epidermal portion consists of a temporary silicone layer, which acts as a mechanical barrier to bacterial invasion.
- Once the neodermis has developed, the silicone layer can be stripped away to accept a split skin graft. When using, excise the burn wound early. Graft with thin SSG. Donor site can be used many times.
- It has been used for post-burns excision and gives a better-quality scar, which is thicker an more supple than following SSG.
- The main problem relates to loss of integra due to haematoma and infection, and meticulous technique is required for success.

Integrins

- Matrix binding cell surface molecules.
- They are the main way that cells both bind to and respond to the extracellular matrix and are involved in a variety of cellular functions, such as wound healing, cell differentiation, homing of tumour cells and apoptosis.
- They are part of a large family of cell adhesion receptors, which are involved in cell–extracellular matrix and cell–cell interactions.

Interferon
See Cytokines.

Interleukin
See Cytokines.

Interosseous muscles

- Four dorsal abduct (DAB) index middle and ring (reference line is middle finger).
- Three palmar adduct (PAD) index ring and little.

Palmar interossei:

- Single muscle belly arising from the anterior aspect of the respective metacarpal on the surface facing the middle finger.
- 1st inserts to ulnar side of index, 2nd to radial side of ring and 3rd to radial side of little.
- They cross palmar to the axis of the MCP joint dorsal to the deep transverse metacarpal ligament.

Dorsal interossei:

- Each arises from 2 metacarpals.
- 1st and 2nd insert into radial side of index and middle finger. 3rd and 4th insert into the ulnar side of middle and ring finger.
- The 1st, 2nd and 4th have superficial and deep muscles with medial and lateral tendons.
- The medial tendons travel under the sagittal band to insert into the lateral tubercle of the

base of proximal phalanx. This abducts and weakly flexes.
- The lateral tendon runs superficial to sagittal band and continues as the lateral band. This flexes the proximal phalanx and extends the IPJs.

Nerve supply: Deep branch of ulnar nerve.

Function:
- All assist MCP joint flexion and PIP and DIP joint extension.
- Also abduction and adduction, digital rotation and centralization of extensor tendon.
- Side-to-side movements of the index finger can be produced with EIP and EDC, but for the others it is solely by interossei. Rotation is important for fine control.
- They also stabilize the digit during pinch grip by preventing MCPJ hyperextension.

Interpolation flap
Similar in design to rotation and *Transposition flap*, but rotates into a nearby, but not immediately adjacent area so it must pass under or over intervening tissue.

Intersection syndrome
- Non-specific tenosynovitis of second dorsal *Extensor compartment*.
- Associated with repetitive trauma of the wrist.
- May mimic *de Quervain's* disease.
- It presents as a tender swelling localized to the region where the APL and EPB muscle bellies crosses ECRB and ECRL 4 cm proximal to the wrist joint.
- Distinct crepitus can be felt in the swelling. *Finklestein test* is positive.
- Most are cured by injection and splintage.
- If symptoms persist the second dorsal compartment is released through longitudinal incision. (see *Green*)
See Tenosynovitis.

Intraluminal endothelial hyperplasia
See Mason's haemangioma.

Intravelar veloplasty
- Technique of muscle apposition during *Cleft palate* repair.

- Kriens described the abnormal orientation of the levator muscles, and the need to detach them from their abnormal insertion and reorientate them in a more transverse direction.

Intrinsic plus/minus
- The intrinsics flex the MCP joint and extend interphalangeal joints – the intrinsic plus position.
- Tight intrinsics will prevent interphalangeal joint flexion if the MCP joint is hyperextended.
- This can happened with tip amputations if the FDP retracts.
- Test for intrinsic tightness by testing passive PIP joint flexion with MPJ extension – the *Bunnell test*.
- With extrinsic tightness IPJ flexion is possible on extension of MPJ.
- Intrinsic minus refers to the absence of intrinsic function as seen in *Ulnar nerve palsy*, resulting in a *Claw hand*.

Inverting papilloma
- A papilloma which usually arises from the lateral wall of the nose.
- It is benign, but can expand within the closed space and cause pressure necrosis of bone.
- SCC may arise from an inverting papilloma. *See Maxilla/Midface.*

Iron
- Essential cofactor for the replication of DNA.
- Also needed for proline hydroxylase used for converting proline to hydroxyproline.
- No studies have definitely linked iron deficiency anaemia with delayed *Wound healing.*

Isolated limb perfusion
- Used in the treatment of *Melanoma* with multiple uncontrollable metastasis confined to the limb from where the primary was excised.
- May be effective for local control.
- The preferred chemotherapy regime is dacarbazine (DTIC), melphalan with platinum and carmustine.

- All agents have demonstrated a 15–30% response rate. The technique has been present since the 60s.
- It involves perfusion with high dose chemotherapy under high oxygenation high pressure and high temperature (40ºC). The limb is isolated with a tourniquet.
- The addition of tumour necrosis factor and interferon is also beneficial.

Ischaemia-reperfusion injury

- Seen following re-establishment of blood flow in free tissue transfer or replant surgery.
- May get tissue injury beyond that caused by ischaemia.

Ischaemia: Causes tissue and cellular hypoxia. Products of anaerobic metabolism, such as

lactate build up, disturbing membrane transport systems resulting in influx of calcium into the cell. Inflammatory mediators are triggered.

Reperfusion: Oxygen is returned and oxygen free radicals are produced by neutrophils – respiratory burst, neutrophils degranulation, and release of pro-inflammatory mediators. *See No reflow phenomenom.*

Ito, naevus of

Same features as the naevus of *Ota*, but in the distribution of the posterior supraclavicular and lateral cutaneous branches to the shoulder, neck and supraclavicular areas. *See Blue naevus.*

J
Jackson pharyngoplasty to Juvara: Septa of

Jackson pharyngoplasty

- Used for the treatment of velopharyngeal incompetence (*VPI*).
- Similar to *Ortichochea* pharyngoplasty, but the flaps are based higher, the tips of the flaps are sutured end-to-end, rather than interdigitated and the lateral ports are not left unsutured.

Jackson's zones

Describe the zones of injury seen in acute *Burns*.

- *Zone of coagulation:* area of irreversible tissue destruction.
- *Zone of stasis:* describes the adjacent at risk tissue with marginal blood flow which without optimal conditions will progress to necrosis.
- *Zone of hyperaemia.*

Jahss manoeuvre

- Technique for closed reduction of metacarpal neck fracture.
- Flexing MCP joint relaxes intrinsics and tightens ligaments.

- The proximal phalanx can thus be used to reduce the fracture with upward force on the flexed PIP joint and counterforce on the metacarpal shaft.

Jeanne's sign

- Clinical test in *Ulnar nerve palsy*.
- Loss of lateral or key pinch of thumb due to paralysis of adductor pollicis muscle, which adducts, flexes at the MCP joint and extends at the IPJ. Get hyperextension of MCP joint.

Jejunal flap

- Used as a free flap principally for oropharyngeal reconstruction.
- The jejunum constitutes the first 2/5s of the 7-m long small bowel from ligament of Treitz to the ileocaecal valve.
- The diameter is 4 cm and the root of the fan-shaped mesentery is 15 cm long.
- On average there are 12–15 branches to the jejunum and ileum.
- The blood supply of the jejunum is supplied by branches of the superior mesenteric artery.

Each branch can support a segment of jejunum up to 24 cm long.

- Usually proximal jejunum is used.
- The first branch is not used because the pedicle length is short.
- Identify the jejunum and isolate the pedicle. Tie off other branches, divide the jejunum, divide the pedicle and transfer the flap. It can be opened out. Position it in an isoperistaltic fashion. Perform proximal bowel anastomosis then revascularize.
- A monitor segment can be fashioned from remaining jejunum and sutured to the neck.

See *Oral cavity reconstruction*. See *Laryngopharyngectomy*. See *Pharynx*.

Joint contracture: hand

Pathology:

- The MCP joint tends to rest extension following injury and swelling.
- The collateral ligaments then shorten. A flexion contracture is therefore caused by extrinsic forces.
- The PIP joint usually becomes stiff in flexion due to restriction of the volar plate.
- Restriction of DIP joint flexion is usually due to extensor adhesions.

PIP joint flexion contractures:

- Expose volar surface through Bruner incision which allows for a Y–V advancement, retract NVB and expose flexor sheath. C1 overlies PIP joint. Lift up C1 to expose flexor tendons.
- Perform tenolysis until FDS and FDP run freely. Retract tendon to expose volar plate with check rein ligaments, which extend from the proximal edge of the volar plate to the margin of the flexor sheath.
- Divide check rein ligaments. Attempt to preserve the vincula which run between them. Gentle force is required to extend the joint.
- If there is still a contracture, gentle blunt dissection beneath the volar plate and/or sharp division of the volarmost fibres of the collateral ligament is undertaken. Enter joint through volar plate in midline and lift up volar plate off bone until joint freed. Hold joint out with K wire for short time before using dynamic splints.

PIPJ extension contractures:

- Require partial ligament resection. Approach dorsally.
- Divide transverse ligaments of Landsmeer. Retract lateral band dorsally.
- Resection part of collateral ligament to allow PIPJ flexion. Begin release dorsally. Assess the extensor hood and release adhesions before dividing collateral ligaments. Immobilize in partial flexion and start protected movement early.
- Occasionally PIP joint movement is restricted by chronic synovitis. Debridement may improve movement. Detach volar plate from one side to gain access to the joint. Debride.

MCP joint flexion contractures: Almost always extrinsic and fully correctable by releasing extrinsic problem.

MCP joint extension contractures:

- Require selective release of the surrounding structures.
- Approach from the dorsal side using a longitudinal incision.
- Retract sagittal bands distally or divided on one side preferably the ulnar side, as it tends to prolapse ulnarly.
- Adhesions between the tendon and capsule are freed. Perform graded release of the collateral ligaments.
- Release dorsal fibres from their origin on the metacarpal head. Release should allow the proximal phalanx to track within the normal axis of joint motion.
- Volar structures can be freed by passing an instrument between volar plate and flexor.

Joint transfers: free

- Free non-vascularized joint transfers over time degenerate and collapse.
- Synovial fluid is required which requires an intact blood supply.
- There is, however, long-term bone and cartilage survival in vascularized joint transfers.
- The first free vascularized toe joint transfer was performed by Foucher in 1976. The alternative is arthrodesis or arthroplasty.
- The best indication for free joint transfers are in children and in young active adults

with normal functioning flexor and extensor tendons. They are also useful when soft tissue is also required.

Anatomy:
- Toe blood supply is from the dorsal and plantar arch with the dominant supply to the 2nd toe from the dorsal arch by the first dorsal metatarsal artery (FDMA).
- The lateral digital artery to the big toe is sacrificed so a paddle of skin from the big toe can also be taken.
- As the growth plate for the metatarsal is distally and the phalanx is proximal if the MTP is taken both growth centres are included, which is important in children, but not in adults.

Outcome:
- Foucher reported 28 joints in 25 patients.
- The average ROM was 35° at the MPJ and 23° at the PIPJ.
- Less than 150 joint replacements have been reported in the world literature.

Joints
- *PIPJ*.
- *DIPJ*.

Joule heating
- Mechanism of tissue destruction seen in *Electrical injuries*.
- Passage of an electrical current through a solid body results in conversion of electrical energy to heat.
- Heat production (Q) is proportional to the square of the current (I), tissue resistance (R) and time of contact (t).

- $Q \alpha I^2 RT$.

Jumping man flap
- Five flap Y–V advancement and *Z-plasty*.
- Useful for releasing contractures on concave regions such as interdigital web space and medial canthal region.
- The central flap advances in a Y–V, while the two Z-plasties on either side are transposed.

Juncturae tendinae
- Tendinous bands connecting ring finger *Extensor digitorum communis* (EDC) to EDC of middle and little fingers.
- They may also connect EDC of index and middle.
- Division of a tendon proximal to a juncturae may result in only partial loss of extension.
- One of the earliest described elective tendon operations was the division of juncturae in harpists to improve independent finger movement.

Juri classification
For male pattern *Balding*.
- *Type 1:* frontal.
- *Type 2:* frontal and crown.
- *Type 3:* vertex.

Juri flap
For *Alopecia*.

Juvara: septa of
See the septa of Legueu and Juvara.

K **Kanavel's signs** to **Kutler V–Y flaps**

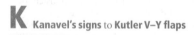

Kanavel's signs
Seen in suppurative *Tenosynovitis* of the flexor tendon sheath.
- Tenderness over the flexor sheath.
- Pain on passive extension.
- Flexed posture.
- Fusiform swelling.

Kapetansky flaps
- Used in the correction of whistle tip deformity following bilateral cleft lip repair.
- Bilateral horizontally orientated V–Y flaps.
- Also a centrally placed upside-down W creates a space into which the lateral flaps will

advance. So they fill the central defect in all dimensions.

See *Secondary lip and nasal deformities*.

Kaplan's cardinal line

- A line drawn on the palm of the hand along the flexor surface of the radially abducted thumb, parallel to the proximal palmar crease.
- The bisection of this line with a line drawn from the scaphoid tubercle to the 3rd web space gives the point of origin of the motor branch of the median nerve. This is also the point where the flexed ring finger hits Kaplan's line.
- The bisection of Kaplan's line with a line drawn from the ulnar border of the abducted ring finger gives the position of the hook of the hamate and Kaplan's line overlies the deep palmar arch.

Kaposi's sarcoma

- A multicentric malignant disorder of vaso-formative tissue. Initially presents with patches of purpura. Later, vascular polyps develop. Chronic lymphoedema occurs and ulceration secondary to RT.
- Described by Hungarian Moriz Kaposi in 1872.
- KS-associated herpes virus (human herpes-virus type 8 [HHV-8]) linked closely with all 4 types of KS.
- HHV-8 appears to interact with the HIV tat protein, excess levels of basic fibroblast growth factor, scatter factor and IL-6.
- Four groups are predisposed to KS including:
  - older men of Mediterranean and Jewish lineage;
  - Africans from areas including Uganda, the Congo Republic, Congo (Brazzaville) and Zambia;
  - persons who are iatrogenically immuno-suppressed;
  - men who are homosexual.
- Endemic African KS has accounted for 10% of cancers and has been seen in a male-to-female ratio of 15:1. In Uganda, KS has caused almost one half (48.9%) of cancer cases in men and 17.9% in women. It is rare in American Blacks.

- For endemic M:F 1:1 in childhood, 15:1 by puberty.

Clinical:
- Multiple vascular nodules. Multifocal though can metastasize. Course may be indolent or fulminant. May occur on oral mucosa and lymph nodes only. Chronic lymphedema may precede KS.
- KS is described in 3 forms including local-ized nodular, locally aggressive, and gener-alized KS. KS typically occurs in these 3 forms and in 6 stages including patch, plaque, nodular, exophytic, infiltrative and lymphadenopathic. Often start in lower extremities.

Causes: HHV-8 linked, but other factors needed. Most important is immunosupression.

Treatment:
- Treatment is based on the extent of disease and the patients immune status.
- Management modalities for KS include non-intervention, surgical removal of skin nodules or severely affected areas (e.g. areas of the extremities, intussuscepted bowel), laser surgery, conventional and mega-voltage radiotherapy, chemotherapy, immu notherapy, anti-viral drugs and cessation of immunosuppressive therapy in iatrogeni-cally immunosuppressed patients.
- Indolent skin tumours in elderly may not need treatment, but systemic vinblastine affects cutaneous and visceral lesions.
- Localized nodular disease responds well to surgery, radiotherapy, intralesional and systemic vinblastine. Vinblastine by both routes is preferable.
- *Taxanes:* e.g. paclitaxel have anti-angiogenic properties and is effective for HIV-KS.
- *Radiotherapy:* good for classic nodular. Conventional RT very effective for localized nodular. Electron beam RT with limited penetration good for superficial lesions. Usually response is complete and better on newer lesions.
- *Laser therapy:* argon laser, beneficial for clas-sic KS.
- *Chemotherapy:* IV vinblastine titred against white cell count. Also intralesional and intra-arterial. Can also use vincristine,

vinblastine, dacarbazine, doxorubicin, and actinomycin D. Alkylating agents (e.g., cyclophosphamide, chlorambucil, bleomycin, doxorubicin, etoposide.

Kaposiform hemangioendothelioma
See _Kasabach–Merritt syndrome_.
- Histologically distinct from haemangiomas.
- Mortality rate of 24% from coagulopathy and local infiltration.
- Treatment as for _Haemangiomas_ with close monitoring of coagulopathy.

Karapandzic flap
- Used for _Lip reconstruction_.
- A modification of the _Gilles' fan flap_, which maintains the neurovascular pedicle in the soft tissue, giving better functional results.
- Can be used for upper or lower lip defects.
- Semicircular incisions are used and facial nerve branches preserved. The commissure rotates.
- Does not import new lip tissue and may give microstomia. The vertical height of the defect determines the width of the flap.
- The incisions are full thickness medially, but at the commissure it is only down to subcutaneous tissue and neurovascular structures are preserved.
- If the defect is central, rotate flaps equally from either side. If more to one side bring more from the contralateral side so as not to distort the commissure.

Kasabach–Merritt syndrome
- Primary platelet trapping is a life-threatening complication of _Haemangioma_-like tumours, specifically kaposiform hemangioendothelioma.
- These tumours are histopathologically distinct from the common haemaniomas of infancy.
- Thrombocytopenia is profound, typically <10 000/mm^3. The prothrombin time (PT) and activated partial thromboplastin time (aPTT) are variably elevated. Low fibrinogen levels and elevated fibrin split products also are detected, usually if tissue necrosis or infection is present.

- An infant with Kasabach–Merritt thrombocytopenia is at risk for intracranial, pulmonary, intraperitoneal or gastrointestinal haemorrhage.
- Also seen rarely with tufted angioma and congenital haemangiopericytoma.

Kazanjian and Converse classification: mandibular fractures
For _Mandibular fractures_.
- _Class 1:_ teeth on bony fragments.
- _Class 2:_ teeth on one bony fragment.
- _Class 3:_ teeth on neither bony fragment.
This relates to the management of the fracture by IMF.

Keloid
- Proliferation of scar tissue outside the border of the scar.
- _Hypertrophic scar_ remains within the borders of the scar.
- 'Chel' means crab claw.
- Can develop over a year after injury.
- More common in dark-skinned people. Autosomal dominant or recessive pattern. Associated with blood group A. Correlates with IgE and allergic symptoms.
- Hormonally related as it appears in puberty and resolves after pregnancy.
- Fibroblast numbers not increased. Both keloids and hypertrophic scars have rich vasculature and thickened epidermal layer. Collagen is fragmented and shortened. Get collagen nodules. Collagen synthesis in both is elevated, but higher in keloids. There is less cross-linkage and more type III. The influence of growth factors is unclear.

Treatment:
- _Surgery:_ high recurrence rate 45–100%. Helpful combined with other treatment.
- _Pressure:_ 60–85% response rate. Wear garments for 18–24 hours/day for 6/12. May work by causing ischaemia, decreasing tissue metabolism and increasing collagenase.
- _Steroids:_ give a variable response of 50–100%. Most effective on younger hypertrophic scars. No steroid has been shown to be more superior. May get skin atrophy, hypopigmentation, necrosis or ulceration. In conjunction with surgery use preoperatively,

then immediately post-operatively followed by weekly injection for 2–5 weeks, then monthly for 3–6/12. Acts by decreasing collagen synthesis.

- *Radiotherapy:* use for scars resistant to other treatment. Need at least 900 Gy. Surgery then RT gives a 76% success rate. Irradiation destroys fibroblasts. Risk of later development of skin cancer which can be reduced by using iridium wires.
- *Silicone materials:* decrease scar volume and increase elasticity in 60–100% of patients. Get mild heat rash. These can be fluid, gel or rubber. Effective in 75–85% after surgery. Wear for 24 hours/day for at least 3/12. The effect is not due to pressure or the difference in O_2 or temperature. It may relate to static electricity and hydration, as keratinocytes need a moist environment to downregulate fibroblasts.
- *Laser:* pulsed dye has the best response with scars being more pliable and less hypertrophic.
- *Cryotherapy:* leads to cellular anoxia. Response rate of 50–70%. Younger scars have a better response.
- *Calcium antagonist:* verapamil has been shown to have some beneficial effect on the control of cell growth and matrix accumulation in keloids. It has been shown to decrease IL-6 and VEGF production.
- *Imiquimod.*

Keratoacanthoma

- Benign self-limiting tumour.
- Occurs in sun-exposed areas and closely resembles *Squamous cell carcinoma*.
- A firm erythematous papule appears and enlarges to up to 2 cm over 2–8 weeks. The central portion of the lesion is filled with a keratin plug. These lesions are mobile over underlying structures. A regressive phase begins when the central plug is expelled and spontaneous resolution occurs.
- *Pathology:* ground glass cytoplasm, cytological atypia, mitoses, margins rounded with no infiltration.
- *Treatment* is excision. The linear scar is preferable to the cicatricial scar, and it may be difficult to distinguish it from an SCC. If it is already large then spontaneous resolution may give a better cosmetic result.

See *Ferguson–Smith syndrome*.

Kernahan classification

Graphical classification of *Cleft lip and palate*. The deformity is likened to a letter Y. Each area is allocated on the Y. Stippling indicates a cleft. Cross-hatching indicates a submucous area. Millard and Jackson have modified the Y classification.

Kienbock's disease

- Kienbock described avascular necrosis of the lunate or lunatomalacia in 1910.
- May result from stress fracture. Negative ulnar variance is more common. Probably have a tenous blood supply, which is disrupted by repetitive loads to the wrist.

Presentation: Usually young adult male with a painful stiff weak wrist. Usually dominant wrist. Rarely a history of acute trauma. Find dorsal wrist swelling, limited wrist movement, but forearm rotation unaffected. Tenderness over lunate dorsally. Diminished grip strength.

Progression: Wrist movement is decreased with progressive radiology, but function is fairly good and symptoms don't correlate with XRs.

Aetiology:
- Relates to vascularity, ulnar variance, lunate fossa inclination, and lunate geometry.
- *Blood supply:*
  ○ *Extra-osseous*: 3 types: 1. single vessel. 2. Several vessels 3. several vessels with anastomosis.
  ○ *Intra-osseous:* Y, I or X shape. Y and I are at risk of losing dorsal or palmar blood flow after trauma.

Ulna variance: refers to the relationship of the distal articular surfaces of radius and ulna. Ulna minus is when the distal radius is longer than the distal ulna. 74% of wrists in Kienbocks are ulna minus, whereas only 23% of normal controls were. This may increase the load on the lunate. Check ulna variance with a neutral rotation PA view. Shoulders abducted 90°, elbows flexed 90° and palm flat on the XR.

Geometry: triangular-shaped lunate concentrates shear forces.

Classification: *by Stahl*.

Treatment:

- Early disease may benefit from intermittent casts or braces, but the wrist pain may be well tolerated for many years.
- Precollapse and negative ulna variance may benefit from joint levelling, by radial shortening.
- Lunate bone grafts and revascularization is being investigated.
- Limited wrist arthrodesis (_Triscaphe_), aim to unload the lunate.
- Proximal row carpectomy provides functional range of pain-free motion, and is useful for stages II and III.
- Wrist arthrodesis for stage IV.

Kite flap
See _Flag flap_.

Kleinmann shear test
- Test for _Carpal instability_.
- Place thumbs on dorsum of pisiform and lunate. The bones usually translate in opposite directions.

Klinefelter's syndrome
- 47, XXY.
- The most frequent abnormality of sexual differentiation.
- Occurs in 1:500 males.
- Get infertility, gynaecomastia, impaired sexual maturation and under-androgenization.

Klippel–Feil syndrome
- _Type I:_ massive continuity of cervical and upper thoracic vertebrae.
- _Type II:_ involvement of only one or two vertebrae, hemivertebrae, scoliosis and occipitalization of the atlas.
- _Type III:_ fusion of both cervical and lower thoracic or lumbar vertebrae.

Clinical features:

- Patients have a short neck, restriction of neck movement (especially rotation), and a low occipital hairline.
- Webbing of the neck, scoliosis, torticollis and, occasionally, Sprengel deformity.
- May have mental retardation.
- 1 in 42 000 births, females > males.
- Associated with cleft palate.
- Cardiac anomalies.

Cause: The process is failure of segmentation of the cervical spine. The cause of this has been postulated to be a lack of midline fusion with disruption of the notochord. A second theory is that the subclavian artery has been disrupted.

Treatment:

- This depends on the extent of the problem, which may consist of cardiac, palatal and skeletal involvement. Anaesthesia may be a problem.
- Spinal fusion should be performed and cord pressure should be decompressed.
- Correction of neck webbing is difficult and consists of resection of excess skin and underlying soft tissue with Z-plasty skin closure.
- The posterior hairline is corrected by expansion of the neck skin with subsequent excision of the hair-bearing area with expanded skin advancement.

Klippel–Trenaunay syndrome
- _Complex combined vascular malformations_ (CLVM) of low flow in limbs.
- Most are sporadic though rarely familial.
- Cutaneous capillary malformation of an extremity, congenital venous abnormalities.
- Limb bone and soft tissue hypertrophy and lateral VVs.
- There may be lymphatic hypoplasia.
- A few patients have a short limb.
- Craniofacial abnormalities include asymmetric facial hypertrophy and microcephaly.

Knight and North classification
For _Zygomatic fractures_, with frequency of occurrence.
- Undisplaced – 6%.
- Isolated arch – 10%.
- Unrotated body – 33%.
- Zygomatic body with medial rotation of ZF suture – 11%.
- Zygomatic body with lateral rotation of ZF suture – 22%.
- Complex – 18%.

Köbner's phenomenon
Skin trauma in _Psoriasis_ resulting in new psoriatic lesions. Can occur with other skin conditions such as lichen planus.

Krukenberg operation

Converts the forearm into prehensile forceps. The flexors and extensors are converted to abductors and adductors. Main indication is for bilateral blind amputees. Also possibly bilateral congenital amputees.

Kuhnt–Szymanowski procedure

A procedure for *Ectropion* correction, which combines a blepharoplasty-type lower lid incision with a wedge resection of the lateral part of the posterior lamella of the lower eyelid.

Kutler V–Y flaps

- For *Fingertip injuries*.
- Two flaps laterally based. Use for transverse or volar amputations at mid-nail level. Debride skin, trim bone. Tip of flap is at DIPJ. Gently spread to divide septa and advance flap. These flaps provide limited advancement.

L Lacrimal duct: trauma to Lymphoedema

Lacrimal duct: trauma

If divided both upper and lower systems should be repaired. Place a tube into the nose to splint the repair. Injury may occur with lacerations around the medial canthus. Also commonly accompanies Le Fort III and naso-ethmoidal fractures. Fixation of the fractures may correct the obstruction. Chronic obstruction will require a dacryocystorrinostomy.

Lacrimal pump

See *Orbicularis oculi*.

Ladder

Reconstructive ladder principle is to perform the simplest effective procedure. The range is:
- Secondary healing.
- Primary closure.
- Split skin graft.
- Full thickness skin graft.
- Local flap.
- Distant pedicled flap.
- Free flap.
- Composite free flap.

Lagophthalmos

- The inability to close the eyelid.
- Causes of lagophthalmos include exoph-thalmos, an impairment of mechanical closure of the lids, e.g. burns of the eyelids, paralysis of orbicularis oculi, leprosy.

Lambdoid synostosis

- True isolated lambdoid synostosis is rare.
- <1% of synostosis.
- <1:10 000 births.
- Get occipital flattening and marked mas-toid bulging. The opposite occiput bulges.

See *Craniosynostosis*.

Landsmeer ligaments
Oblique retinacular ligament (ORL)

- The ORLs are attached proximally to the distal metaphysis of the proximal phalanx at the distal bony attachment of the A2 pulley.
- The ligaments run distally under the trans-verse retinacular ligament to join the lateral band.
- Each ORL lies volar to the axis of PIP joint motion and through the attachment to the conjoined tendon passes dorsally to the DIP joint. FDP initiates flexion at the DIP joint, which tightens the ORL, which increases flexion at the PIP joint giving synchronized flexion. It helps to prevent hyperextension of the PIP joint during extension.
- At the level of the PIPJ, ORL holds in place 7 tendons – central slip of extensor tendon, 2 lateral bands, 2 slips from the central slip to the lateral bands and 2 slips from the lat-eral bands to the central slip.

Transverse retinacular ligament:
- Short wide fibres extend along the lateral side of the PIP joint superficial to the collateral ligament. They originate from the volar plate and the flexor tendon sheath in the area of the A1 pulley. They extend dorsally where they attach to the lateral margin of each lateral band.
- The transverse retinacular ligament pulls the lateral bands volarly during digital flexion. During extension they limit the dorso-medial displacement of the lateral bands. They play an important role in preventing swan neck deformity.

See *Retinacular system*. See *Haines–Zancolli* test.

Langer's lines
Lines of *Skin* tension demonstrated by cutting circles in cadaveric skin and noting direction of the ellipse. They do not relate to the line of collagen fibre orientation. Wrinkle lines lie perpendicular to the long axis of facial muscles. There are no Langer's lines across the sternum.

Langerhan's cells
Located within stratum spinosum of the epidermis. Front line immune system. They process foreign antigens and present them to T lymphocytes.
See *Skin*.

Laryngopharyngectomy
- Circumferential resection is most often required in cancer, but also in lye ingestion and trauma.
- Without reconstruction, speech and oral nutrition are lost.
- Gastric pull-up and pectoralis major flaps have been used for proximal defects, but have significant morbidity, with up to 40% fistula formation and operative mortality of up to 20%.
- *Free jejunal transfer* is the procedure of choice. The biggest problem remains fistula and stenosis, which occur in about 20% of patients. Excessive length may cause swallowing difficulties.
- *Voice restoration*.

Larynx carcinoma
The larynx is divided into 3 parts for staging of malignancies.
- *Supraglottic larynx:* extends from superior tip of epiglottis to apex of laryngeal ventricle.
- *Glottic larynx:* bounded superiorly by the apex of the laryngeal ventricle and inferiorly 1 cm below the ventricle apex or 5 mm below the free edge of vocal cord.
- *Subglottis:* extends from inferior edge of glottis to inferior aspect of cricoid cartilage.
- There are certain barriers to tumour spread, which may enable a less extensive resection. Metastasis to the neck varies depending on site with supraglottic being the highest risk.

Laser
- Based on Einstein's theory of Light Amplification by Stimulated Emission of Radiation. Developed by Maimon in 1960.
- Monochromatic collimated coherent light is produced. All light is part of the electromagnetic spectrum. Surgical lasers are between near infrared and ultraviolet, which includes visible light. Similar to a fluorescent light. The medium is a solid, liquid or gas, which when excited by absorbed energy causes the atom to be elevated to a higher energy state. Atoms in an excited state are a fixed energy level above ground state. As the atom returns to ground state the energy is released as an emission of radiation as photons.

Components:
- Active medium in a resonator. Parallel mirrors at each end. Energy supplied by an energizer pump. Energy is absorbed causing population inversion. Energy is amplified by the reflecting mirrors. The radiation each atom emits is in phase with the radiation in the tube. The radiation is allowed to escape through a small unsilvered hole in the mirror. Monochromatic collimated coherent light escapes.

Light measurements:
- Used routinely in laser applications include energy, fluence, power and irradiance.
  - energy is proportional to the number of photons and is measured in joules (J);

○ *power* is the rate of delivery of the energy, measured in watts (W), where 1 W = 1 J/S;
○ *irradiance* is the power per unit area, measured in W/cm^2.
○ *fluence* is the energy delivered per unit area, measured in J/cm^2.

Electromagnetic spectrum: Range from gamma rays to radio waves. Most clinical lasers are in the visible portion (400–700 nm).

Mode of delivery:

• Variety of delivery methods.
• *CW or continuous wave:* uninterrupted without pulses.
• *Pulsed mode:* light is delivered in single pulses or a train of pulses.
• *Superpulsed mode:* extremely high-peak powers with each pulse. Pulses are brief and repetition rate may be varied.
• *Q switching:* when one of the resonating mirrors is non-reflective for an interval of pumping. When this occurs the stored energy is emitted as a pulse of light 10 billionths of a second in length.

Tissue action and interactions:

• On contact with tissue, laser light is scattered, reflected, transmitted, but mostly absorbed. Kinetic energy converts to heat which ablates tissue.
• The chromophore of the tissue determines which wavelength is absorbed.
• *Thermal:* the tissue effect is primarily thermal. The extent of the effect depends on the degree of absorption of light and diffusion to adjacent tissues. Key factors are the energy density, pulse duration and heat conduction.
• *Mechanical:* if pulse duration is shorter than thermal relaxation, then thermo-elastic expansion will occur. This change is sudden and generates acoustic waves.
• *Selective photothermolysis:* this theory has two components:
○ wavelength determines absorption of energy;
○ exposure time (pulse width) limits thermal diffusion if the pulse width is less than the thermal relaxation time of the tissues.

• *Thermal relaxation time:* the time required for a specific tissue to absorb and transmit thermal energy. To minimize thermal injury, the appropriate *pulse width* is chosen. Pulse width is the duration of pulse. Laser therapy has been refined by matching pulse widths to thermal relaxation time. Clinical result is maximized when laser passes through tissue and is absorbed by the target. The target substances are called chromophores.
• Primary chromophores are haemoglobin, melanin and water. They may also come from external sources such as tattoo pigments. Laser techniques have been limited by thermally induced damage. Getting the wavelength right reduces this. Cooling with cryogen spray can protect epidermis when treating vascular lesions.

Laser systems:

• CO_2 (10 600 nm): the most frequently used. As the beam is invisible it is coupled with a visible beam of HeNe. Can be delivered as CW, pulsed CW, which has less thermal injury.
• *Flashlamp-pumped pulsed dye (FLPD):* dye lasers contain fluorescent dyes, which are dissolved in solvents such as water or alcohol. These absorb light at one wavelength and emit at another. By changing the dye they can be tuned over a wide band (400–1000 nm). Laser is delivered in short single pulses at high peak powers. So 585 nm wavelength is absorbed well by haemoglobin and a pulse duration of 450 ms matches the thermal relaxation time of blood vessels making it suitable for cutaneous vascular lesions. It penetrates to depth of 0.75 mm. In dark skin can lead to damage to melanocytes, leading to hypopigmentation.
• *Long-pulse dye laser:* for larger calibre vessels, a longer pulse width is required. 595–600 nm for 1.5 ms. Promising results with leg veins.
• *YAG lasers:* several types (neodymium Nd, erbium Er). The common denominator is a crystal of yttrium-aluminium-garnet. This is doped with an ion. Doping is the process where the crystal is grown with an impurity. Nd:YAG has a wavelength of 1064. There is no particular chromophore for this

wavelength so its effect is coagulation and haemostasis. Effective for diffuse thermal injury such as deep vascular tumours. Q-switched Nd:YAG used for tattoos. KTP:YAG has a wavelength of 532 nm. Good for oral mucosa. Er:YAG has a wavelength of 294 nm close to that of water. Therefore little heat transferred. Good for skin resurfacing.

- *Q-switched Alexandrite:* chromium-doped BeAl2O4. Tune from 701 to 826 nm. Good for tattoo greens and blues.
- *Argon:* one of the first used. Two wavelengths of 488 and 514 nm so it is absorbed by haemoglobin and melanin. Can give hypertrophic scars and depigmentation.
- *Copper vapour:* 578 and 511 wavelength. 578 is oxyhaemoglobin and 511 is melanin. Used for *Port wine stains* and telangiectasia.
- *Ruby:* first laser developed. Initially CW then Q-switched. 694 nm – melanin. Useful for pigmented lesions and tattoos. Long-pulse ruby penetrates deeper and has been used for hair removal. May get pigment changes.

Safety: CO_2 laser is in the invisible infrared spectrum. Protective plastic eyewear required. Glass may shatter. Patients require frosted metal scleral protectors with lubrication.

Clinical applications:

- *Vascular lesions:* the pulsed dye is most commonly used. Continuous wave lasers may be effective for large-diameter vascular lesions including nodular *Port wine stains*.
- Pigmented lesions: blue, green, red and near infrared wavelengths can be used. Q-switched ruby Q-switched alexandrite and Q-switched Nd:YAG can be used to treat dermal lesions. Epidermal lesions respond to the green pulsed dye laser, frequency doubled Q-switched Nd:YAG, and the Q-switched ruby lasers.
- Benign naevi *Naevus of Ota/Ito*, *Café au lait macules*, *Naevus spilus*, *Becker's naevi*, *Melasma* have a variable response. Dysplastic naevi should not be treated and treatment of congenital naevi is controversial.
- *Tattoos:* The *Q-switched laser*, Nd:YAG, alexandrite and green pulsed dye lasers are all employed in tattoo removal. Each laser

enables removal of specific colours of ink; however, none of these can remove all ink pigments. Multicoloured tattoos, especially fluorescent inks, are difficult to treat. Irreversible blackening of some inks has occurred with Q-switched lasers. CO_2 laser vaporizes the tattoo and the defect left to re-epithelialize resulting in a scar.

- *Laser resurfacing:* good for Fitzpatrick skin type 1 and 2. Type 3 can get pigment abnormalities. Continuous wave CO_2 lasers were used, but resulted in significant scarring. Ultrapulsed laser limits damage with a high power for short duration. The ER:YAG lasers were the next to be used for resurfacing. Vaporization leads to re-epithelialization. Darker skin may hyperpigment. If so, treat with hydroquinone, hydrocortisone and tretinoin. Post-operatively the area can be dressed with an occlusive dressing or vaseline.
- *Laser depilation:* does not provide a permanent solution, but rather a hair-free interval. Use long pulsed alexandrite or Nd.YAG. Six treatments gives an 80% reduction in hair.
- *Others:* Lasers have also been used in the treatment of warts, in incisional surgery and for actinic cheilitis.

Laser Doppler flowometry

Can be used to record blood flow in a small area or scan over a large area. It measures Doppler shift of light. These changes are produced by movement of macromolecules within vessels. The depth of penetration is limited to 1.5 mm.

Lateral arm flap

- Initially described as a free flap, it can also be pedicled proximally or distally. Fasciocutaneous flap based on septal vessels.
- The flap is supplied by the posterior radial collateral artery arising from the profunda brachii.
- Pedicle can be 8 cm long. The vessel diameter is 1.2 mm.
- The flap is supplied by the lower lateral cutaneous nerve of the arm which arises from the radial nerve and passes through triceps. The posterior cutaneous nerve runs through the flap.

- The flap can be sensate and can measure 14 X 30 cm.

Operative procedure:

- Flap outlined on the distal 1/3 of lateral aspect of arm. Extend over lateral epicondyle. Flap axis and proximal incision is traced along a line between acromion and epicondyle. Incise deep fascia with skin and release posterior half from triceps until septum is seen. Septum separated anterior from posterior compartment and contains the vessel. Anteriorly separate fascia from brachialis, brachioradialis and extensors. Proximally separate deltoid from triceps to expose the pedicle and radial nerve. Ligate descending anterior branch. Identify two nerves – one to flap, the other going through it. Incise septum to release the flap. Ligate vessels distally.

See Oral cavity reconstruction.

Lateral femoral cutaneous nerve decompression

- T12.
- The lateral femoral cutaneous nerve runs along the inside of the iliac bone on iliacus and passes through transversus and through inguinal ligament at variable point 1–6 cm medial to the anterior superior iliac spine. Decompress through a tranverse incision overlying the lateral 1/3 of the inguinal ligament and identify the nerve by dissecting through fascia inferior to ligament.
- Delineate nerve and split inguinal ligament and tendinous transversus tendon until completely released.

Lateral plantar flap

- Sensate flap below the lateral malleolar area along the lateral side of the foot.
- Pedicled on the lateral calcaneal artery, a terminal branch of the peroneal artery.
- Rotates to the Achilles tendon and lateral malleolar area.
- Can be raised as an adipofascial flap.

Lateral plantar nerve

S1–2: Supplies the lateral forefoot.

Lateral pterygoid

Origin: Two heads. Upper from infratemporal crest, lower head from lateral surface of lateral pterygoid plate.

Insertion: Upper head into capsule of joint and articular disc. Lower head into neck of condyle.

Action: Upper portion pulls medially and forward. External portion pulls the condyle downward medially and forward.

Latissimus dorsi flap

Origin: Spinous processes T7–12, L1–5, posterior superior iliac crest, ribs 9–12.

Insertion: Into humerus.

Blood supply: Dominant pedicle, thoracodorsal artery, and segmental pedicles, posterior intercostals and lumbar artery perforating branches – type V muscle. The thoracodorsal artery comes off the subscapular artery. Mean length 9 cm, increase by 2 cm by following up subscapular artery. Usually a single artery and vein. The vessels usually bifurcate into an upper transverse branch and a lateral vertical branch. It is possible to raise the muscle based on reverse flow from serratus anterior when the main pedicle has been cut.

Nerve supply: Thoracodorsal nerve from the posterior cord of the brachial plexus.

Function: Shoulder adduction, arm medial rotation and extension. Pulls the trunk forward. After raising flap there is no significant difference in shoulder power. Scar contracture causes up to 30% reduction in shoulder movement in 1/3 of patients (Laitung/Peck). No occupational problems.

Skin paddle: Many options for raising skin as there are multiple perforators. More numerous in the proximal 2/3 of muscle. Elevate whole of muscle. Increase arc of rotation by dividing branch to serratus and dividing insertion.

See Trunk reconstruction, Breast reconstruction, Chest wall reconstruction.

Le Fort fractures

René Le Fort was a French surgeon at the end of the 19th century. He looked at the fractures of skulls dropped from upper-storey windows. Fracture lines travel adjacent to thicker areas of bone. Maxillary fractures had the following patterns.

Alveolar fractures: Fractured due to direct force or indirect force transmitted from the mandible. Usually reduce and fix with palatal splint.

Le Fort 1 – transverse:
- Also called Geurin fracture.
- Get two segments – the lower floating palate contains the alveolus, palate and pterygoid plates.
- The fracture line passes transversely across:
  o base of piriform aperture;
  o base of maxillary sinus;
  o pterygoid plates.

Le Fort 2 fracture – pyramidal:
- The fracture line passes:
  o across the nasal bones;
  o into the medial wall of the orbit;
  o diagonally downwards and outwards through the maxilla;
  o through the pterygoid plates.
- The bony fragment contains lacrimal crests, bulk of maxilla, piriform margin, alveolus, palate.

Le Fort 3 fracture – craniofacial dysjunction:
- The fracture line passes:
  o through the nasofrontal suture;
  o across the orbital floor to the NF suture;
  o through the zygomatic arch and pterygoid plates.

This results in detachment of the entire midfacial skeleton from the cranial base. They are often asymmetrical. The midface is held to the skull only by soft tissues.

Vertical or sagittal fracture: The maxilla is split longitudinally along the junction of maxilla with vomer.
See *Maxillary fractures*.

Le Fort osteotomy

Le Fort I: The most commonly used osteotomy. Perform 4–5 mm above the roots of the teeth. Go across maxilla below infra-orbital foramen. Through lateral and medial maxillary walls below nasolacrimal duct. Separate septum from vomer. Perform osteotomy between the maxillary tuberosity and the pterygoid plate of the sphenoid. Bone grafts are used.

Le Fort II: This is the true total maxillary osteotomy. It is indicated in occasional cleft patients with severe maxillary hypoplasia involving the nose and infra-orbital rims and in Crouzon's disease without exorbitism, Binder's syndrome and patients with hemifacial microsomia, where the naso-ethmoid complex is deviated to the affected side.

Le Fort III: This enlarges the orbital cavity and advances the maxilla. As the degree of exorbitism and retromaxillism may not correlate, the goal of this operation is to correct the bulging eye. A Le Fort I can also be performed to correct the malocclusion. See *Maxilla*. See *Maxillary osteotomy*.

Le Mesurier–Hagedorn cleft lip repair

Cleft lip repair with a rectangular flap from the cleft side is inset into a releasing incision on the non-cleft side to create an artificial Cupid's bow.

Ledderhose's disease

Plantar fibromatosis associated with *Dupuytren's contracture*. Large tender nodules occur on the instep. Rarely get flexion contracture in the toes.

Leddy and Packer's classification of FDP avulsion

Classification for *Closed avulsion* of FDP. Based on the level at which the tendon lies.
- *Type I:* retracts to palm, vincula are disrupted.
- *Type II:* retracts to PIPJ after disruption of the short vincula. Tendon nutrition is preserved so it can be repaired up to 3/12 after injury. However, delay can convert it to a type I injury.
- *Type III:* bony fragment that doesn't pass the A4 pulley. Both vincula are preserved.

Leeches

Leeches are worms of the Annelid phylum, which feed on blood extracted from the host. The most common type used is *Hirudo medicinalis* from Southeast Asia and Europe. They were used 3500 years ago in Egypt. Also in India. They were used in the Middle Ages and extensively in the 19th century for bloodletting. They have been used since 1960 in plastic surgery. In 1981 there was a reported success rate of 60% artery-only digit replants.

Indications: Venous congestion may lead to oedema, reduced capillary and arterial flow, and venous and arterial thrombosis. Leeches may assist in flap salvage. They may be used to decongest replanted parts. If there is a good arterial inflow and poor venous outflow consider leech therapy. Venous competence is usually restored by day 4–5 for digits and 6–10 for free flaps.

Action:
- The front sucker conceals cartilaginous cutting plates that make a 2-mm incision. In 30 minutes a leech can ingest 10 times its own body weight or 5–15 ml of blood.
- Hirudin, an anticoagulant is injected. This inhibits the conversion of fibrinogen to fibrin. It also blocks platelet aggregation in response to thrombin. As thrombin is the final common pathway it is regarded as the most potent anticoagulant.
- Leech saliva also contains a local anaesthetic, hyaluronidase and a histamine like vasodilator.

Complications:
- Infection with *Aeromonas hydrophila*, which is found in the gut of the leech. This is a Gram-negative rod and may infect up to 20% of patients. Give prophylaxis with third generation cephalosporin aminoglycoside.
- May cause significant blood loss.

Application: May prick the flap to encourage the leeches to feed. Direct the head (narrow end) to the flap. If they fail to feed it is a poor prognostic indicator for flap survival. They feed for about 30 minutes.

Leg ulcers

Aetiology: Venous ulceration accounts for most cases of ulceration. 27% of adults have venous insufficiency, with 1.5% having ulceration. (*Venous hypertension*, *Venous ulcers*).

Differential diagnosis: is extensive, including:
- Vascular disease.
- Tumours.
- Metabolic disease.
- Vasculitis.
- Haematological.
- Infectious.
- Insect bites.
- Drugs.
- Radiation.
- Frostbite.
- Weber–Christian disease.
- Lichen planus.
- Trophic ulcers.
- Self-induced.

Pneumonic – VATIMAN:
- *Venous.*
- *Arterial.*
- *Trauma:* insect bites, trophic, frostbite, radiation.
- *Infection:* bacterial, fungal TB, syphilis.
- *Metabolic:* DM, necrobiosis lipoidica, pyoderma gangrenosum, porphyria, gout.
- *Autoimmune:* lupus, RA, polyarteritis nodosa.
- *Neoplasia:* SCC, BCC, Kaposi sarcoma, lymphoma.

Investigations: To determine the cause of the ulcer – wound swab, ABPI – normally 1.2. Venous duplex scanning and arterial studies. XR, biopsy.

Management: Is tailored to the underlying cause of the ulceration. Arterial inflow deficiency will require arterial reconstruction, see *Venous ulcers* for their management.

Non-operative treatment: Elevate, hygiene, compression.

Surgery: Subfascial ligation of perforating vessels, skin graft, flap reconstruction.

Plantar forefoot ulcers: Usually over the metatarsal heads. Exposes bone and tendons and require digital amputations. Metatarsal head resection, conservative for big toe, resections for 2–4 and amputation for 5th. Plantar V–Y advancement flaps, islanded toe flaps, or distally based muscle flaps.

Heel ulcer: Wide osseous debridement. Local rotation/advancement flaps, instep island flaps, turnover muscle flaps and free flaps.

Sickle cell ulcers: Occur in 25–75% of homozygous sickle cell disease. They are chronic, recurrent, painful and disabling. Minor trauma causes sickling and thrombosis, ischaemia and further ulceration. Skin grafts are not helpful as they do not bring in any new blood supply. Free flaps are the procedure of choice. The ischaemia is not inevitably detrimental. Perform exchange transfusion, maintain haematocrit at 31–35%, washout flap with warm heparinized saline-dextran, give dextran and aspirin, warm, antibiotics, oxygen.

Legueu: septa of

- The septa of Legueu and Juvara originate from the palmar fascia at the level of the proximal edge of the flexor tendon sheath and pass dorsally between the lateral surfaces of the A1 pulleys and the digital neurovascular bundles.
- They attach to the deep transverse metacarpal ligament at the point of insertion of the volar plate of the MCP joint.

See Retinacular system

Leiomyomas

- Benign cutaneous tumours consisting of smooth muscle proliferation.
- Multiple cutaneous leiomyomas occur in widely varying numbers.
- Frequently they harden and become painful on pressure or application of cold. They may arise from arrectores pilorum muscles.
- Solitary angioleiomyomas are seen mainly on the legs. They may be sensitive to pressure and cold and may arise from venular smooth muscle.
- A third variety is found in the scrotum, labia majora, or nipple area.
- Treatment is by excision, but recurrence is frequent.

Lentigo

- Pigmented flat lesions that increase with age and are frequently found on the face and neck.
- They contain increased numbers of melanocytes. They persist in the absence of sunlight. Three types:
  ○ *lentigo simplex*: young and middle aged;
  ○ *lentigo senilis*: elderly;
  ○ *solar lentigo*: occurs after sun exposure.
See Naevus.

Lentigo maligna

- Also Hutchinson's melanotic freckle.
- Elderly patients, sun-exposed areas of face and extremities.
- It is a melanoma *in situ*.
- Slow radial growth phase of 10–15 years. Mottled.
- Transformation to *Melanoma* occurs in 30–50%.
- Treat by excision.

LEOPARD syndrome

- May be due to a mutation in the stem cell pool of the neural crest giving cutaneous and neurological defects. It is a rare condition.
- Small dark macules.
- Lentigines.
- Electrocardiographic conduction abnormalities.
- Ocular hypertelorism.
- Pulmonary stenosis.
- Abnormalities of genitalia.
- Retardation of growth.
- Deafness.

Leprosy

Leprosy affects primarily the skin and peripheral nerves, producing characteristic deformities – the lepra facies, reconstruction for leprosy are:

- The commonest peripheral neuropathy is ulnar nerve palsy followed by median nerve palsy. Treatment may require tendon transfers.
- Common deformities that are typical of the face in leprosy:
  ○ megalolobule of the external ear;
  ○ loss of eyebrows;
  ○ nasal deformity;

- ○ sagging and wrinkled redundant facial skin;
- ○ lagophthalmos.

Lesion

When examining a lesion, remember S^3C^2M
- Site.
- Size.
- Shape.
- Colour.
- Consistency.
- Mobility.

Leucoplakia

- White patch, found on oral, vulval, vaginal mucosa.
- In the mouth it is often seen in older men, linked to smoking, poor-fitting dentures and poor oral hygiene.
- Microscopically get hyperkeratosis and acanthosis. Get cellular atypia in epidermal layer and inflammatory infiltrate in dermal layer.
- 15–20% undergo malignant transformation. The _Squamous cell carcinoma_ that develop are much more aggressive than those associated with _Solar keratosis_.

Levator palpabrae superioris

- Arises from roof of orbit in front of optic foramen and above superior rectus muscle. Passes forward for 40 mm to end just behind the septum as an aponeurosis.
- Close to the origin of the aponeurosis the muscle sheath is thickened above the muscle to form a band – Whitnall's ligament. This may be a definite structure or a more diffuse thickening. It inserts into the trochlea medially, and the capsule of the lacrimal gland and orbital wall laterally. It acts as a fulcrum for the action of the levator.
- The levator aponeurosis descends into the lid and the septum inserts onto its anterior surface as a thickened band 8 mm below Whitnall's ligament and 3 mm above tarsus. The angle formed contains the pre-aponeurotic fat pad. As the aponeurosis descends it becomes thinner and fans out. It inserts anteriorly into orbicularis muscle at the skin crease and below into the lower anterior surface of the tarsal plate.

Levator veli palatini

Origin: Inferior surface of petrous temporal bone and medial rim of Eustachian tube.

Insertion: Palatine aponeurosis.

Action: Elevates, retracts and laterally deviates the soft palate. It may open the Eustachian tube on swallowing.

Nerve supply: Pharyngeal branch of vagus nerve with motor fibres from the cranial accessory nerve. See _Cleft palate_.

Lhermitte sign

- Sudden painful or electrical sensation on flexing the neck.
- Spreads to the lower cervical or lumbosacral spine into the limbs.

Seen in multiple sclerosis, cervical myopathy or after head injury.

Ligamentotaxis

- Refers to the maintenance of traction distal to an injured joint during a period of healing.
- This distal traction force on the periarticular ligaments and palmar plate attachments results in reduction of some articular fracture fragments, and any associated joint dislocation with realignment of the joint surface.

Lignocaine

Local anaesthetic: Maximal dose plain is 3 mg/kg. With adrenaline is 7 mg/kg, e.g. 70 kg man and 2% lignocaine plain = $70 \times 3 \div 20 =$ 10.5 ml; 80 kg man with 2% with = $80 \times 7 \div 20$ = 28 ml.

Limberg flap

See _Rhombic flap_.

Linburg's sign

Flexion of index DIP joint when thumb IPJ is flexed. Present in 30% of people due to adhesions in the carpal tunnel between FPL and FDP index. May cause a problem in musicians.

Linburg's syndrome

Symptomatic restrictive thumb-index flexor tenosynovitis with hypertrophic tenosynovium between FPL and FDP. Forearm pain is aggravated when index DIP joint is blocked when the thumb is flexed.

Treatment: Rest, NSAIDs, steroids. Surgery involved exploring the distal forearm and wrist and dividing any tendinous interconnections.

Lingual flap

Dorsal lingual flap:

- Must not cross the median raphe. Elevated at 8 mm thickness to include mucosa, submucosa and superficial muscle.
- Posteriorly based can be used for retromolar triangle. Anteriorly based can repair cheek and commissure. Transverse flaps can repair floor of mouth (FOM) defects.

Lingual tip: Perimeter flaps can be raised.

Ventral surface flaps: Used for FOM with skin graft to donor.
See *Oral cavity reconstruction.*

Linton flap

- Used in the treatment of *Venous ulcers.*
- Aims to divide the perforators between the superficial and deep system.
- Incision is parallel and 2 cm posterior to the medial tibial border from medial malleolus to midcalf.
- Deep fascia is divided and all perforating veins are ligated. It can be performed endoscopically.

Lip anatomy

Important landmarks are the commissure, philtral columns, Cupid's bow.

Muscles:

- *Orbicularis oris:* provide oral competence. Originate lateral to the commissure (modiolus) and insert into the opposite philtral column:
  - horizontal muscle fibres compress the lips;
  - oblique fibres evert the lip; these fibres travel upward and medially from the modiolus to insert at the anterior nasal

spine, nasal septum, and anterior nasal floor.

- *Levator labii superioris* muscle originates from the inferior and medial orbital margin and curves around the alar base to insert into the orbicularis oris fibres and the philtral column on the ipsilateral side.
- *Levator anguli oris* muscle arises just below the lateral edge of the LLS.
- *Zygomaticus major* muscle extends from the malar eminence and inserts into the modiolus.
- *Nasalis* muscle has three components, which arise from bone below the piriform aperture.
- *Depressor septi* muscle is the most medial muscle. This paired muscle arises from the periosteum over the central and lateral incisors to insert into the footplates of the medial crura. It depresses the tip of the nose and lifts the upper central lip.
- *Mentalis* muscles elevate the lower lip. They originate from alveolar periosteum just below the vestibular sulcus and descend obliquely to insert into the skin of the chin.
- *Depressor labii inferioris* (quadratus) arises from the lower border of the mandible. The fibres pass upward and medially, to join orbicularis oris. It depresses the lower lip.
- *Depressor anguli oris* (triangularis) arises inferior to the quadratus muscle and continues upward to the modiolus. It draws the angle of the mouth downward and laterally.

Innervation:

- *Motor:* buccal and zygomatic branches of facial nerve for upper and mandibular for lower lip.
- *Sensory:* superior labial nerve from infraorbital branch of trigeminal nerve for upper and inferior alveolar nerve from the mental nerve for lower lip.

Vascular: Facial artery arises between mandible and anterior border of masseter, divides at commissure to form the superior and inferior labial artery.

Lymphatics: Drain to submandibular and submental nodes.

Vermilion border: Also white roll, transition between mucosa of the lip and skin. Alignment important.

Lip carcinoma

Diagnosis:
- Most tumours of the upper lip are BCCs and of the lower lip SCCs.
- 5% of SCCs occur on the upper lip. 2% affect the commissure, which is difficult to reconstruct and has a high metastatic potential.
- If nodes are present, disease survival drops from 90 to 50%.

Treatment: T1 and T2 surgery and RT equally effective.

See *Head and neck cancer*

Lip reconstruction

Reconstructive principles:
- ¼ to ⅓ of lip length can be excised and primarily sutured. Preserve sensation, and ensure anatomic alignment. Major problem is reduction of size of the mouth. The lower lip has a less complex shape and can be reduced without cosmetic compromise.

Vermilion reconstruction:
- Vermilion is a modified mucosal surface. It is the most visible portion of the lip. It is very sensitive.
- Lip shave procedure performed for widespread field change particularly of the lower lip. Primary closure may be possible. If there is too much tension perform a buccal advancement by releasing mucosa in the deep sulcus and elevated deep to salivary glands just superficial to muscle. This bipedicled flap is then advanced.
- *Tongue flaps* in two stages give a poor cosmetic colour match and have a feminizing effect on men. It also has fine papilla. If less than ⅓ of lip width excised, an advancement flap of vermilion is performed.
- *Vermilion switch flap* can be used.
- *Notch deformities* of vermilion: Perform excision, Z-plasty, V–Y advancement.

Commissure reconstruction

Lower lip reconstruction:
- Anaesthesia with *Mental nerve block*. For the region below the labiomental fold also need local premandibular infiltration or bilateral inferior alveolar nerve blocks

along the medial border of the mandibular ramus.
- *Wedge excision*: for tumour avoid simple V incision as this will not give adequate tumour clearance towards the apex of the V. Instead perform a W incision.
- *Step ladder technique (Johanson):*
- *Abbé flap*: for lower lip place flap at junction of mid and lateral thirds to spare the philtrum and commissure. If the incision is placed in the philtrum the scar will occur in a naturally occurring ridge.
- *Estlander flap*: a laterally based switch flap pedicled on the labial artery.
- *Karapandzic flap*: a modification of the Gilles' fan flap, which maintains the neurovascular pedicle in the soft tissue giving better functional results.
- *Bernard operation*: advancement of full thickness flaps with triangular excision.
- *Webster modification* of Bernard operation: excises skin only in the Burow's triangles.
- *Gilles' fan flap*: fan-shaped rotational advancement flap based on the superior labial artery.
- *McGregor flap*: rectangular-shaped flap, based on superior labial artery, which is rotated around the commissure without reducing the size of the stoma.
- *Schuchardt flap*: the defect is excised as a rectangular defect and the incision is extended around the labiomental fold to the submental region on each side to allow lip to slide into the defect.

Defects over 65%:
- Depends on the availability of tissue. Bilateral cheek advancement or composite flaps, otherwise free flaps.
- *Free flap*: for very large defects. Radial forearm flap with palmaris longus tendon attached to the modiolus enables the flap to act as a dam. Ensure harvest of enough tissue to act as a sulcus. Antebrachial nerve can be co-apted to mental nerve. Usually the lip remains immobile and insensate.
- *Upper lip*: more difficult to reconstruct because of the more complex shape:
  ○ Small defects can be closed directly.

- *Medium defects*: <u>*Abbé flap*</u>. Excision of per-iled crescents may enable a decrease in defect size to accommodate the Abbé flap.
- *Large defects:*
  - reverse <u>*Karapandzic flap*</u>;
  - <u>*Bernard*</u> procedure for large defects perform an inverted;
  - total reconstruction depends on the available tissue; bilateral cheek advancement, nasolabial flaps or innervated composite flaps can be used;
  - composite radial forearm flaps with palmaris longus or bone may be used.
- *Vascularized scalp island flap:* to replace particularly burned upper lip with hair bearing skin in the male. An island of scalp centred over the posterior branch of the superficial temporal artery is designed high enough in the parietal scalp to allow for adequate rotation. The Dopplered vessels are dissected to anterior tragus and passed through a tunnel.

Lipodermatosclerosis

See <u>*Venous ulcers*</u>. Brawny oedema seen in venous ulceration.

Liposuction

History:

- The beginnings of liposuction occurred in 1921 when Dujarrier attempted to reduce the fat from the knees of a ballerina. Injury to the femoral artery resulted in amputation.
- Curettage was commenced again in the 1960s by Schrudde, following which suction was added.
- Liposuction is the aspiration of fat by cannulae attached to high vacuum. The skin shrinks, the stroma with vessels and nerves remains intact.

Ultrasound-assisted liposuction:

- Ultrasound energy is transmitted to a piezo-electric transducer, which transforms sounds waves to mechanical vibrations that are transmitted to a titanium probe. This induces tissue cavitation and melting.
- It is more effective and easier, but is more traumatic and slower than conventional liposuction.

Power-assisted liposuction: Non-ultrasonic. Maximize fat removal while reducing the effort.

Tumescent infiltration:

- All areas to be liposucked are first injected with dilute lignocaine and adrenaline until turgid. Vasoconstriction occurs after 10 minutes.
- Recipe for tumescent injection
- 2% lignocaine   25 ml
- 1:1000 epinephrine 1 ml
- Lactated Ringer's solution   1000 ml
- Gives 1026 ml of 0.05% lignocaine with 1:1 000 000 epinephrine
- IV fluid replacement may not be necessary as fluid is absorbed Expansion eases the passage of the cannula. Doses of lignocaine exceed those recommended but absorption into the circulation is slow.

Aspiration: Use multiple access incisions. Pinch thickness should be 1–3 cm. A visual reduction should be apparent.

Complications: Contour irregularities, damage to adjacent structures, paraesthesia, haemorrhage, fluid shifts, death – a few have been reported, mostly due to PE.
See <u>*Fat anatomy*</u>.

Littler neurovascular island flap

- For large volar thumb defects to bring sensation to thumb.
- Skin and subcutaneous tissue from the ulnar side of long or ring finger is transposed across the palm as a neurovascular island flap.
- Digital nerve fascicles are dissected from common digital nerve in the palm. Preserve a cuff of tissue around the pedicle to preserve venous drainage. Perform a digital Allen's test.
- Probably the middle finger should preferably be used as it is also median nerve.
See <u>*Fingertip injuries*</u>.

LOAF

Mnemonic for innervation of muscles by the median nerve in the hand –
- *L:* 2 radial lumbricals.
- *O:* opponens brevis.

- *A:* abductor pollicis brevis.
- *F:* superficial head of flexor pollicis brevis.

Local anaesthetics

History:
- *Cocaine* (an ester) was the first to be used but was addictive and dangerous.
- Procaine was used in 1905.
- Two groups esters and amide. *Lignocaine* was discovered in 1948. True allergic reaction of amides is extremely rare.

Action:
- Reversibly prevent nerve conduction by blocking sodium channels.
- The rate of metabolism of local anaesthetics is related to the number of additional carbon atoms on the aromatic or the amine side of the molecule.
- Potency and toxicity are determined by the structure of the aromatic and the amine group.
- Anaesthetic potency is determined primarily by the degree of lipid solubility.
- The onset of action is primarily due to the pKa.
- They exist in anionic non-ionized and cationic ionized form. Preparations are acidic so have more cationic. The anionic form penetrates the nerve membrane. Adding sodium bicarbonate increases the anionic form and speeds onset. Also decreases discomfort.

Duration:
- Duration of action is related to the degree of binding to a protein receptor in the sodium channel and the vasodilatatory effect. Metabolism is affected by age, liver failure and CCF.

Systemic:
- The CNS is more sensitive to toxicity and is made more sensitive by hypercarbia, hypoxia and acidosis.
- Patients may experience dizziness, tinnitus, circumoral numbness, loss of consciousness and fitting.
- After CNS excitation get depression and respiratory arrest.
- LAs prolong conduction time in the heart and produce a long PR interval. High concentrations will depress the sinus node and lead to sinus bradycardia and sinus arrest. They also exert a direct myocardial depressant affect.
- Bupivicaine can produce VF.
- The CVS toxic dose compared with the CNS toxic dose for lignocaine is 7× and for bupivicaine is 3.5×.

See Tumescent technique.

Long posterior flap below-knee amputation

- The rationale for this flap is that the anterior skin has the least good blood supply and the posterior skin is supplied by perforators through gastrocnemius/soleus.
- This muscle mass retains knee flexion.
- Tibia sectioned 10–12 cm below tibial plateau. Mark circumferential line at this level. Mark axial lines extending distally.
- The posterior flap should be rather more than ⅓ of the circumference of the limb – less will reduce vascularity, more will increase the dog ears. Anterior incision cuts to bone. Anterior compartment muscles divided at this level. Ligate anterior tibial vessels and divide nerve. Incise interosseus membrane. Divide peroneal muscles. Transect fibula high. Divide tibia 2 cm below anterior skin incision. Transect tibialis posterior. Extend skin incision distally cutting along gastrocnemius/soleus. Remove specimen. Cut muscle to give smooth slope. Resect muscle medially and laterally. Some suggest soleus should be completely resected. Ligate vessels. Fold over flaps and trim muscle and skin. Suction drain. Suture aponeurosis to anterior tibial periosteum. Suture skin without tension.
- An alternative which gives a better stump shape is the skew flap.

Longitudinal arrest: congenital hand

- Congenital hand anomaly with digital skeletal elements.
- Fit prosthesis activated by digits:
  - complete: hand on trunk;
  - *proximal:* forearm on trunk;
  - *distal:* hand on humerus.

Lop ear
- Also cup ear or constricted ear.
- Encircling helix seems tight like a purse string with helical and scaphal hooding.
- 1:10 of prominent ears.

Treatment:
- Determined by the height of the lop ear in comparison to the normal side.
- Reshape existing tissues or supplement skin and cartilage.
- May need to excise overhanging cartilage and may require cartilage grafts or repair as for microtia.

See Ear reconstruction.

Louis–Bar syndrome
Also called ataxia-telangiectasis.
- A neurovascular disorder.
- Autosomal recessive inheritance that appears at 3–6 years of life.
- Telangiectasis occur on the nasal and temporal area and then on the upper half of the body.
- Cerebella ataxia also begins in early childhood, followed by progressive neuromotor degeneration.
- Also get endocrine dysfunction, chromosomal instability, immunologic deficiencies, and growth retardation.
- Death usually occurs in the 20s from recurrent sinopulmonary infections and bronchiectasis or from lymphoreticular malignancy.
- Heterozygous carriers of the gene also may be at significantly increased risk for cancer.

Love's sign
- Clinical test seen with *Glomus tumour*.
- The presence of one very painful localized spot on palpation.

Lower limb anatomy
Thigh:
- *Femoral triangle:* bounded by: inguinal ligament, medial border of adductor longus, lateral border of sartorius. *Roof:* fascia lata. *Floor:* psoas, illiacus, pectineus, adductor longus. *Contents:* femoral nerve, artery and vein, deep inguinal nodes.
- *Anterior thigh muscles:* rectus femoris, vastus lateralis, medialis and intermedialis, sartorius
- *Adductors:* adductor magnus, adductor longus, adductor brevis, gracilis.
- *Hamstrings:* biceps femoris, semimembranosus, semitendinosus.
- *Fascia lata:* deep fascia of the whole of the thigh. Tensor fasciæ latæ is inserted between its layers. Attachments are the sacrum and coccyx, inguinal ligament, iliac crest, superior ramus of the pubis, inferior ramus, tuberosity of the ischium and sacrotuberous ligament. Forms iliotibial band which attaches to the lateral condyle of the tibia.
- *Blood vessels:* femoral artery; profunda femoris, and its lateral and medial circumflex branches; muscular branches. Femoral vein, great (long) and short saphenous veins,
- *Nerve supply to muscles:*
  - obturator: adductors (magnus, longus and brevis), gracilis;
  - *femoral:* quadrates femoris, pectineus, sartorius, iliacus, superior gluteal, TFL;
  - *sciatic:* semitendinosus, semimembranosus, biceps femoris, adductor magnus.
- *Cutaneous nerve supply:* cutaneous branches of femoral nerve (medial, intermediate, lateral and posterior), cutaneous branches of obturator nerve.

Lower leg:
- *Anterior compartment:* contains extensor muscles, tibialis anterior, extensor hallucis longus, extensor digitorum longus. Anterior tibial artery and deep peroneal nerve.
- *Lateral compartment:* peroneus longus, brevis and tertius. No artery, but a superficial peroneal nerve.
- *Posterior superficial compartment:* contains soleus and gastrocnemius.
- *Posterior deep compartment:* tibialis posterior, flexor digitorum longus, flexor hallucis longus. Contains posterior tibial artery, peroneal artery and posterior tibial nerve.
- *Nerves:*
  - Sensory supply:
    - *sural:* lateral midfoot;
    - *posterior tibial:* heel/plantar midfoot;
    - *deep peroneal:* first web;
    - *superficial peroneal:* dorsal midfoot;
    - *saphenous:* medial ankle.

Lower limb reconstruction

Indications: Required for fractures, chronic wounds, unstable scars, sarcoma, diabetes, radiation, osteomyelitis, ischaemia.

Methods: Local muscle advancement flaps, fasciocutaneous flaps and distant flaps.

Hip:
• To cover exposed metalwork or pressure necrosis.
• TFL has little muscle bulk.
• Vastus lateralis has good muscle and a skin paddle with little functional loss.
• Rectus femoris can be used similarly, but with not so much bulk.
• Extended deep inferior epigastric flap is a good alternative for large hip defects. This is essentially a VRAM with an adjacent random element. It may extend up to the knee (pennant flap).
• Lat dorsi free flap is the best free tissue transfer.

Mid-thigh:
• Gracilis, but not much bulk.
• Vastus medialis is supplied by perforators along its length so it can't be rotated. It can be transposed medially.

Knee:
• Gastrocnemius, but may not cross to other side of knee or superiorly.
• Distally based vastus lateralis is not reliable distally.
• Saphenous fasciocutaneous flap may be useful.
• Extensive defects require a free flap.

Proximal tibia:
• Medial and lateral gastrocnemius (shorter than medial).
• Fasciocutaneous flaps including saphenous flap.
• Free flap.

Mid-tibia:
• Turnover flap of tibialis anterior for small defects.
• Soleus muscle useful for larger defects.
• Fasciocutaneous flaps.
• Free flaps.

Ankle/distal tibia:
• Extensor digitorum brevis for small defects.
• Lateral fasciocutaneous flap for larger defects.
• Dorsalis pedis flap.
• Distally based fasciocutaneous flaps including the sural flap.

Foot:
• Classification: Hidalgo and Shaw.
• Small muscle flaps, but rarely useful.
• Sural artery flap.
• Free flap.

Achilles tendon and malleolar area:
• Local fasciocutaneous flaps.
• Lateral calcaneal flap can be sensate with a flap length of up to 14 cm if delayed.
• Dorsalis pedis flap can provide sensate coverage.
• The extensor digitorum brevis is the most useful local muscle flap, based on the lateral tarsal-dorsalis pedis pedicle.
• Temperoparietal flap and radial forearm free flap may provide thin coverage.

Heel and mid-plantar foot:
• Tissue needs to be able to withstand shear forces. Durability and sensory loss important.
• Can use muscle flaps with skin grafts or fasciocutaneous flaps.
• The flap should fit well, not be too thick and underlying bony problems should be corrected.
• For the neuropathic foot, ulcer may need to be debrided with the underlying bone.
• Medial plantar flaps can be raised with plantar nerves.

Distal plantar and forefoot: Most require free tissue transfer.

Dorsum:
• If tendons are exposed then vascularized coverage is required.
• Fascial free flaps such as TPF provide thin coverage, which allows tendon gliding.

Cross-leg flap:
• Involving raising a flap from the contralateral leg and leaving attached for 3–5 weeks.

- Very few indications as the patient suffers discomfort and stiffness although it is better tolerated in a child.
- The posterior thigh may be used and neurorrhaphy performed with the inferior gluteal nerve.

Tarsal tunnel syndrome:

Amputation:

- Primary amputation for trauma if limb survival and function are unlikely. Sciatic/posterior tibial function important.
- Use mangled extremity severity score (*MESS*), and *Gustilo score* for open fractures.
- *Absolute indications:* unreconstructible NV, skeletal or soft tissue injury.
- *Relative indication:* when function or appearance of the limb will be inferior to a prosthesis.

Replantation:

- frequently not performed as unable to restore neurology and good function from prosthetics.
- More favourable outcome in a child.
- Consider if a clean cut with short ischaemic time. If replantation is not going to be performed, consider using limb for grafts.

Papineau technique:

Free flaps:

- Successful in fresh wounds >95%, less successful in infected wound (80%).
- Godina advocates early free flap within 3 days of an open fracture.

Nerve repair:

- Sharp lacerations require immediate repair. If there is extensive contusion, wait 2–3 weeks. Prognosis varies and depends on distance.
- *Femoral nerve palsy:* unable to fully extend the knee giving a significant disability when walking uphill. Should be explored as some recovery should occur.
- *Sciatic nerve injuries:* get better recovery in the tibial than the peroneal distribution. Repair in the buttock may give some plantar flexion and some plantar sensation. High lesions often have severe vasomotor and trophic changes. Peroneal return does not usually occur.

- *Tibial nerve injuries:* are very disabling as the terminal branches supply plantar sensation and also sympathetic supply. Partial recovery of motor and sensation should occur following repair.
- *Common peroneal nerve:* the most frequently injured peripheral nerve as it is so superficial. Post-operative results are the poorest. Loss leads to foot drop and equino varus.

Lower limb trauma

Classifications:

- *Gustilo score.*
- *MESS.*
- *Hidalgo classification.*
- *Byrd and Spicer.*
- *Arnez and Tyler classification.*
- AO classification.

History: Establish mechanism of trauma to give an indication as to the amount of energy transferred.

Examination:

- ATLS principles, with neurovascular assessment.
- Size of defect, degloving, associated injuries, segmental injuries, imprints.

Management: Debride, lavage, fracture stabilization, 2nd look, soft tissue cover.

Lumbosacral back flap

- Used for the coverage of *Pressure sores*.
- Based on contralateral lumbar perforators, L1–5.
- Covers medium-sized pressure sores of the sacrum, but only with skin.

Lumbrical muscles

- Worm like. Four lumbricals. Flex MPJ and extend IPJs.
- The work horse of the extensor apparatus.
- The only muscles with no bony attachment.

Origin:

- Arise from radial side of FDP tendons and pass volar to the intermetacarpal ligaments.
- 1st and 2nd are attached to index and middle FDP whereas 3rd and 4th are attached to 2 adjacent FDPs of middle and ring, and ring and little.

- They run on the radial side of the digits. A narrow flat tendon emerges from the muscle at the MCP joint to join the radial edge of the extensor aponeurosis at an angle of 40°.
- The radial 2 lumbricals join the dorsal interossei, whereas the ulnar two join the palmar interossei.

Insertion: The lateral slip of the extensor tendons.

Nerve supply: Radial two are median and ulnar two are ulnar nerve.

Function: Extension of IPJs in any position of MCP joint. They are important in balancing flexors and extensors. Relaxation of FDP decreases the antagonistic force and so decreases the resistance on the extensor apparatus.
See *Claw hand*.

Lunate: fracture
- Uncommon.
- Two patterns:
  - impaction from axial load between capitate and radius;
  - dorsal avulsion or impaction caused by impingement on the dorsal edge of the radius.
- Get mid-dorsal wrist pain. This may predispose to *Kienbocks Disease*.
- Treat non-displaced fractures with immobilization.
- If displaced, perform open reduction through a dorsal approach.

Lund and Browder chart
Used to accurately assess the size of *Burns*, which allows for age group differences.

Lunotriquetral compression test
- Loads lunotriquetral joint along ulnoradial axis by palpating within the ulnar snuffbox.
- Direct pressure causes pain with lunotriquetral instability, synovitis, degenerative disease, partial synchondrosis.

Lunula
White arc of *Nail* distal to eponychium. Due to persistence of nuclei in cells of germinal matrix. Nail becomes transparent as they disintegrate.

Lupus vulgaris
- Rare form of cutaneous tuberculosis.
- Destruction of soft tissues followed by atrophic scarring.
- Active areas of disease are studded with lupus nodules.
- It needs to be distinguished from cold abscess.

Treatment:
- Anti-tuberculosis chemotherapy.
- Scarring may require excision.
- Previous attempts to treat with radiotherapy led to SCCs within the lupus.

Lymph node levels in head and neck cancer
Level I:
- *Submental:* between anterior belly of digastrics and above hyoid.
- *Submandibular* between anterior and posterior belly of digastric and mandibular angle.

Level II:
- *Upper jugular:* from skull base to bifurcation of carotid or hyoid. Posteriorly is the SCM, anteriorly is the sternohyoid.
- The lymphatics of the anterior triangle course along the internal jugular vein. They are embedded in the carotid sheath and most lie anterolaterally to the vein.
- Level II nodes are often extracapsular and XI nerve must be sacrificed to clear them.

Level III:
- *Middle jugular:* from inferior border of level II to omohyoid.
- Level III drain the middle part of the aerodigestive tract, larynx, pharynx and hypopharynx.

Level IV:
- *Lower jugular:* from inferior border of level III to clavicle.
- Level IV drain thyroid, oesophagus and trachea

Level V:
- *Posterior triangle:* around lower portion of spinal accessory nerve, along the transverse cervical vessels. Bounded by a triangle formed by the clavicle, posterior border of SCM and anterior border of trapezius.
- The nodes in the posterior triangle course along the spinal accessory nerve. They are not often involved in oral cancers. Small nodes along the transverse cervical vessels are more frequently involved with chest primaries.

Level VI:
- *Anterior compartment:* from hyoid to suprasternal notch. Lateral border is medial border of carotid sheath. Includes parathyroidal and paratracheal lymph nodes and those along the recurrent laryngeal nerves.
See *Head and neck cancer*. See *Neck dissection*.

Lymphangioma circumscriptum
Cutaneous *Lymphatic malformations*, which can often can be resected totally and the defect closed with a split-thickness skin graft.

Lymphangiosarcoma
- Rare consequence of long-standing *Lymphoedema*.
- Most are post-mastectomy with long-standing obstruction.
- Aggressive, metastasize early and non-responsive to chemo- and radiotherapy.
- Limb amputation is advised.
- Average survival 19 months.
- When it is related to post-mastectomy oedema it is called Stewart–Treves syndrome.

Lymphatic malformations
- They can be described as either microcystic, macrocystic or combined forms.
- Previously microcystic was called lymphangioma and macrocystic was called cystic hygroma.
- They never involute, but expand and contract depending on the ebb and flow of lymphatic fluid.
- Most are seen at birth or within 2 years, but they can occur in the older child or the adult.

- Dilated lymphatics in the skin present as vesicles which form red nodules with bleeding.
- Those in the face are usually combined *Vascular malformations*, and cause facial asymmetry and possibly cause airway obstruction.
- It may be confused with a VM or it may be a combined LVM.

Treatment:
- Sudden enlargement is usually due to bleeding or cellulitis. Treat with antibiotics and NSAIDs.
- Large cysts can be treated with aspiration of lymphatic fluid and instillation of sclerosant agents, for example, pure ethanol, sodium tetradecyl sulphate.
- Resection is the only way to remove a LM.
- Surgical guidelines are:
  o focus on a defined anatomic region;
  o define the duration of the procedure;
  o limit the acceptable blood loss;
  o perform as thorough a resection as possible, given anatomic restrictions.
- Transected lymphatic channels regenerate after subtotal excision leading to recurrence.

Complications: Immediate post-operative complications include prolonged serous drainage, haematoma and cellulitis.
See *Lymphangioma circumscriptum*.

Lymphatics
Function:
- Endothelial-lined channels, which transport fluid, proteins and particles from the interstitial compartment to the vascular system.
- Also presents foreign matter to the immune system.
- In the intestines they also transport triglycerides and chylomicrons.

Anatomy:
- Embryologically the lymphatics develop from the venous system.
- They do not have well-defined basement membranes.
- Epidermal lymphatics have no valves, dermal lymphatics have small valves.
- A cutaneous network of valveless channels drain into valved vessels in the subdermal

layer. These join to follow the major veins. These drain to nodal basins *en route* to the right and left subclavian veins.

- In the abdomen the lumbar lymphatic trunks join to form the cisterna chyli – a thin walled sac lying in front of the L1–2 vertebrae.
- This becomes the thoracic duct, which enters the left subclavian vein.
- The right lymphatic duct drains into the right sublcavian from the arm, chest and head and neck.
- Lymphatics are not present in CNS, muscle, tendon, cartilage, bone.

Action: Lymph is propelled by external muscle compression, helped by valves, pulsations from vessels, and intra-abdominal and intra-thoracic pressures. Smooth muscle in the lymphatics regulates calibre.
See *Lymphoedema*.

Lymphoedema

- The accumulation of protein-rich fluid in the interstitial space leading to enlargement. The protein activates inflammation, but phagocytosis is impaired. Collagen deposition is increased in response to injury. Get thickened fibrosed channels which work ineffectively. Stasis predisposes to infection, which can worsen the lymphoedema. Mainly *Strep.* and *Staph.* No medical or surgical cure exists.
- Goals of treatment are reduction of fluid accumulation, reduction of complications, and improved limb function. Typical history is of gradual oedema unilaterally.

Anatomy:
- If there is no particular insult, 77% of lymphatics are hypoplastic and 15% are aplastic. 8% are hyperplastic with tortuous lymphatics with valvular incompetence.

Malignant change: *Lymphangiosarcoma*.

Classification: Traditionally divided into primary and secondary. However, it may be that it is a spectrum with severe disease being manifested at birth and less severe disease being manifested at a variable time after birth depending on the type of insults and the ability to compensate.

Primary lymphoedema:
- A diagnosis of exclusion. Classify into congenital, early and late.
- *Lymphoedema congenita* is 15% of primary lymphoedema and 15% are familial (Milroy's disease, F:M 2:1, lower extremities).
- *Lymphoedema praecox* (early primary lymphoedema) accounts for 75% of lymphoedema and onset is before 35 years. More common in women and in the lower extremities.
- *Lymphoedema tarda:* after 35 years.

Secondary lymphoedema:
- Results from damage to lymphatics. In developed countries mainly due to metastatic tumour and lymphadenectomies. In developing countries, filiariasis by the organism *Wuchereria bancrofti* produces elephantiasis.
- Five Is.
- *Invasion:* primary lymphatic tumours, secondary tumours.
- *Infection:* filariasis, lymphogranuloma, TB.
- *Inflammation:* snake bites, insect bites.
- *Irradiation.*
- *Iatrogenic:* lymph node dissection, varicose vein.

Imaging:
- On CT and MRI get honeycomb appearance.
- Lymphangiograms are rarely performed as they are time-consuming, potentially dangerous and give little useful information.
- Lymphoscintigraphy with technetium-99 radiolabelled colloid is useful for identifying sentinel nodes.

Conservative treatment:
- Elevation, compression stockings, mechanical pump compression. Skin hygiene, diet for obesity.
- Coumarin reduces lymphoedema possibly by increasing the number of macrophages and by increasing the rate of macrophage mediated proteolysis.
- Micronized diosmin has had some success in treatment of ulcers from venous insufficiency and may also be effective with lymphoedema. It decreases capillary permeability.
- *Diuretics:* may be beneficial early in the disease. As diuretics do not clear the protein then the protein levels will actually rise and possibly lead to more fibrosis.

Restorative surgery:
- Many attempts have been made to improve lymphatic drainage, but none have been universally accepted.
- *Lymphangioplasty:* attempts to create new drainage pathways with silk, nylon, Teflon.
- *Buried dermal flaps (Thompson technique):* dermal flaps in muscle in an attempt to communicate between superficial and deep compartments. No evidence that it works and significant complication of flap necrosis and wound infection.
- *Omental transposition:* attempts to bring in functioning lymphatics. Poor long-term results.
- *Enteromesenteric bridge:* bowel denuded of mucosa is transposed. Encouraging results, but no long-term trials.
- *Lymph node-venous anastomosis:* implant transacted lymph node end-to-side with a vein. Results are short-lived.
- *Microlymphaticovenous anastomosis:* variable results, but best when 2 or 3 anastomosis are performed early for secondary lymphoedema.
- *Microsurgical lymphatic grafting:*

Excisional surgery:
- These are presently the most successful. Indicated to reduce the weight and accompanying fatigue, and to reduce the lymphangitis and cellulitis.
- <u>*Charles operation* radical excision:</u> excises all tissue down to muscle and applies skin grafts. Gives a poor result with insensate easily traumatized skin.
- *Homans technique:* longitudinal segment of skin and subcutaneous tissue is removed and the incision edges are sutured.

- *Staged subcutaneous excision:* remove subcutaneous tissue while keeping skin flaps. Less radical than Charles operation and is the most reasonable treatment for the symptoms of lymphoedema. 80% of the lymphatics fluid is carried in the superficial lymphatic system. The theory is to removed diseased lymphatics while preserving the dermal lymphatic plexus. Can give long-term improvement and minimize complications. Plan to remove as much skin and subcutaneous tissue while achieving primary closure. Perform in 2 stages separated by 3 months. Use a TQ. Raise medial flap 1.5 cm thick to mid-sagittal plane of calf. All subcutaneous tissue is removed. Sural nerve is preserved. Deep fascia is excised. Remain superficial to deep fascia at the knee and ankle. Redundant skin is excised. Suction catheter. Laterally the same procedure is employed though deep fascia is preserved.
- *Liposuction:* can be used in primary and secondary lymphoedema with volume reduction of 8–25%. Best when skin elasticity is preserved. Temporary measure.

Genital lymphoedema: Two systems of lymphatic drainage to the genitalia. Superficial lymphatics go to superficial inguinal nodes. A deeper network drains urethra and corpus spongiosum. Genital lymphoedema generally only involves the superficial system. Therefore, treatment involves excision of skin down to Buck's fascia from coronal sulcus to scrotum. Apply meshed graft to scrotum and non-meshed graft to penis.
See <u>Lymphatics</u>.

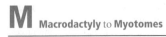
M Macrodactyly to **Myotomes**

Macrodactyly
Nerve territory-orientated macrodactyly.
- Enlargement of all structures in the finger. Distinguish from haemangiomas, vascular malformations, Ollier's disease.

- In 70% an adjacent digit is affected. Index finger is the most commonly affected.
- The enlarged area often corresponds to specific nerve distribution.

Classification:
- *Static or progressive:*
  - *static macrodactyly:* the enlarged finger grows in proportion to the rest of the child;
  - *progressive macrodactyly:* the enlarged finger grows out of proportion to the rest of the child.
- *Syndromic or isolated:*
  - Syndromes include Ollier's, Maffucci, Klippel–Trenauney–Weber syndrome.
- *Type I–IV*
  - Type I: gigantism and lipofibromatosis. Occur in the distribution of a peripheral nerve.
  - Type II: gigantism and neurofibromatosis.
  - Type III: gigantism and digital hyperostosis. Rare. Often bilateral. Nodular due to osteochondral masses.
  - Type IV: gigantism and hemihypertrophy. Rare.

Treatment: Surgery is complicated by delayed healing. Treat by amputation, growth plate ablation, osteotomies and debulking.

Macrophages

Important in _Wound healing_. They infiltrate the wound during the inflammatory phase. They remove debris and orchestrate the events of wound healing. A primary source of _Growth factors_.

Mafenide

- A sulpha medicine, particularly indicated for _Burns_ involving cartilage.
- A broad antibacterial spectrum, though limited activity against MRSA *Staph. aureus.*
- It penetrates eschar well and also cartilage, so it is good for ears and noses. It is applied 12-hourly. It is painful to apply.

Maffuci's syndrome

- Multiple _Enchondromas_ associated with soft tissue vascular malformations.
- Even higher frequency of malignant transformation than _Ollier's_ disease (which is 25% by aged 40 years).
- The vascular lesions are complex venous in type; they can occur in the subcutaneous

tissue, bones (particularly the limbs), the leptomeninges, or the gastrointestinal tract. Patients may develop spindle cell haemangioendotheliomas. See _Complex combined vascular malformations_.

MAGPI

Meatal Advancement and Glansplasty:

- Used in true glanular _Hypospadias_.
- If used for subcoronal meatus get retrusive meatus.
- Essentially the meatus is opened vertically and closed transversely, and the glans is opened transversely and closed vertically.
- Vertical incision of transverse mucosal bar distal to meatus. Close this transversely to advance the dorsal lip of the meatal mucosa out toward the tip of the glans.
- Glansplasty achieved by midline approximation of lateral glanular wings after freeing them from corporal tunica. Closure of the glans flaps moves the meatus towards the glans tip. Close glans in two layers.
- It does not lengthen the urethra and does not correct chordee.

Malignant fibrous histiocytoma

- Present as firm cutaneous or subcutaneous lesion in elderly patients.
- Pathological diagnosis can be difficult, but histochemical analysis for alpha-1-antitrypsin can be helpful.
- Consists of fibroblast like cells with pleomorphic giant cells.
- Two major types, myxoid and inflammatory, latter being the poorer prognosis.
- Associated with leukaemia, neurofibromatosis, Paget's and RT.
- Local recurrence rates are 70%. Propensity for lymph node metastasis.
- Give adjuvant RT.

See _Pseudosarcomatous lesions_. See _Sarcoma_.

Mallet finger

Loss of continuity of extensor tendon with DIP joint with flexion of DIP joint. Left untreated the mallet can become a _Swan neck_ deformity.

Classification:
- *I:* rupture of tendon insertion.

- *II:* tendon laceration.
- *III:* loss of skin and tendon.
- *IV:* avulsion fracture of distal phalanx.

Treatment:
- *I:* splint or closed reduction and fixation with a K wire.
- *II:* tendon repair and splint.
- *III:* soft tissue repair with tendon repair or graft OR DIP joint fusion.
- *IV:* controversial. XR and reXR with splint. If well reduced continue splintage. If the joint is subluxed and the fragment displaced then ORIF.
- *Mallet thumb* is rarer than mallet finger. Surgery is usually indicated as there have been no reports of successful conservative treatment and there is often a large gap at operation. The thicker EPL tendon holds sutures better than the EDC tendon.

Mammography
- UK national screening programme involves mammography every 2–3 years between 50 and 65 years.
- The American Cancer Society suggests annual screening from 40 years. The benefit of screening between 40–50 years is controversial.
- Perform younger if there is a family history, but the diagnostic accuracy is less.
- Mortality reduction between 20 and 45% has been reported.
- Suspicious lesions are fine microcalcifications, masses, architectural distortion. A mass with microcalcifications is the most suspicious.
- Suspicious lesions should be biopsied following needle localization.

See *Breast cancer.*

Manchot

1889: described cutaneous territories based on blood supply.

Mandible
The strongest bone in the facial skeleton. Thick bicortical structure. L-shaped with a horizontal portion (body and symphysis) and two vertical portions (rami). The angle, coronoid process, symphysis and condylar neck provide the sites of muscular attachment. The alveolar supporting processes and condyle provide articulation.

Mandibular fractures
Symptoms and signs:
- Present with pain, trismus, malocclusion, crepitus, bruising.
- Palpation may reveal a step along the mandibular border or in dentition.
- Paraesthesia may be present in the distribution of the inferior alveolar nerve.

Location:
- Condyle 36%.
- Body 20%.
- Angle 20%.
- Symphysis 14%.
- Alveolus 4%.
- Ramus 3%.
- Coronoid process 3%.

Common patterns:
- Always exclude a second fracture as double fractures are common, particularly.
- Angle and contralateral body.
- Parasymphysis and contralateral subcondylar region.
- Symphysis and both condyles.

Classification:
- *Closed or compound:* compound through skin, buccal mucosa or tooth socket.
- *Kazanjian and Converse.*
- *Favourable and unfavourable:*
  - *Unfavourable:* slope upwards and anteriorly from lower border of mandible, slope anteriorly and inwards in a transverse plane. They are inherently unstable because of the pull of masseter, digastric and pterygoids, which distract the fragments at the fracture site.
  - *Favourable:* Fractures in the opposite direction are stable as the muscle action compresses the fracture. Teeth in fracture segment may stabilize the fracture.

Radiology: Perform OPG, PA, lateral oblique and reverse Towne's view to see condyles. CT doesn't help much.

Management:

- *Conservative:* for most condylar fractures and for stable undisplaced fractures with normal occlusion.
- *Intermaxillary fixation (IMF):* teeth of maxilla and mandible are wired together – called IMF as mandible used to be called inferior maxilla. Fix with wires, arch bars or cap splints. Don't attach to incisor or canine as their single root makes them unstable. Leave for 3–6 weeks. It is not rigid, oral hygiene is difficult, eating is difficult and there is potential airway obstruction. If enough teeth are present on either side of the fracture, a splint can be made without the need for bimaxillary fixation.
- *Open reduction and internal fixation:* the preferred method for most mandibular fractures. Use mono or bicortical fixation. Bicortical risks damaging tooth roots. Use Champy's principle of tension band plating. He noted that muscular forces distract upper and compress lower border, so a plate on the upper border acts as a tension band compressing the lower border – place between gum and nerve. Often used for fractures posterior to the mental foramen. Anterior fractures are treated with upper and lower bicortical plate fixation. Perform via an intra-oral approach where possible.
- *External fixation:* rarely used, but indicated with extensive bony defects and osteomyelitis.
- *Condylar fractures:* controversial. If immobilized, intracapsular fractures are prone to ankylosis. Options are:
  - conservative with a soft diet
  - closed reduction and IMF
  - ORIF – use:
    - when the condylar head is dislocated from the TMJ;
    - when the condyle is laterally displaced 30º or more from the axis of the ascending ramus;
    - in bilateral fractures associated with shortening of the ascending ramus and anterior open bite;
    - if adequate occlusion cannot be achieved by closed reduction;
    - if there is a foreign body in the TMJ.

See *Facial fractures*.

Mandibular hypoplasia

Classification: Prozansky and Murray and Mulliken.

Treatment:

- *Distraction osteogenesis:* at operation, a corticotomy is performed at the angle. Screws are inserted in front and behind the corticotomy. These fit to the distraction device. Start distraction on the 5th day and continue for around 3–4 weeks. Leave for further 6–8 weeks until new bone is seen on XR.
- In grade I hypoplasia, 12–18 mm elongation is achieved.

Micrognathia: The deformity is bilateral and both the ramus and body is affected. Bilateral and bidirectional distraction is required. Two corticotomies are performed, one vertical in the mandibular body and the other horizontal in the ascending ramus. A bidirectional device is used on each side.
See *Ilizarov technique*. See *Hemifacial microsomia*.

Mandibular nerve

V3 of the trigeminal nerve exits the foramen ovale and branches to form the buccal, lingual, inferior alveolar and mental nerves. Block with a needle into the retromolar fossa parallel to the mandibular teeth at 45º angle. Provides anaesthesia for the lower face, mandible, teeth and anterior 2/3 tongue.

Mandibular reconstruction
Defects following resection:

- *Anterior mandibulectomy:* Andy Gump deformity named after the chinless character in the popular comic strip. Get loss of height and width of lower face due to resection of the anterior mandibular arch. Gives problems with oral competence, speech, swallowing and mastication.
- *Lateral mandibulectomy:* less severe than with central defects. Get cheek contour deformities, deviation of the symphysis and upward pull of the remnants.
- *Mandibular swing:* lateral segments used to be left unreconstructed. Unopposed muscle pull causes a swing to the resected

side leading to significant cross bite. Gives a flattened concave appearance, dental wear.

- *Lip and chin ptosis:* anterior arch defects even when reconstructed often produce lip and chin ptosis where the soft tissue slides off the reconstructed arch. As bone is resected, the depressors are detached and the elevators are unopposed so the mandible rides up, not limited by occlusion in patients with no teeth. The soft tissue become ptotic after detachment. Lower branches of the facial nerve may be destroyed in the neck dissection and scar may pull down soft tissue.

Goal of reconstruction:
- Primary wound healing, cosmetic, functional. Best achieved with immediate reconstruction.
- Conventional reconstructive techniques: free bone graft, alloplastic materials, freeze-dried allografts, pedicled flaps. All have unpredictable results.
- Use non-vascularized bone grafts for small defects or condylar defects in children.
- Use reconstruction plates if there is good soft tissue cover and patients with poor prognosis.

Reconstruction:
- *Condyle:* vascularized bone flaps can be used, shaped to fit into the glenoid fossa. If disease-free the condyle can be placed onto bone graft or a prosthetic condyle screwed on.
- *Osseo-integrated implants:* for dental restoration. Can be performed with the mandibular reconstruction or delayed. May get delayed healing in irradiated bone.
- *Plate:* mould the plate to the mandible prior to resection then shape the bone to the plate.
- *Radial forearm osseocutaneous flap:* can give up to 14 cm of straight unicortical bone with good pliable skin. Skin can cover external and internal on separate paddles. Can use nerves, and has good pedicle. However, the radius may fracture, there may be skin graft loss, visible donor site. Fracture can be reduced by limiting the amount of bone harvested and by avoiding perpendicular

osteotomies. Fracture rates as high as 67% have been reduced to 3%.

- *Iliac crest osseocutaneous flap:* provides thick bone with natural curve and good for osseo-integration. However, the soft tissue is bulky and the skin paddle unpredictable.
- *Scapular osseocutaneous flap:* can provide 14 cm of straight bone with a separate skin paddle and minimal donor site morbidity, but the soft tissue is bulky, osteotomies can devascularize bone and cannot be raised at the same time as the resection.
- *Fibular osseocutaneous flap:* Gives up to 25 cm of bicortical bone, with minimal donor site morbidity, but has an unreliable skin paddle, delayed mobilization and neuropraxia.

Mandibular osteotomy
Sagittal splitting is the most versatile ramus osteotomy because it can be used for both mandibular prognathia and retrognathia.

Mandibular swing
- To gain access for oral tumour surgery.
- The lip is split in the midline. The straight line stops at the deepest part of the chin cleft then curves around the chin prominence to reach the midline below. The mandible is divided between the mental foramen and the insertion of anterior belly of digastric to increase exposure. A straight bony cut is performed. This approach divides the lingual mucosa and the mylohyoid muscle. The insertions of genioglossus, geniohyoid and anterior digastric muscles are preserved. See *Head and neck cancer*.

Mannerfelt syndrome
- Spontaneous rupture of FPL in RA. Most common flexor to rupture. Due to carpal irregularities such as spurring of the volar surface of the scaphoid.
- Treat by tendon transfer, tendon graft or arthrodesis of the IPJ.
- Carpal spur should be excised and exposed bone covered with fascial flap.

Marcaine
- Maximum safe dose 2 mg/kg.

• Marcaine plain or with adrenaline the same maximum dose, e.g. 60 kg woman with 0.5% marcaine = 60 × 2 ÷ 5 = 15 ml.

Marchac dorsal nasal flap
Good for closing defects 2.5 cm or less in diameter. Based on cutaneous perforating branches of the lateral nasal artery in the area of the medial canthus. Design the flap at the medial canthal region of the opposite side, drawing a line to the glabella with a backcut. See *Hatchet flap*. See *Rieger flap*.

Marcus Gunn jaw-winking
• Rarely seen in some patients with upper eyelid *Ptosis* due to a congential synkinesis between pterygoid muscles and levator palpebrae superioris.
• Ask patient to move jaw to the side opposite to the ptotic upper lid or open the mouth wide. The lid will lift if jaw-winking present.

Marcus Gunn pupil
• Get paradoxical pupillary dilatation when light is shone into the affected pupil.
• This occurs with injury to the optic nerve and suggests a partial lesion.
• First shine a light in the affected eye – get minimal or no response. Shining a light in the opposite eye causes constriction of both. Now shining in the affected eye causes dilatation.

Marfan's syndrome
• Disorder caused by genetic defect of connective tissue.
• Autosomal dominant inheritance.
• The defect itself has been isolated to *FBN1* gene on chromosome 15, which codes for the connective tissue protein, fibrillin.
• Develop *Arachnodactyly* with hyperextensibility.
• Also lens subluxation, aortic dilatation, mitral valve regurgitation, pes planus and protrusio acetabuli.

Marjolin's ulcer
• *Squamous cell carcinoma* arising in traumatized area such as burn scar, fistula tracts, osteomyelitis sinus.

• Described by Marjolin in 1828.
• Aggressive tumours with a poorer overall survival.
• There is a metastatic rate of 61%.
• The usual time to appearance is 25 years, but it can be as short as 3 years.

Marlex mesh
See *Polypropylene*.

Martin–Gruber anastomosis
• Branches from the median nerve to the ulnar nerve in the forearm carrying all motor nerves to the ulnar nerve.
• Division of the ulnar nerve above the level of anastomosis will result in preservation of motor function whereas median nerve division causes a simian hand.
• Occurs in 23% of subjects. 5% send ulnar fibres to the median nerve.
See *Riche–Cannieu anastomosis*.

Maruyama flap
• A retrograde dorsal metacarpal artery flap based on communicating web-space perforators that penetrate from the palmar arches through to the dorsal surface of the hand at the level of the metacarpal neck.
• These palmar perforators anastomose with the dorsal metacarpal arteries located above the fascia of the dorsal interosseous muscles between each metacarpal.
• The skin paddles are centred between the bases of the metacarpals on the dorsum of the hand.
• The skin paddle can measure 2–3 cm, but becomes unreliable proximal to the wrist.
• The dorsal metacarpal artery is ligated proximally and the flap elevated in a proximal fashion. The pedicle can be dissected back to the level of the metacarpal neck where the palmar communicating perforators emerge from the volar surface between the metacarpals. Dissect the pedicle with a safe cuff of investing fascia. It can be used to cover defects up to the level of the PIPJ. The donor site can be closed directly or with a skin graft.
See *Foucher flap*, *Flag flap*.

Mason's haemangioma
- Also called intraluminal endothelial hyperplasia.
- Less common than _Vascular leiomyoma_.
- It occurs on the fingers. It presents as a small dark subdermal lesion. It is a vascular lesion, but is clinically solid.
- It is benign though histologically resembles angiosarcoma.

Masquelet's test
- Ballottement test of lunotriquetral joint.
- Both hands used to apply shear force across articulation.
- Dorsal pressure applied to lunate and triquetrum with thumb and counter pressure with index finger.

See _Reagan's_, _Carpal instability_.

Masse's sign
- Clinical test in _Ulnar nerve palsy_.
- Loss of hypothenar elevation due to paralysis and wasting of _opponens digiti quinti_.

Masseter

Origin: Zygomatic bone and zygomatic arch.

Insertion: Lateral surface of ramus and inferior mandible at the angle.

Nerve supply: Anterior division of mandibular nerve (V).

Action: Elevator, pulls mandible up and forward.

Mastocytoma
- May be present at birth, but can develop in early childhood.
- It initially starts as a recurring blistering patch with a persistent red-brown discolouration.
- In time, the patch becomes raised and may be 1 cm or more in diameter.
- When solitary they are generally benign and resolve spontaneously. Rarely they are generalized and very rarely malignant.

Mastopexy
See _Breast_

Matrix metalloproteins
These are responsible for the degradation of extracellular matrix. Imbalance between the active enzyme and their natural inhibitors may be seen in a number of diseases. They are zinc and calcium dependent.

Mathes and Nahai classification
Vascular classification of _Musculocutaneous flaps_.
- _Type I:_ single pedicle (TFL, gastrocnemius, small muscles).
- _Type II:_ dominant pedicle with minor pedicles (gracilis, biceps femoris, SCM, soleus, trapezius).
- _Type III:_ dual dominant pedicles (gluteus maximus, pectoralis minor, rectus abdominis, serratus, temporalis).
- _Type IV:_ segmental (flexor hallucis longus, sartorius and tibialis anterior).
- _Type V:_ dominant and segmental (internal oblique, latissimus dorsi, pectoralis major).

Maxilla
Consists of a body and 4 processes – frontal, zygomatic, palatine and alveolar. The body contains the maxillary sinus. The bone thins to eggshell thickness. The alveolar process is thick as long as teeth are present.

Maxilla/midface tumours
- Maxillary sinus is an invagination of nasal mucosa into the maxillary bone. Ethmoid frontal and sphenoid sinuses do the same. They are air-bearing cavities.
- Disease within them is not recognized early. Most expand slowly giving nasal obstruction. Most tumours are large by the time they are discovered. The most common is the SCC.

Risk factors:
- Smoking, wood, nickel, chromium, radium.
- It may be associated with an _Inverting papilloma_.
- Tumours below _Ohngren's line_ have a better prognosis, but are uncommon.
- Suprastructure tumours that involve the roof of the sinus are seen more commonly.
- Treatment usually involves maxillectomy and post-operative radiotherapy. Radiotherapy can give nerve problems, bone necrosis and trismus, and should be carefully planned.
- If there is lymph node involvement the mortality is 90%.

Tumour management:
- *Tumour grade:* if low grade usually treat with surgery alone. Reconstruct with skin graft and dental appliance. Usually higher grade and may require orbital exenteration, craniotomy, RT and CT.
- *Stage:* location as well as size is important.

Surgical approaches:
- *Lateral rhinotomy* (Weber Ferguson), which can be extended into the lip.
- *Total rhinotomy* provides access to the midline, cribiform plate and ethmoid.
- *Midface degloving*, which avoids a facial incision by making a large gingivobuccal incision.

Surgical operations:
- *Medial maxillectomy:* commonly used for benign tumours that involve the lateral wall of the nose. The main complication is stenosis of the nasolacrimal duct.
- *Suprastructure maxillectomy:* addresses tumours in the sinus that involve the orbit and may have an intracranial extension.
- *Infrastructure maxillectomy:* is the least common procedure. Used for tumours confined to the antrum, hard palate or superior alveolar ridge. It can be performed intra-orally and lined with a SSG.
- *Maxillectomy with preservation of the orbital contents:* if tumour extends to orbital floor it is removed and the floor reconstructed with skin graft. If peri-orbital is involved the exenteration is performed.
- *Radical maxillectomy:* for advanced tumours. Includes maxilla, ethmoid sinus, pterygoid plates and orbit.

Reconstruction:
- Many operations don't require reconstruction other than plating of osteotomies used to gain access.
- Reconstruction of radical maxillectomy is now performed using a free flap.
- If there is intracranial extension, muscle is transferred to seal the dura.
- Reconstructing the bony floor of the orbit requires vascularized bone. Scapula or fibula is useful. Two flaps may be required.

See Oral cavity reconstruction. See Le Fort.

Maxillary fractures
- Maxillary fractures are less common than mandible, zygoma or nasal.
- The maxilla is reinforced by 3 vertical and 3 horizontal buttresses.
- The vertical buttresses include the:
  - nasomaxillary buttress lying along the junction of cheek and nose;
  - zygomatico-maxillary buttress, which passes through the body of the zygoma and upwards towards the zygomatic arch;
  - pterygopalatine buttress, which passes posteriorly.
- The horizontal buttresses pass through the:
  - infra-orbital rims;
  - zygoma;
  - alveolar arch.
- The maxilla is designed to absorb the forces of mastication and provide a vertical buttress for occluding teeth. Fractures are usually due to direct impact to the bone. The pattern and distribution depend on the magnitude and direction of the force. Upper *Le Fort fractures* may injure the nasolacrimal canal. Higher fractures may involve the cranial fossa, with dural lacerations and fistulae. Fractures are caused by frontal or lateral impact.

Symptoms and signs: These include:
- *Bruising and swelling:* usually superficial to the peri-orbital region and cheek and intra-orbital.
- *Battle's sign:* bruising over the mastoid process.
- Changes in dental occlusion.
- Epistaxis.
- Enopthalmos.
- Diplopia.
- Paraesthesia in the distribution of the inferior alveolar nerve.
- Palpable step in bone with dish-face appearance from displacement downwards and posteriorly.
- *Mobility of the maxillary segment:* pathognomonic of Le Fort fracture:
  - if alveolus alone suggests Le Fort 1 fracture;
  - alveolus and nasofrontal suggests Le Fort 2;
  - alveolus, nasofrontal and ZF suture suggests Le Fort 3.

Radiology: Plain XR – Pa, Waters' views for sinus, CT and 3D CT.

Treatment:
- Establish an airway, control haemorrhage, close soft tissue wounds and fix fractures. ORIF is the preferred method. Gain access through:
  - bicoronal incision for nasofrontal, orbital walls, ZF suture and zygomatic arch;
  - lower eyelid incision for orbital floor and infra-orbital rim;
  - upper buccal sulcus incision for lower part of maxilla.
- Reduce fragments with Rowe's distraction forceps. Apply IMF to stabilize maxilla. Apply plates across maxillary buttresses. Bone grafting may be required.

Complications: Haemorrhage, airway compromise, CSF rhinorrhoea with infection, blindness (from nerve transection or haematoma), reduced nasal passage and rarely non-union.
See *Facial fractures*.

Maxillary osteotomies for malocclusion
- *Wassmund procedure:* premaxillary osteotomy to correct marked overbite/overjet (see *Teeth*).
- *Schuchardt procedure* is a posterior maxillary osteotomy with intrusion of the osteotomized segment into the maxillary sinus, usually done to correct an anterior open bite or extruded maxillary teeth because of the absence of their maxillary counterparts.

Mayer–Rokitansky–Küster–Hauser syndrome
See *Vaginal agenesis*.

McGregor flap: cheek
- A lateral orbital transposition flap used for *Eyelid reconstruction*.
- For a lower lid defect of >60% of lid margin.
- The flap extends from the lateral canthal tendon upwards to the lateral temporal hairline. A Z-plasty is made laterally. A canthotomy is performed and the lid advanced medially.

McGregor flap: lip
- Used for lower *Lip reconstruction* to reconstruct the entire lower lip.
- Modification of *Gilles' fan flap* it is adynamic and insensate.
- Rectangular-shaped flap based on superior labial artery, which is rotated around the commissure without reducing the size of the stoma.
- The width of the flap equals the height of the defect, the length of the flap equals the width of the defect and the width of the flap. A mucosal advancement is required.

Medial plantar nerve
L4–L5: Supplies the medial forefoot.

Medial pterygoid
Origin: Pterygoid fossa from lateral pterygoid process.

Insertion: Medial surface of ramus and angle of the mandible.

Action: Upward, medial and forward traction on the mandible.

Median nerve
- In hand supplies, lumbricals (radial two), opponens pollicis, abductor pollicis brevis, flexor pollicis brevis (superficial 1/2). See *LOAF*.
- In the forearm the median nerve runs between FDS and FDP. It innervates PT, FCR, PL and FDS.
- The anterior interosseus nerve arises from the dorsal ulnar aspect of the median nerve at the distal end of the cubital fossa. It travels along the interosseous membrane terminating in PQ. It supplies FDP and FPL.
- In the wrist the median nerve lies deep to PL, and between it and FCR.
- Palmar cutaneous branch arises 5–7cm proximal to the wrist on the radial side along FCR. It runs superficial to TCL to supply proximal palm.
- The median nerve enters the carpal tunnel superficial to the tendons. It divides into its terminal branches at the distal end of the tunnel.

- The digital nerves supply thumb, index, middle and radial half of ring finger.
- _Motor branch_ arises from the radial side, but there are many variations. It pierces the fibrous septum separating the mid-palmar from the thenar space. It supplies superficial head of FPB, APB and OP.
- The common digital branches run deep to the superficial palmar arch but superficial to the vessels at the base of the digits. The digital branch to radial side of index supplies 1st lumbrical and the common digital nerve to ulnar side of index and middle supplies the 2nd lumbrical.

Median nerve compression

- From proximal to distal, the sites of compression are:
  - distal 1/3 of humerus beneath projecting supracondylar process;
  - _Ligament of Struthers_;
  - lacertus fibrosis;
  - bicipital aponeurosis.
- In the forearm the potential sites are:
  - between the humeral and ulnar heads of pronator teres;
  - the arch of FDS.
- In the wrist:
  - carpal tunnel.

Pathophysiology: Primary lesion is vascular embarrassment. Get anoxia and venous congestion, oedema and a worsening of venous obstruction. Long-standing compression leads to fibrosis, and impaired axonal transport and demyelination.

Median nerve motor branch

Three main variations. Called Lanz variations:

- ½ _of patients:_ branches distal to the carpal tunnel with a recurrent course into the muscles.
- ⅓ _of patients:_ branches in the carpal tunnel, but follows the same course.
- ⅕ _of patients:_ branches inside the carpal tunnel and pierces ligament to supply the muscles.

Also:

- Accessory variations of the thenar branch at the distal carpal tunnel. Multiple branches

may arise distally and travel parallel to the thenar muscles.

- _High division:_ with the thenar branch dividing in the forearm, but running the same course with the median nerve separated by a persistent median artery.
- _Accessory variation of the thenar branch in the carpal tunnel:_ these are branches that course superficial to the ligaments and supply the thenar muscles. These may be confused with a cutaneous branch. Sometimes they rejoin the main nerve distally.

Medpor

High-density porous polyethylene. Replacing silicone as the most commonly used material for facial augmentation. Pore sizes allow stabilization of the implant through bone and soft tissue in growth. Minimal foreign body reaction.
See Alloplasts.

Meibomian glands

Sebaceous glands, which drain directly onto the skin, found in the labia, penis and tarsus.

Meissner corpuscles

- _Sensory receptors_ only found in the hand.
- Rapidly adapting myelinated A fibres, which mediate moving touch and vibration.
- They are encapsulated mechanoreceptors in the dermal papillary ridges of the skin. They range from 20 on the finger tip to 5/mm^2 on the palm.

Melanin

Melanoctyes in the basal layer produce melanosomes containing melanin, which is synthesized from tyrosine. These are transferred to keratinocytes – they fan around the nucleus superficially. Melanin protects skin from UV radiation. Malignant transformation leads to melanoma. _See Skin._

Melanocytes

- Derived from neural crest and usually located in the stratum germinatum.
- Spindle-shaped clear cells with a dark nucleus and dendritic processes. They synthesize melanin from tyrosine. Melanin accumulates in melanosomes, which pass to

surrounding cells via the dendritic processes where they fan around the nucleus superficially.

- The number of melanocytes is the same between races, but the amount of melanin production varies.
- Melanin production is stimulated by sunlight and by the pituitary hormone melanocyte-stimulating hormone (MSH).
- When melanocytes move from epidermis to dermis they become naevus cells. These are round, do not have dendritic processes and congregate in nests.

Melanocytic naevi

- Classify benign lesions into those containing naevus cells and those containing melanocytes – they become naevus cells when they migrate to the dermis.

Naevus cell naevi

- *Congenital:* giant and none.
- *Acquired:* junctional, compound, intradermal.
- *Special:* Spitz, dysplastic, halo.

Melanocytic naevi

- *Epidermal:* ephelis, lentigo, café-au-lait patch, Becker naevus, Albrights.
- *Dermal* – blue naevus, Mongolian blue spots, naevus of Oto and Ito.

See Naevus.

Melanoma

Incidence:

- Accounts for 3% of all cancers. Incidence has doubled since 1970. The rapid rise might be levelling off.
- The lifetime risk for a Caucasian in Australia is 1 in 14.
- In USA and UK it is 1 in 80.

Risk factors:

- *Genetic:* 5–10% have family history. Alterations of *CDKN2*, a tumour suppressor gene for the protein p16 have been found in 50% of melanoma prone families. Mutation in N-*ras* oncogene found in ⅓ of patients.
- *Sun exposure:* exposure to <u>Ultraviolet radiation (UV)</u>, mainly UVB, but also UVA. Sunscreen blocks are mainly to UVB so they increase exposure to UVA and may increase

the risk of melanoma. Main risk factor is intermittent exposure, rather than chronic exposure.

- *Pigment traits:* blue eyes, red hair, pale complexion have increased risk.
- *Skin reaction to sunlight:* skin with <u>Fitzpatrick skin types</u>, which burns easily and tans poorly is at risk.
- *Freckling:* relates to poor sun tolerance.
- *Benign melanocytic naevi:* number of naevi not size. Dysplastic naevi have higher risk. Patients with dysplastic naevus syndrome have a 12 times greater risk of melanoma.
- *Immunosupression:* renal transplants and cancers, such as lymphomas.

Clinical presentation:

- Very rare in children. Most cases occur in giant congenital naevi. Transplacental has been reported. 3 major and 4 minor signs.
- *Major indicators:* change in size, shape, colour.
- *Minor indicators:* (DISC) diameter >5 mm, inflammation, sensory change (itch), crusting or bleeding.
- Also ABCDE.
- Asymmetry.
- Border notching.
- Colour variegation with black, brown, red or white hue.
- Diameter >6 mm.
- Elevation.

Types:

- All have horizontal growth phase and vertical growth phase. As no blood vessels in epidermis get no metastatic spread in horizontal phase.
- *Lentigo maligna melanoma:* 4–10%, head, neck arms, elderly. Lentigo maligna present for 10–15 years before malignant change.
- *Acral lentiginous melanoma:* 2–8% in Caucasians, but most common type in dark skins. Palms or soles, or beneath nail plate. Not all melanomas in these sites are acral lentiginous except in dark skins.
- *Superficial spreading:* 70%. Upper back in men and women, legs in women. Growth is radial without he propensity to metastasize.
- *Nodular:* 20%. Legs and trunk. Get rapid growth without radial growth phase. Can get ulceration and bleeding. The most aggressive.
- *Amelanotic melanoma.*

Stage	TNM classification	Histological/ clinical features	5-year survival rate (%)
0	Tis N0 M0	intra-epithelial/*in situ* melanoma	100
IA	T1a N0 M0	≤1 mm without ulceration and level II/III	≥95
IB	T1b N0 M0	≤1 mm with ulceration or level IV/V	89–91
	T2a N0 M0	1.01–2 mm without ulceration	
IIA	T2b N0 M0	1.01–2 mm with ulceration	77–79
	T3a N0 M0	2.01–4 mm without ulceration	
IIB	T3b N0 M0	2.01–4 mm with ulceration	63–67
	T4a N0 M0	>4 mm without ulceration	
IIC	T4b N0 M0	>4 mm with ulceration	45
IIIA	T1–4a N1a M0	single regional nodal micrometastasis, non-ulcerated	63–69
	T1–4a N2a M0	primary 2–3 microscopic positive regional nodes, non-ulcerated primary	
IIIB	T1–4bN1a M0	single regional nodal micrometastasis, ulcerated	46-53
	T1–4bN2a M0	primary 2–3 microscopic regional nodes, non-	
	T1–4a N1b M0	ulcerated primary single regional nodal macro-	
	T1–4a N2b M0	metastasis, non-ulcerated primary 2–3	
	T1–4a/b N2c M0	macroscopic regional nodes, no ulceration of primary in-transit met(s)* and/or satellite lesion(s) *without* metastatic lymph nodes	30–50
IIIC	T1–4b N2a M0	single macroscopic regional node, ulcerated	24–29
	T1–4b N2b M0	primary 2–3 macroscopic metastatic regional	
	Any T N3 M0	nodes, ulcerated primary 4 or more metastatic nodes, matted nodes/ gross extracapsular extension, or in-transit met(s)/ satellite lesion(s) and metastatic nodes	
IV	Any T any N M1a	distant skin, subcutaneous, or nodal mets with normal LDH levels lung mets with normal	7–19
	Any T any N M1b	LDH All other visceral mets with normal LDH or any distant mets with elevated LDH	
	Any T any N M1c		

- *Multiple primaries.*
- *Desmoplastic melanoma:* found in the head and neck. They contain a malignant desmoplastic spindling stromal. May present as non-pigmented nodules or plaques. They recur locally and invade along nerves.

Prognosis: Depends on:

- *Tumour thickness and depth of invasion:* <u>Clark</u> determined 5 levels of microinvasion. <u>Breslow</u> measured the maximal vertical height of the tumour. This avoids the confounding effect of the variable thickness of the reticular dermis. More precise at predicting the risk of metastatic disease. The groupings for prognosis are 1, 2 and 4 mm.
- *Ulceration:*
- *Lymphocytic infiltration:* favourable prognostic factor.
- *Mitotic rate:* correlates inversely with survival.

- *Anatomic site:* extremity lesions have better prognosis.
- *Gender:* women survive better than men.
- *Age:* elderly have worse prognosis.

Histology: Stains are S100 and HMB45.

TNM Staging:
- *Tis: in situ* melanoma.
- *T1:* depth <0.75 mm, Clark II.
- *T2:* depth 0.75–1.5 mm, Clarkb III.
- *T3:* depth 1.5–4 mm, Clark IV.
- *T4:* depth >4 mm or satellite lesions, Clark V.
- *N1:* node <3 cm or <3 in-transit metastases >2 cm from lesion.
- *N2:* node >3 cm or >3 in-transit metastases >2 cm beyond lesion.
- *M0:* no metastases.
- *M1:* distant metastases.

Clinical staging:

Stage 1A	T1N0M0	10-year survival 95%
Stage 1B	T2N0M0	90%
Stage 2A	T3N0M0	65%
Stage 2B	T4N0M0	45%
Stage 3A	Any TN1M0	15–40%
Stage 3B	Any TN2M0	
Stage 4	M1	5%

AJCC groupings based on TNM classification:
- *T classification (thickness):*
  - *T1a:* 1 mm without ulceration and level II or III.
  - *T1b:* 1 mm with ulceration or level IV or V.
  - *T2a:* 1.01–2 mm without ulceration.
  - *T2b:* 1.01–2 mm with ulceration.
  - *T3a:* 2.01–4 mm without ulceration.
  - *T3b:* 2.01–4 mm with ulceration.
  - *T4a:* Greater than 4 mm without ulceration.
  - *T4b:* Greater than 4 mm with ulceration.
- *N classification:*
  - *N1:* 1 node positive for metastasis.
  - *N1a:* 1 node positive for micrometastasis.
  - *N1b:* 1 node positive for macrometastasis.
  - *N2:* 2–3 nodes positive for metastasis.
  - *N2a:* 2–3 nodes positive for micrometastasis.
  - *N2b:* 2–3 nodes positive for macrometastasis.
  - *N2c:* intransit met(s) or satellite(s) without metastatic nodes.
  - *N3:* 4 or more metastatic nodes or matted nodes or intransit metastases or satellite(s) with
  - metastatic node(s).
  - *Note:* micrometastases are diagnosed after elective or sentinel lymphadenectomy. Macrometastases are defined as clinically detectable nodal metastases confirmed by therapeutic lymphadenectomy or when nodal metastasis exhibits gross extracapsular extension.
- *M classification:*
  - *M1a:* listant skin, subcutaneous, or nodal metastases, normal LDH level;
  - *M1b:* lung metastases, normal LDH level;
  - *M1c:* all other visceral metastases or any distant metastases with an elevated LDH level.

Treatment:
- *Primary excision:* 2 mm margin. Perform incision biopsy with a large lesion requiring major reconstruction, lentigos and subungal lesions.
- *Secondary surgery:* wider excision. Excise skin and subcutaneous tissue down to fascia:
  - Veronesi, 1988 <2 mm depth, no difference between 1 and 3 cm margin;
  - Balch, 1995, 1–4 mm depth, no difference between 2 and 4 cm margin.
- *Recommended margins:*
  - *melanoma in situ:* 5–10 mm;
  - *<1 mm:* 1 cm margin;
  - *1–2 mm:* 1–2 cm;
  - *2–4 mm:* 2 cm;
  - *>4 mm:* 2–4 cm.
- *Palpable nodes:* FNA or open biopsy.
- *Positive nodes:* CXR, LFTs, USS/CT/MRI. Block dissection.

Controversies in treatment:
- *ELND.*
- *Sentinel node biopsy:*

Palliation:
- *DTIC* (dacarbazine) has a 20% response rate. A prolonged course in more effective. It is not associated with nausea and is cheap. Can occasionally cause hepatic veno-occlusive disease.
- *Combination:* (DTIC, cisplatin, BCNU, Tamoxifen) has a 44% response rate. It can be effective with liver disease. The overall survival is the same as DTIC. Some patients have a dramatic response, others have none.
- *Adjuvant interferon:* the Kirkwood study looked at patients with a Breslow depth of >4 mm. High-dose interferon was administered. The side-effects are flu like symptoms, hepatotoxicity. It costs £10 000 per patient. The relapse-free and overall survival was improved at 1 year. The WHO trial for LN involvement showed no benefit, and other trials showed improvement in disease free survival, but not overall survival.
- *EORTC study:* used a tumour vaccine against ag GM2 ganglioside. It may be augmented by interferon.
- *Other chemotherapy:* fortemustine can be used against intracranial mets and temozolomide can be given orally with a similar response to DTIC.
- *Isolated limb perfusion.*

Metastasis: As well as lymph node and distant metastasis, get satellite and in-transit metastasis that occur in 2–20% of patients. These are found within the dermis or blood vessels. Satellites occur within 5 cm of the original tumour, in-transit are further than 5 cm. Distant sites are LN, cutaneous then lung, liver, brain, bone. As the disease progresses, CNS mets become more common. May perform surgical resection if possible. The 1-year survival with brain mets is 30%.

Moles with malignant potential: May arise *de novo* or in melanocytic naevi, Dysplastic naevi and melanoma *in situ*. All congenital naevi have a malignant potential though the degree of potential is unknown. Large congenital naevi >20 cm^2 have a malignant potential and should either be excised excised by 6 months to 2 years if possible, or should be placed under regular surveillance and suspicious areas biopsied.

Intraoral melanoma: <10% of melanomas arise from mucosa. 50% are intra-oral. Most common in the elderly male and most are on the palate. They have often spread extensively at the time of presentation. Treatment is wide excision with neck dissection if involved. Survival is 15% at 5 years. See Head and neck cancer.

Important trials:
- *ECOG trial 1684 (Eastern Co-operative Oncology Group):* demonstrated improved overall survival in patients with high-risk melanomas treated with high dose IF alpha 2b. It suggested that IF may have a role as an adjuvant therapy for melanoma.
- *WHO trial: Lancet* 1998. No benefit from ELND.
- *ECOG trial 1690:* no increase in survival with IF alpha 2b casting doubt on the use of IF.
- *Koops:* 1998 – no survival benefit from ILP.

Melasma
- An acquired, hormonally influenced hyperpigmentation.
- Histologically the pigment may be located in either the epidermis or the dermis, or in both locations.
- Lasers may be effective in clearing pigments, including the Q-switched ruby, green pulsed dye, and Nd:YAG laser, but repigmentation is common.
- Additionally, hyperpigmentation following laser treatment may occur.

Meleney's gangrene
Streptococcal Necrotizing fasciitis.

Melolin
Gauze with polyethylene backing. See Dressings.

Mental nerve block
- The mental nerve is the continuation of the inferior alveolar nerve, and it emerges from the mental foramen on the chin. located approximately 2.5 cm from the midline of the face in the midpupillary line, in line with the canine.
- It provides sensation to the chin, lower lip, mucosa, and gingiva of the lower lip.

- It is a branch of the mandibular division of the trigeminal nerve (V3).
- To block the nerve cutaneously, the foramen should be palpated and a wheal of anaesthesia placed. Then, the needle should be reinserted and advanced to the vicinity of the mental foramen but not into it. Approximately 1–3 ml of anaesthetic should be injected into the area.
- To block the nerve intra-orally, the foramen should be palpated with the middle finger of one hand and the lip lifted by the thumb and index finger of the same hand. The needle should be inserted at the inferior labial sulcus at the apex of the first bicuspid and 1–3 ml of anaesthetic injected. It may be locate by rolling the lower lip outward and stretching the mucosa away from the canine root.

Merkel cell

- Present in the epidermis and thought to be a pressure receptor.
- Rare and only seen by electron microscopy.
- They are connected to keratinocytes by desmosomes.
- A slowly adapting mechanoreceptor which mediates constant touch and pressure through myelinated fibres.

See Skin, Sensory receptors.

Merkel cell tumour

- Resemble Basal cell carcinoma histologically.
- Occurs as single tumour in older people.
- Tumour may be epidermal, dermal or subcutaneous.
- Microscopically get irregularly anastomosing trabeculae and rosette arrangement of basophilic uniform cells.
- They contain small granules similar to the neurosecretory granules of epidermal Merkel cell. Cytokeratin 20 stain.
- They resemble small cell carcinoma and a chest XR should be performed to exclude a secondary from a lung primary.
- They are aggressive and metastasize to nodes, viscera and bone.

Treatment:

- Cure is difficult.

- Excise with wide margin and consider adjuvant radiotherapy to the tumour bed and draining lymph nodes.

Mesh

- Used for Abdominal wall reconstruction. Most commonly used as an inlay graft attached to the fascial edges. Also used retrorectus placing the mesh in the space between rectus abdominus and peritoneum.
- Marlex: polypropylene. first used in the Vietnam War for open abdominal wounds. 100% extrusion rate with a graft over the mesh, but useful in the short term and less extrusion with flaps over the mesh.
- Prolene: lower extrusion rate, but still around 40%. Greater pliability.
- Gortex: fewer adhesions.
- Vicryl: absorbed by 8 weeks. Provides temporary support. Retains the shape.

Mesodermal tumours

- Acrochordon.
- Dermatofibroma.
- Dermatofibrosarcoma protuberans.
- Neurofibroma.
- Granula cell tumour.

MESS

Mangled Extremity Severity Score. Consider amputation with a MESS score of over 7.

Skeletal/soft tissue injury:	low energy	1
	medium energy	2
	high energy	3
Limb ischaemia: (double score if >6 hours)	near-normal	1
	pulseless, poor refill	2
	cold insensate	3
Shock:	BP >90 mmHg	1
	Transient hypotension	2
	Persistent hypotension	3
Age:	<30	1
	30–50	2
	>50	3

See Lower limb reconstruction. See Lower limb trauma.

Metacarpalphalangeal joint dislocation

Finger:

- *Anatomy:* mobility is unique with lateral movement in extension, but stable in flexion. Looking laterally the shape is condylar and looking end on trapezoid being wider volarly. MCP joint contributes to finger convergence on flexion. Volar plate is firmly attached to proximal phalanx, but loosely to metacarpal allowing hyperextension. They are also stabilized by the deep tranverse metacarpal ligament, which attaches to volar plates. Collateral ligaments originate dorsal to the axis of rotation on the metacarpal head and insert volarly on the proximal phalanx. ACLs insert into volar plate. The shape of the head and dorsal origin keeps them taut in flexion.

- *Dislocation:* rare and dorsal more common due to forced hyperextension. Most common in index finger. Hyperextension most commonly causes subluxation. Both entail proximal rupture of the volar plate, which is still in position in subluxation, but folded into the joint in dislocation. Dorsal dislocation is usually irreducible closed due to the noose formed around the neck by the flexor and lumbrical.

  o *Operation:* attempt closed reduction but if this fails, open reduction through a dorsal or volar incision for dorsal dislocation (where base of proximal phalanx is dorsal to metacarpal head). Clear the joint and repair ligaments.

  o *Subluxations are reduced closed:* don't apply longitudinal traction and hyperextension. Instead, flex the wrist, and apply pressure dorsally. Place in an extension-blocking splint for 3 weeks.

- *Collateral ligament injury:* uncommon, mainly in middle, ring and little. Caused by sudden deviation of the digit in flexion.

  o *Operation:* most are sprains. Treat conservatively. If unstable they will require repair through a dorsal incision. Reattach the ligament with a pull-out suture and hold in flexion.

- *Locked MPJ:* get rigid loss of extension. Can be confused with triggering. It may be degenerative or spontaneous. Degenerative – >50,

usually middle finger. Caused by osteophytes or changes around the joint capsule. Spontaneous – <50, usually index. No XR changes. Due to abnormal bands within the joint, loose bodies, capsular tears or irregular articular surfaces.

  o *Operation:* occasionally the joint can be freed under LA, but otherwise exploration is required.

Thumb

- *Anatomy:* stability important for power grip and precision grasp. ROM 5–100°. The metacarpal head is wider than the fingers and the sesamoid bones are incorporated into the volar plate. FPB and AP partial insert into these and provide additional support as do the other surrounding tendons.

- *Dislocation:* usually due to hyperextension. Much more common than the fingers as more exposed. Volar plate usually ruptures distal to sesamoid bones. There is no lumbrical so entrapment doesn't occur. Open reduction may be required.

  o *Operations:* closed reduction by flexing with traction. Open reduction is through a palmar incision. Some surgeons recommend volar plate repair. Sesamoid fracture can be held with a circular suture or removed. Volar dislocation is less common.

- *Collateral ligament injury*.

Metastatic bone carcinoma

- The most common malignant *Bone tumours* and the 3rd most common site for metastasis.
- Most affect the axial skeleton. 20% are in the upper limb but uncommon in the hand. Mimics infection.
- In the hand, most occur in the distal phalanx.
- *XR:* aggressive radiolucent lesion with periosteal reaction.

Treatment:

- Depends on many factors including life expectancy. Surgery is only indicated for impending fracture. Also use radiotherapy. These patients have a poor prognosis so treatment is usually palliative.
- In the hand, ray amputation is often the best treatment.

Methylmethacrylate

- Self-curing acrylic resin used for securing joint components to bone.
- Has minimal adhesive properties.
- Can be preformed or mouldable.
- Body response is minimal. Get exothermic reaction which may damage tissues. Cardiac arrest has been reported.
- Used in orthopaedics as a bone cement and neurosurgery for reconstructing _Cranial_ defects. Useful in thoracic surgery for _Chest wall reconstruction_, where it is placed between a Marlex mesh. It is used for dental prostheses.
- It does not biodegrade or become replaced by functional bone. It is associated with chronic inflammation.

See _Alloplasts_.

Metopic synostosis

- The metopic suture is the first cranial suture to fuse, occurring at approximately 2 years of age.
- Lack of growth in the frontal bones, producing a keel-shape deformity – trigonocephaly.
- Relatively uncommon and accounts for less than 10% of isolated suture, non-syndromic craniosynostoses.
- Brain development is usually normal.
- Hypotelorism occurs with upward slanting of both lateral canthi and the lateral portions of the eyebrows, as well as flattening of the supra-orbital ridges.

Operative procedure:

- A bifrontal craniotomy is performed, and the frontal and parietal bones are removed as a single bone graft.
- The orbital rims are advanced.
- Remodelling of the bifrontoparietal bone graft is performed using a shaping burr and radial osteotomies.

See _Craniosynostosis_.

MHC

Major histocompatibility complex:

- The most important antigens contributing to rejection.
- Found on chromosome 6 and are called different things in different species.
- Called HLA in humans. Two major classes:

  o Class I antigens have 3 loci in humans, HLA A, B and C, and are found on most nucleated cells;
  o Class II antigens in humans are HLA DR, DP and DQ, found on vascular endothelium and lymphocytes and macrophages; matching of HLA-A, B and DR are the most important.

- _Other antigens:_ important for transplant are blood group, minor histocompatibilty and skin specific antigens.

See _Transplant immunology_.

Micropenis

Insufficient androgen stimulation. Usually caused by primary hypogonadism or hypothalamic or pituitary dysfunction. It is 2.5 standard deviations below the mean length.

See _Embryology_.

Microsurgery

History:

- _1950s:_ The first binocular microscope was developed by Carl-Zeiss.
- _1962:_ Malt and McKhann, first limb replant.
- _1964:_ Buncke in performed the first successful ear replant.
- _1968:_ Komatsu and Tamai first digit replant.
- _1968:_ Cobbett first toe-to-hand transfer.
- _1969:_ free omental flap to scalp.
- _1972:_ temporal free flap in Japan by Harii and Ohmori.
- _1973:_ Daniel and Taylor free groin flap.

Patency: Acland described 5 important factors – surgical precision, size of the vessel, blood flow, tension, and the use of anticoagulant and anti-thrombotic medication.

Thrombus formation.

Anastomosis techniques: As well as suturing, a number of other techniques have been tried. Vein cuffs and polyglycolic acid tubing have been used to produce the sleeve anastomosis. A coupler system is in use and laser has been used to weld the vessels. Laser has good patency rates, but develop stenosis and micro-aneurysms.

Complications and prevention:

- _No-reflow phenomenom._
- _Ischaemia-reperfusion injury._

- *Vasospasm:* the best management is prevention. Keep patient warm and well perfused. Dilatation and application of lignocaine, papaverine or verapamil. *Heparin*, *Dextran*, *Aspirin*.

Management of non-flowing anastomosis: Apply anti-spasmotic like 5% lidocaine with warm gauze. Make sure patient is warm, well hydrated, good blood pressure and no vasoconstrictors. Leave anastomosis. Look at pedicle for twist or compression. If thrombosis redo. Consider thrombolytic treatment e.g. Streptokinase.
See Free flap.

Microtia

- Hypoplasia of the external ear, ranging from small to absent ear. Most commonly vertical sausage ear.
- Incidence: 1:7000.
- M:F 2:1.
- Rt:Lt:Bilat 5:3:1.
- Inner ear rarely involved, but have conduction block.
- Middle ear is not reconstructed unless bilateral. Possibly due to stapedial artery occlusion. 50% associated with hemifacial microsomia, also Treacher Collins.

Non-surgical treatment: Prosthetic – glue on or osseointegration.

Surgery: Around school age when rib growth is sufficient and the ear is almost fully grown. Requires:
- Construction of cartilage framework.
- Dissect vestigial ear and place framework.
- Lobule transposition.
- Tragal construction.
- Helical rim elevation.
See Ear reconstruction.

Milia
See Epithelial cysts.

Millard cleft lip repair
A rotation advancement. A curved incision on the cleft side releases lip tissue bringing the Cupid's bow into alignment. Lateral lip element is brought in to the gap caused by the rotation.
See Cleft lip.

Millesi classification of brachial plexus injury
Classification of brachial plexus *Injury*.
- *I:* supraganglionic.
- *II:* infraganglionic.
- *III:* trunk.
- *IV:* cord.

Milroy's disease
Familial *Lymphoedema* congenita.

Minoxidil
- A powerful peripheral vasodilator that perhaps stimulates the passage of *Hair* from telogen to anagen phase.
- It causes hair growth or stops hair loss in 39% of men who use it for 1 year. It is more effective in men younger than 40 with recent hair loss limited to the crown area.
- It does not help the receding hair line. Efficacy plateaus at 1 year.
See Hair transplantation.

Mirault–Blair–Brown cleft lip repair
See Cleft lip. Lip length increased on the cleft side by a triangular flap taken from the non-cleft side. The Cupid's bow is destroyed.

Mirror hand
See Ulnar dimelia.

Moberg flap
- Volar advancement flap uses the entire volar surface of the digit. Mainly used for thumb defects.
- Flap will include both NVBs. Maximum length gain is 1 cm.
- Preserve branches to dorsal nerve and dorsal vessels otherwise can get dorsal skin loss. Get finger stiffness.
- Proximal NVBs can be dissected to increase length and a large V–Y advancement created. Begin active extension by 10–14 days.
See Fingertip injuries.

Moberg pick-up test
- Stereognosis is the ability to recognize objects based on touch.
- Ten objects are picked up and identified first visually then blindfolded.

- Less useful for an isolated ulnar nerve lesion as the object can be identified using the intact median nerve.
- If median nerve is being tested, ring and little fingers are taped.

See Sensation testing.

Mobile wad
Muscles of brachioradialis, ECRL and ECRB. Innervated by the radial nerve proximal to the bifurcation.

Möbius syndrome
- Developmental disorder with bilateral facial paralysis.
- Involves 6th and 7th cranial nerves and possibly the 3rd, 5th, 9th and 12th.
- 25% have limb abnormalities and 15% have abnormal pectoral muscles.
- The paralysis may occasionally be unilateral.

Reconstruction: Aim for functioning nasolabial folds. Bring motor nerves – partial spinal accessory or trigeminal possibly with nerve grafts. Then provide muscle with a free transfer. *See Facial re-animation.*

Moh's surgery
- First described in 1941, who used zinc chloride paste on tumours to evaluate surgical margins. The paste caused a severe inflammatory reaction.
- Currently, it involves frozen-section technique to immediately examine the microscopic margins. Immediate feedback is given about positive margins which are then re-excised until clear.
- Useful for infiltrative BCCs, verrucous carcinoma of the mouth, genitalia or feet, keratoacanthomas, dermatofibrosarcoma protuberans, malignant fibrous histiocytoma, atypical fibroxanthoma, extramammary Paget's, sebaceous carcinomas which often affect the eyelid, adenoid cystic carcinoma and granular cell tumours.
- The cure rate is 99% for BCCs and 95% for SCCs.

Procedure:
- Usually LA. First debulk the tumour with a curette. A scalpel blade is used to remove the tissue in a horizontal fashion with the scalpel held at a 45° angle to the skin.

All clinically visible tumour is excised in saucer-like layers.
- Marks are placed on the tissue and patient, and a reference map is created. Horizontal frozen sections from the underside are performed and any tumour extensions are re-excised.

Mongolian spot
- Variably sized bluish-black patch over the lower back and buttocks in infants, occasionally over upper back and rarely in other sites.
- Usually present at birth, more common in Asians and blacks, rare in whites. 96% of Africans have these lesions and 10% of white infants.
- May be multiple. Usually regress in early childhood.

See Naevus.

Monocryl
Poliglecaprone 25. A monofilament synthetic suture. Similar absorption to *Vicryl*. Less prone to bacterial colonization.

Morley's compression test
- Test for *Thoracic outlet syndrome* producing tenderness at the root of the neck with pressure over the plexus in the interscalene groove causing neurological symptoms.
- Perform with patient sitting, feeling neck from behind. Feel the postero-lateral edge of the sternomastoid muscle. Slip fingers under the edge of the muscle at the root of the neck above the clavicle and feel the anterior scalene muscle. Roll fingers postero-laterally to feel the interscalene groove and then the scalenus medius.
- The plexus is felt on the interscalene groove, and reproduction of symptoms is diagnostic. Palpate for masses, listen for bruit. Fullness in the supraclavicular fossa is usually a cervical rib.

MRC grading of nerve function
Motor function
- *M0:* no contraction.
- *M1:* flicker.
- *M2:* movement with gravity eliminated.
- *M3:* movement against gravity.
- *M4:* movement against gravity and resistance.

- *M5:* normal.
See Sensory function

MRI

- Tissue is excited by a high-powered magnet. The energy emitted from the hydrogen ions in water and fat is measured.
- Upon the emission of energy, nuclei are said to relax, indicating that they assume a lower energy state by realigning with the applied magnetic field. The rate at which relaxation occurs is determined by two tissue properties, the T1 or longitudinal relaxation time and the T2 or transverse relaxation time.
- These relaxation times determine the amount of energy received from different tissues and are the basis for image contrast in MRI.
- *T1:* these images show anatomic detail and 'crisp' appearing anatomy. Fat-containing tissues will appear brighter (have higher signal) on T1-weighted images. These are sometimes referred to as FAT images. Structures with high H2O content will appear darker (muscle, CSF).
- *T2:* These images appear slightly 'grainy' or 'pixely'. This sequence is designed to show fluid collections, can detect tumour infiltration of marrow, infection, acute fractures with haemorrhage or other pathological conditions that usually have with them associated oedema. CSF will be bright on this imaging sequence.
- Stir films are modified T2 images with the fat signal suppressed:
  - ○ gadolinium enhancement is taken up by pathological tissue and looks white, so it is best seen on a T1 image where the fluid is black;
  - ○ *positive points:* good for soft tissues, can view in any plane.
- *Negative points:* poor for bone, takes a long time, expensive, metallic objects.
- *NB* Fluid black and white – T1 and T2.

Mucous cyst

Subdermal cyst usually over the dorsum of the DIP joint. Cyst fluid arises from the joint and associated with *Heberden's nodes*. Excise if there is pain, enlarging cyst, infection or nail involvement. XR shows degenerative change with diminished joint space and osteophytes.

Treatment: If excision is indicated, perform through an H incision. Often overlying skin requires excision. Excise cyst down to joint. Remove any osteophytes, close the capsule, and perform a local flap to close the defect.

Muir and Barclay Formula

For burns resuscitation.
- TBSA% × Wt kg/2 = one ration:
  - ○ give one ration 4-hourly in first 12 hours;
  - ○ give one ration 6-hourly in next 12 hours;
  - ○ give remaining ration over 12 hours.

Muir-Torre syndrome

- Multiple internal malignancies.
- Cutaneous sebaceous proliferation.
- Keratoacanthomas.
- *Basal cell carcinoma* and SCC.

Muller's muscle

Smooth muscle with sympathetic innervation. Situated in the posterior lamellar of the upper lid and attaches to levator and tarsus.

Origin: Posterior border of levator.

Insertion: Superior border of tarsus. It is 10–12 mm long and 15 mm wide. It is adherent to conjunctiva.

Mulliken and Glowacki classification

- Classification for vascular malformation (1982).
- Vascular abnormalities are classified as *Haemangiomas* or *Vascular malformations*.
- Vascular malformations are subcategorized based on predominant channel type and flow characteristics:
  - ○ *slow flow:* capillary (CM) and telangiectases, lymphatic (LM), venous (VM);
  - ○ *fast flow:* arterial and arteriovenous.

Histology:
- Each of the four major subcategories of vascular malformation has a particular histopathological appearance. Flat, quiescent lining endothelium is characteristic of all dysmorphic vascular abnormalities.
- *Capillary malformation (CM):* comprised of uniform, ectatic, thin-walled capillary- to venular-sized channels located in the papillary and upper reticular dermis.

- *Lymphatic malformation (LM):* has walls of variable thickness, comprised of both striated and smooth muscle, with nodular collections of lymphocytes in the connective tissue stroma.
- *Venous malformation (VM):* thin-walled with irregular islands of smooth muscle. The dysplastic venous networks drain to adjacent veins, many of which are varicose and deficient of valves.
- *Combined lymphaticavenous malformation (LVM):* occurs particularly in the craniofacial region; microscopic thromboses also are seen in these combined slow-flow anomalies.
- *Arteriovenous malformations:* The arteries in AVM are dysplastic, consisting of thickened fibromuscular walls, fragmented elastic lamina and fibrotic stroma. The veins in an immature AVM appear 'arterialized' (reactive muscular hyperplasia).

Munro classification of hypertelorism

Classifies <u>Hypertelorism</u> by shape of the orbit.
- *Type A:* parallel medial orbital walls.
- *Type B:* ballooning of anterior interorbital tissue.
- *Type C:* central portion of medial wall balloons.
- *Type D:* wide posterior ethmoidals. C and D are most difficult to correct.

Muscle

When injured, muscle can either form a scar or regenerate. Skeletal muscle usually regenerates, smooth and cardiac muscle do not.

Anatomy: Each cell is circumscribed by its sarcolemma consisting of cell membrane, basement membrane, and endomysium. Bundles of fibres are fascicles, surrounded by perimysium and the whole muscle is covered with epimysium.

Injury: When cut the cell retracts leaving sarcolemma empty. This is filled with clot, which includes fibrin. Get inflammatory cell and fibroblast migration. By the 3rd day, the basal lamina are lined by macrophages. Fibroblasts proliferate and collagen is laid down (type III then type I).

Regeneration:
- Occur from small satellite cells on the basal lamina of the sarcolemma. These satellite cells only occur in skeletal muscle. Only satellite cells can mitose.
- Satellite cells become myoblasts and fill the injured area. These fuse to produce multinucleated cells which then produce contractile proteins. These mature and finally become reinnervated. So fibroblasts produce the framework for muscle cells to regenerate. Excessive scar will block regeneration.

Treatment: Mobilization accelerates revascularization but may cause more disruption. 5 days of immobilization is sufficient to prevent re-rupture of muscle in the rat model.

Muscles: upper limb
Extrinsic muscles:
- *Extensors – superficial:* 4 muscles, <u>EDC</u>, <u>EDM</u>, <u>ECU</u> and anconeus. They all share a common origin on the lateral epicondyle.
- *Extensors – deep:* 4 muscles, <u>APL</u>, <u>EPB</u>, <u>EPL</u>, <u>EIP</u>
- *Extensors – lateral:* supinator, <u>Brachioradialis</u>, <u>ECRL</u>, <u>ECRB</u>. The latter 3 form the <u>Mobile wad</u> of Henry.
- *Flexors – superficial:* <u>PT</u>, <u>FCR</u>, <u>PL</u>, <u>FCU</u>. All from medial epicondyle.
- *Flexors – intermediate:* <u>FDS</u>.
- *Flexors – deep:* <u>FPL</u>, <u>FDP</u>.

Intrinsic muscles:
- <u>Interossei</u>, <u>Lumbricals</u>.
- *Of thumb:* <u>APB</u>, <u>FPB</u>, <u>OP</u>, <u>AP</u>.

Musculocutaneous/muscle flaps
- The motor nerve is always accompanied by a vascular pedicle, which is often the major source of circulation. There are often collaterals.
- A *dominant* pedicle can sustain an entire muscle.
- A *minor* pedicle can sustain only a portion of muscle. Some muscles have several *segmental* vessels each supplying a portion of muscle. Muscles with a single dominant pedicle are most useful as flaps.

Classification:

- <u>Taylor</u>: by nerve supply – for dynamic transfer.
- <u>Nahai and Mathes</u>: by vascular supply.
- Most are type II. Those with a dominant pedicle would be the most reliable.
- Skin in a musculocutaneous flap is supplied by perforators that are usually terminal branches of musculocutaneous perforators though there can be direct cutaneous perforators. Improve chances of survival of skin by having a broad-based skin paddle with bevelled edges, which is proximal to pedicle. Doppler or better colour duplex can assist in determining perforators.
- Neovascularization occurs particularly over the cutaneous area so a musculocutaneous flap will become pedicle independent much quicker than a muscular flap.

Function preservation: If a portion of muscle is left with intact origin, insertion and innervation. Examples would be a hemisoleus or part of a distally based latissimus.

Skin territory:

- The skin territory of each superficial muscle is defined anatomically as that segment of skin extending between the origin and insertion of the muscle and located between its edges along the course of the muscle. If fascia is included, the skin island may be extended beyond muscle dimensions in certain musculocutaneous flaps.
- Generally, the more narrow muscles (i.e. gracilis) have a greater limitation in skin territory because of the decreased number of perforating vessels to the overlying skin and the increased importance of septocutaneous vessels to the skin territory in proximity to the muscle.

Segmental flap: A type 3 muscle such as gluteus maximus can have part of the muscle raised so that some functioning muscle remains. Type IV muscle have to be raised segmentally as the rest of the muscle would not survive.
See Flaps.

Mustardé flap

- Used for <u>Eyelid reconstruction</u>.
- Lower lid is reconstructed with composite graft and cheek advancement.

- For upper eyelid perform lateral canthotomy and elevate the whole of the lower eyelid to switch to upper eyelid.
- The arc of rotation passes just below the lateral brow. Keep a wide base. It can be elevated subcutaneously or below SMAS.
See Cheek rotation flap.

Mustardé lid switch

- A laterally based transverse flap of the lower eyelid is transposed to the upper lid.
- It may be possible to directly close the lower lid. If not, it can be reconstructed using one of the techniques described in <u>Eyelid reconstruction</u>.
- The transposition flap is divided at a second procedure.
- Also total lid switch.

Mycobacteria
Tuberculosis:

- 2% of infected patients have involvement of the upper limb.
- Get a cold abscess. XR show osteopenia with lack of bone destruction. Slight periosteal reaction and joint narrowing. Aspiration may be diagnostic. Biopsy may be necessary. Growth on Lowenstein–Jensen medium at 37°C. Some atypical mycobacteria grow at 30–32°C.
- Treat by aggressive debridement. Wound closure is acceptable.

Atypical mycobacteria:

- Incidence is increasing. Delay in diagnosis is common as they have an indolent course.
- *Mycobacterium marinum* with aquatic exposure.
- *M. terrae* with farm exposure.
- *M. avium* particularly in immunocompromised patients.
- Treat with aggressive debridement and long-term antibiotics. Minocycline or combination therapy.
See Infection.

Mycosis fungoides

- Cutaneous T-cell lymphoma, or mycosis fungoides, is a cutaneous form of lymphoma.
- Presents with pruritic erythematous scaly patches, infiltrated plaques, and irregular skin nodules and ulcers.

- Diagnosed histologically.
- Extensive skin involvement precludes any definitive operative treatment.
- Topical nitrogen mustard or psoralen _Photochemotherapy_ utilizing the photoactive psoralen drugs followed by long-wavelength ultraviolet irradiation (UVA) can be utilized.
- Patients who are unresponsive to these treatments can be treated with electron beam therapy. In most instances when irradiation ulcers have occurred, the extent of the disease and the extent of the previous electron beam therapy preclude the availability of adjacent tissues for pedicle flaps. Although mycosis fungoides is sometimes a fatal disease, in some cases the course is prolonged.
- New treatments include extracorporeal photophoresis.

Myeloma
See _Bone tumours_.
- The most common primary bone malignancy.
- Occurs in >40s.
- Most produce monoclonal immunoglobulins.
- Bone involved contain red marrow, e.g. vertebral bodies, ilium, ribs.
- Long-term survival averages 4 years.
- _XR:_ radiolucent punched out lesions.
- _Treatment:_ very sensitive to chemo- and radiotherapy. Surgery is only indicated if there is a risk of fracture.

Myofascial dysfunction
See _RSD_.
- Myofascial dysfunction trigger points are often present in RSD.
- This is a clinical diagnosis.
- Specific proximal trigger points are found in muscle or fascia, which elicit immediate referred pain or numbness at distant sites.
- The trigger point is often a palpable lump. In the absence of treatment, trigger points become a chronic condition that does not spontaneously resolve.
- Treatment varies, but use muscle stretch and vasocoolant icing to inactivate trigger points.

Myofibroblast
Resembles a fibroblast but contains cytoplasmic filaments of α-smooth muscle actin. It is also found in smooth muscle. They are responsible for wound contraction. The number of fibroblasts in a wound is proportional to the contraction. Increased numbers are found in Dupuytren's disease.

Myoglobinuria
See _Electrical injuries_.
- Released from muscle following destruction.
- It is a monomer containing a haem molecule.
- Following electrical injury is indicative of rhabdomyolysis secondary to muscle destruction.
- If not treated, get intratubular deposition of pigments and acute renal failure.
- Treat with:
  ○ forced diuresis with mannitol;
  ○ alkalize the urine with 88–132 mEq/L sodium bicarbonate.

Myotomes
Upper limb
- _Shoulder:_
  ○ _abduct:_ C5;
  ○ _adduct:_ C6,7,8.
- _Elbow:_
  ○ _flex:_ C5,6;
  ○ _extend:_ C 7,8.
- _Forearm:_
  ○ _pronate:_ C6;
  ○ _supinate:_ C6.
- _Wrist:_
  ○ _flex:_ C6,7;
  ○ _extend:_ C6,7.
- _Fingers and thumb:_
  ○ _flex:_ C7,8;
  ○ _extend:_ C7,8.
- _Hand (intrinsics):_ T1.

Lower limb:
- _Hip:_
  ○ _flex:_ L2,3;
  ○ _extend:_ L4,5.
- _Knee:_
  ○ _extend:_ L3,4;
  ○ _flex:_ L5,1.
- _Ankle:_
  ○ _dorsi-flex:_ L4,5;
  ○ _plantar-flex:_ S1,2.

Naevus

Naevi are the commonest tumours. A naevus refers to abnormal growth, an ectodermal *Hamartoma*.

Junctional naevus:
- Cell nests confined to the dermoepidermal junction.
- Flat or slightly raised pigmented area, variable colours between lesions, but evenly pigmented, occasionally darker in the centre.
- Usually a transient phase in children prior to becoming compound naevi. They may remain junctional in the palms, soles and mucosae.

Intradermal naevus: Cells confined to the dermis. Rare in children.

Compound naevus:
- Cells in both locations.
- The junctional component may transform though this is rare. A raised plaque or papillomatous lesion with variable colour.
- They increase in thickness during late childhood and adolescence, when they may cause concern.
- May be associated with coarse hairs.

Solar lentigo: Not a naevus cell lesion, but consists of a smooth, dark brown patch measuring up to 1.5 cm in diameter in which there are increased numbers of normal melanocytes. In middle-aged or older people. They can be removed by excision or cryotherapy.

Freckles: Also called ephelis.
- Multiple flat pigmented lesions resulting from increased melanocytic activity.
- Benign.
- Can be destroyed with liquid nitrogen.

Multiple lentigines syndrome

(LEOPARD syndrome):

Neural naevus: A *Type C* intradermal naevus. The cells are similar to Schwann cells. Smooth, lobulated and hairless. Commonly found within congenital giant naevi and there may be a high association with malignancy.

Dysplastic naevus: Histologically has a discontinuous radial growth of dysplastic cells.
Blue naevus.
Halo naevus.
Congenital naevus.
Dysplastic naevus syndrome.
Lentigo Maligna.
Naevus of Ota and Ito.
Mongolian spot.
Spitz naevus.
Naevus spilus.
Epidermal naevus.
Sebaceous naevus.
Café au lait patch.
Becker's naevus.

Naevus sebaceous of Jadassohn
- Superficial skin lesion, present at birth in head and neck and more rarely trunk and limbs.
- Well-circumscribed, irregularly raised plaque, usually solitary.
- Yellowish waxy appearance with no hair.
- In puberty it thickens and becomes verrucous.
- It is a hamartomatous conglomerate of sebaceous glands and defective hair follicles.
- Large lesions are associated with epilepsy.
- Naevus sebaceous syndrome includes naevus sebaceous, ocular dermoids, mental retardation, epilepsy and skeletal abnormalities.
- 15–20% rate of malignant transformation usually to *Basal cell carcinoma*. Also to *Syringocystadenoma papilliferum*, KA and SCC. Rarely occurs before early adulthood.
- Complete excision before puberty is recommended.
- Extensive lesions may require tissue expansion.

Naevus spilus
- Sharply demarcated brown patch speckled with smaller areas of black pigmentation.
- Get a background of *Café au lait macules* and multiple junctional nevi.
- Quite common and found on the trunk and extremities.

- Treat by observation. Response to Q-switched pulsed _Lasers_ is variable.

Nager's syndrome
Bilateral hemifacial _Microsomia_.

Nahai–Mathes
Classification of _Fasciocutaneous flaps_.
- A: direct perforator.
- B: septocutaneous perforator.
- C: musculocutaneous perforator (indirect).

Nail
Anatomy:
- *Entire nail unit:* perionychium consists of nail plate, proximal nail fold (eponychium), lateral nail fold (paronychium), distal edge of nail (hyponychium) and germinal matrix. Nail plate is multilayered of cornified cells derived from anuclear onychocytes from the germinal matrix of the nail bed.
- *Nail bed:* soft tissue below the nail plate. The germinal matrix (proximally) forms the early developing nail, the overlying fold contributes the smooth surface and the sterile matrix (distally) adds bulk. The entire nail bed including the overlying eponychial fold contributes material to the developing and growing nail lunula, which is a white arc of nail distal to eponychium due to persistence of nuclei in cells of germinal matrix. Nail becomes transparent as they disintegrate. The sterile matrix epithelium does not undergo _Parakeratosis_.
- *Keratinization:* there are three modes.
  - germinal matrix forms the main substance of hardened nail plate with stratified layers of onychocytes;
  - sterile matrix produces semi-rigid keratin, which also acts as an adhesive, sticking the nail to the nail bed;
  - external sheen is produced by epidermoid keratinization from the dorsal roof, nail bed is anchored to the periosteum.
- *Nail fold:* houses the proximal nail plate. The nail wall tapers distally to form the eponychium. Continuity of nail fold is required for nail growth. At the hyponychium the nail plate becomes non-adherent and extends over the tip of the finger. A build up of cells occurs under the distal nail,

which acts as a barrier. The nail bed has a rich vascular supply.

Growth: 1 mm per week or around 0.1 mm per day. Stress or illness can inhibit growth and trimming can increase growth.

Avulsion: Nail avulsion will take surface epithelium and keratinous solehorn (keratin produced by the sterile matrix). Blood and plasma exudate creates a scab. Lateral nail folds and hyponychium provide reparative epidermis. This layer is hyperkeratotic but provides protection. New nail plate starts to regenerate in 2–3 weeks. Get a rolling front of advancing nail plate. Replacement of reparative epithelium with bed epithelium is synchronous with the progression of new nail plate. Both come from germinal matrix.

Traumatic nail deformities: It is easier to manage nail bed wounds acutely than perform secondary reconstruction. Anatomic alignment is crucial. If poorly aligned, nail will not adhere to the scar tissue. The nail should be removed and the nail bed examined and repaired following which the nail is replaced.

Subungal haematoma: Caused by bleeding under the nail plate. How much bleeding requires exploration is not clear. Perhaps >50% haematoma should be explored. Pain requires release of the haematoma using a hand-held cautery. Residual haematomas migrate distally with the nail.

Simple and stellate lacerations: Usually due to a localized blow with compression. Requires debridement and accurate suture. Nail bed may need to be undermined to allow closure. Nail is replaced as a splint. If the nail is lost a splint should be put in its place. If the germinal matrix is involved the dorsal roof is lifted through lateral incisions.

Crush injuries: Have a poorer prognosis. Repair what is possible. Avulsed nail bed can be removed and replaced with free grafts using split sterile matrix. Associated fractures may require a K wire.

Avulsion injuries: With partial or total loss of nail bed. Nail bed adherent to the nail can be replaced as a graft. If the germinal matrix is avulsed it should be replaced under the eponychial fold. Split sterile matrix graft can be taken from the uninjured part of nail. Otherwise use big toe grafts. Take germinal matrix as well to prevent nail growth where there is no sterile matrix. A defect of germinal matrix requires a full thickness graft, but sterile matrix requires only a split graft. Harvest with a size 15 scalpel blade. Replacing a sterile matrix with SSG will not allow nail adherence.

Composite grafts: Hyponychium and nail bed are unique structures. In children under 10 years composite grafts should be replaced. In older children and adults convert the composite graft into a full thickness skin graft. Defat the tissue and preserve nail bed.

Reconstruction: Always less effective. Wait for at least a year.

Non-adherent nail: Due to scarring of the nail bed. As the growing nail hits the scar tissue it becomes non-adherent. This catches and leads to trauma under the nail. Treatment involves trimming nail back to normal sterile matrix. Excise scar and close primarily or with split sterile matrix grafts. Non-adherence may be due to hyperkeratosis and requires scraping of the sterile matrix.

Split nail: Often due to an axial scar, which divides the nail plate. It may also be caused by scarring of the dorsal roof or defect of the germinal matrix. Longitudinal scars may be excised or Z-plasty to change the direction of the scar. Larger scars require split grafts. Germinal matrix loss requires full thickness germinal matrix graft. Dorsal roof scarring may require a split sterile matrix graft. Cover grafts with a silicone sheet.

Hook nail: A nail that grows over the tip of the finger. Due to loss of structural support. The nail is sensitive and catches. Reconstruction involves recreating the injury and restoring bony and soft tissue support using Atasoy or Kutler flaps. Apply split nail bed graft. Bony support is more difficult and may require a composite toe flap.

Linear ridging: Often associated with underlying bone or soft tissue abnormality. CT may be required to establish the cause. Treatment is the same as split nail.

Reconstruction of the eponychium: Most common with burns. Also friction injury. Get an irregular nail or a notched deformity. Can use a composite graft from toe. Dorsal skin may be rotated or transposed. A split sterile matrix graft is sutured to the undersurface to restore dorsal root bed.

Pincer nail deformity:
• *Biconvex shape:* the nail folds and the contour of the phalanx contribute to overall shape. With a pincer nail this shape is lost. It may be related to loss of lateral integrity of the distal phalanx. It is unsightly and may be ingrown and more prone to paronychia. Reconstruction involves dermal grafts laterally to restore contour. A tunnel is made laterally into which the dermal graft is inserted.

Nail lengthening
Can be used in fingertip reconstructions when nail sterile matrix has been destroyed. Eponychium is slid more proximally by de-epithealizing a strip of skin just proximal to the eponychial fold to allow it to move proximally. This gives more nail show. Described by Bakhach.

Nalebuff classification
Thumb deformity in RA. *See RA.*
• *I:* Boutonnière deformity most common, MPJ flexion, IPJ extended.
• *II:* Boutonnière deformity with adduction. Rare. Combined I and III – MPJ flexion with IPJ hyperextension and subluxation of CMC.
• *III:* swan neck deformity with dislocated CMC, MPJ extended and IPJ flexed.
• *IV:* UCL incompetence with CMCJ subluxation.
• *V:* like III, but not adducted. Due to stretching of the MCP joint volar plate.

Narakas classification
Of *Obstetric brachial plexus* injury.
• *Group 1:* C5,6: paralysis of shoulder, absent elbow flexion – spontaneous recovery in >80%.

- *Group 2:* C5,6,7: As above with wrist drop – good hand, good shoulder and elbow in 60%.
- *Group 3:* All: complete paralysis – good hand in most, good shoulder and elbow in 30–50%.
- *Group 4:* All: complete paralysis, Horner sign, limb atonic – full recovery very rare.

Nasal fractures

Anatomy:
- The nose is comprised of 5 bones, the frontal process of maxilla, the nasal process of frontal bone, nasal bones, vomer and ethmoid.
- *Nerve supply:* trigeminal nerve – V1 (ophthalmic) infratrochlear and anterior ethmoidal. V2 (maxillary) – infra-orbital and nasopalatine.
- *Rhinion:* the middle third of the nose which is the junction of the upper bony part and the lower cartilaginous part. At the rhinion the upper lateral cartilage overlaps the nasal bone and the lower lateral cartilage overlaps the upper lateral. Fracture of the rhinion may dislocate the upper lateral cartilages and cause a saddle deformity.
- *Blood supply:* from both internal and external carotids, but mainly from the external carotid via the maxillary artery and also the facial artery. The internal carotid contributes to the nose superior to the middle turbinate.

Fractures:
- Mainly occur in the thinner distal part of the paired nasal bones. Fractures may cause injury to the nasolacrimal system and epiphoria. Severe blows may cause widening of the interorbital distance.
- Most commonly fractured facial bone. Lateral impact results in deviation of nasal bones and septum to the opposite side. Frontal impact results in splaying of the nasal bones, buckling or dislocation of the septum, collapse of the nasal dorsum.

Classification: <u>Stranc and Robertson</u>.

Symptoms and signs:
- Bruising and swelling.
- Obvious deformity.
- Look intransally for septal haematoma, which should be drained at their most dependent portion to prevent pressure necrosis.

Treatment:
- Simple fractures may be treated by closed reduction.
- Ashe's forceps relocate the nasal septum.
- Walsham's forceps relocate nasal bones.
- The nose is packed and an external splint applied.
- Secondary rhinoplasty may be required.

See <u>Facial fractures</u>.

Nasal reconstruction

History: Surgical reconstruction of the nose evolved along three basic lines:
- Indian method, using forehead flaps.
- French method, with lateral cheek flaps.
- Italian method, involving arm flap.

Nasal subunit:
- *9 units:* dorsum, tip, columellar and paired sidewalls, alae and soft triangle. These subunits need to be respected during reconstruction.
- If a defect fills more than 50% of a subunit then the entire subunit should be replaced, to place scars in subunit boundaries. The tissue filling the defect should be of the same thickness. Contour is important.

See <u>Aesthetic units</u>.

Assessment for reconstruction:
- The goal of reconstruction is aesthetic and functional with a patent airway. Always analyse what is missing and what is available for reconstruction.
- The nose has skin that varies from thick stiff skin on the tip to thin smooth skin on the dorsum. There is a bone and cartilage framework and thin vascular mucosa inside. All structures that are missing require replacement.
- If cheek, lip and nose are missing, first reconstruct cheek and lip and rebuild nose once the other is healed, thus allowing a stable platform. Reconstruct according to the units missing. Reconstruction can be prefabricated.

Soft tissue:
- Upper $^2/_3$ skin is thin and mobile, lower $^1/_3$ thick and adherent.
- *Grafts:* full thickness skin grafts are good for the upper nose and dorsum. The thicker skin of tip and alar is not as well served with a graft. <u>Composite grafts</u> can be used for rim

defects, harvested from the root of the helix. Their size should be limited to 1.5 cm and the margins made oblique to increase the contact with the graft bed.

- *Banner flap:* transposition flap.
- *Bilobed flap:* Defects less than 1.5 cm over the tip can be reconstructed with a local flap, such as a bilobed flap.
- *Cheek advancement flap:*
- *Nasolabial flap:* the flap can be raised on the superiorly or inferiorly based pedicle, and rotated into position. It can be islanded and tunnelled to reach the alar rim. It can be turned over on itself to also provide lining. For alar base lesions it can be advanced as a V–Y flap. It may become rounded on healing and support can be given with a strip of cartilage.
- *Dorsal nasal flap:*
- *Rintala flap:*
- *Forehead flap:* design on either the right or left supratrochlear vessels. Design a template, use a narrow pedicle. The flap can extend into hair bearing skin. The flap should be vertical and then delay is not necessary. *See Gullwing flap.*
- *Scalping flap:*
- *Tagliacozzi flap:*
- *Radial forearm flap:* the first choice for tissue transfer as the skin is thin, the pedicle long. It can be prefabricated with lining and bone.

Support:

- The nasal skeleton is in thirds. The upper ⅓ is bony. These overlap the upper lateral cartilages and these overlap the lower lateral cartilages.
- The aim of support is to act against gravity and external forces, create nasal tip projection, form subcutaneous hard tissue, which acts against trapdoor contraction, recreate nasal subunit.
- Even if an entire subunit of skin is replaced, usually only a partial subunit of cartilage reconstruction is required. As the skin on top is thicker than the normal skin, the skeleton size should be reduced.
- Septal cartilage can be used. An 8-mm wide L-shaped dorsum and caudal strut must be maintained to support the nose after harvesting a septal graft. Ear concha rib is used

for dorsal support and lateral support sliced in thin slices. Requirements include:

- Septal or conchal cartilage replaces alar cartilage. These are sutured to the stump of medial crura. Tip projection with tip grafts on top of the alar cartilage domes.
- Rib graft or ethmoid perpendicular plate shaped in trapezoidal fashion positioned on the side wall to replace upper lateral cartilage
- 4–6 mm wide batten of conchal or septal cartilage from alar base to nostril apex. This fixes the alar rim in position.
- A flying buttress of septal cartilage grafts, conchal cartilage or rib graft along the dorsum.
- Can also use an L strut, a hinged septal flap, a septal pivot flap or a cantilever graft.

Lining: A thin mucosal layer except in the vestibule where it is keratinized. Reconstructions most often fail because of lack of lining. They must be vascular enough to support the cartilage grafts and supple enough to conform to the shape and thin enough not to obstruct the airway. It may be placed at the same time as external cover or the flap may be prelaminated. The options are:

- Use residual nasal lining. It can be advanced 2–3 mm.
- *Turn-in nasal flaps:* local hinge over flaps: turn over skin and scar adjacent to a healed nasal defect. The main disadvantage is an unreliable blood supply. These flaps should be kept short.
- Nasolabial flaps have been used, but are always too thick. Vascularity is tenous and cartilage grafts are risky.
- *Septal hinge flap:* the technique involves removal of septal mucosa ipsilateral to the defect and dissection of an appropriately sized flap of septal cartilage. This septal 'door' is made to open on a dorsal hinge toward the reconstructive side, so that the septal mucosa on its far side bridges the wound and lines the airway. The technique promises more than it delivers.
- *Prefabricated skin graft and lining:* cartilage and graft can be placed on the forehead flap and transferred once they have survived. However, the cartilage retains the shape of the concha or septum, and is fixed by scar so that it is difficult to alter the shape.

- *Folding forehead or nasolabial flap:* this is not a good option. Doubling the flap increases donor site morbidity with a large flap and diminishes distal blood supply, increasing the risk of necrosis, and producing thick shapeless and unsupported alar margins.
- *Intranasal lining flaps:* significant amounts of lining remain in the residual nose. Lining flaps from the vestibule, middle vault and septum are thin.

Columella:
- Difficult to reconstruct.
- Use nasolabial flaps (unilateral or bilateral) on superior pedicles. They can be tunnelled under the alar base.
- Upper lip forked flaps may be useful in the elderly patient with a long lip.
- Forehead flaps and chondrocutaneous grafts are secondary options.

Total nasal reconstruction:
- First described in 600 BC by Sushruta in the Hindu book of Revelation using forehead and cheek flaps. Tagliacozzi used lateral arm in the 16th century.
- Turnover flaps for lining.
- Harvest whole of concha using anterior incision around rim of concha leaving curve in place. Take to external auditory meatus. Cut into 2 strips to make medial and lateral crus of lower lateral cartilage. Use Tebbitt spanning sutures to create curve.
- Suture to nasal septum or columella strut. Other pieces of cartilage can be used to augment nasal tip.
- *Costal cartilage:* for woman do inframammary incision then cut straight down onto cartilage. Incise onto rib and use periosteal elevator to get around. Use Doyen rib elevator to isolate segment of rib.
- For columella strut cut groove lengthways to sit in nasal septum and to step 'mast'. Extra bits of cartilage can be used as non-anatomical cartilage in alar margin.
- *Forehead flap:* make accurate template. Raise very thin over hairline then through fascia then at orbital margin take periosteum. Angle base to enable rotation. Thin, but be careful to include vessel. Cut out hair follicle roots. Inset flap. Close defect leaving any small area to granulate.

Naso-ethmoidal fractures
Caused by trauma to the interorbital region. They often occur in conjunction with other fractures and involve the root of the nose, medial wall of orbit and ethmoidal air cells. Suspect brain trauma.

Symptoms and signs:
- Bruising and swelling.
- A palpable bony step.
- *Telecanthus* – if the medial canthal tendon is detached from its bony origin.
- Enopthalmos.
- Diplopia.
- CSF leak.

Treatment:
- Usually ORIF.
- Access is obtained via lacerations, bicoronal incision or medial orbital incision (Lynch incision). Nasal bones are elevated. A bone graft may be required to reconstruct the dorsum of the nose. The nasomaxillary buttress is reconstructed with plates and screws. The medial canthal tendon is reconstructed.
  See Facial fractures.

Nasolabial flap
- Blood supply based on perforators from the facial and angular arteries passing through underlying levator labii and zygomatic muscles.
- Position flap just lateral to the nasolabial fold.
- Use inferiorly based flaps for buccal and FOM defects of 2.5–7 cm. The flaps including muscle may be transposed further. Small defects of the nasal ala can be reconstructed with a superiorly based flap. An inferiorly based flap can reconstruct lip above vermilion.
- Flaps can be pedicled and transposed, tunnelled, islanded, turned over for lining, V–Y advancement.
  See Oral cavity reconstruction.

Natatory ligaments
Composed of transverse fibres, which run distal to the superficial transverse ligament at the palmar surface of the interdigital commissure. The proximal border extends from the ulnar border of the little finger to the radial border of the index finger. It occasionally extends to

the thumb. Contracture results in limitation of abduction.
See *Retinacular system*.

Neck dissection

Types of neck dissection:

- *Radical neck dissection:* or comprehensive. The internal jugular, accessory nerve, and sternocleidomastoid muscle are sacrificed. In addition, other structures such as skin, strap muscles, and external carotid may be resected.
- *Extended radical neck dissection:* as well as 5 levels, also paratracheal and mediastinal nodes, and parotid gland.
- *Modified radical neck dissection:* all lymph nodes are removed but at least one of the non-lymphatic structures removed in the radical dissection are spared:
  - *type 1:* accessory nerve preserved;
  - *type 2:* accessory nerve and SCM preserved;
  - *type 3:* accessory nerve, SCM and IJV preserved.
- *Functional neck dissection:* means different things to different authors and should not be used.
- *Selective neck dissection:* where not all of the levels are removed:
  - *suprahyoid:* submandibular triangle and submandibular gland with lymph nodes;
  - *supraomohyoid:* contents of the submandibular triangle, jugulodigastric, and mid-jugular lymph nodes together with nodes from the posterior triangle along the accessory chain are removed (this procedure is a staging operation in a clinically negative neck with a suspicion of metastasis rather than a therapeutic procedure; if the jugular nodes are negative, involvement of the accessory group is unlikely);
  - *anterolateral:* level 2–4; often for laryngeal and hypolaryngeal tumours;
  - *anterior:* level 2–4 and tracheo-oesophageal nodes, for thyroid tumours;
  - *posterior:* level 2–5, posterior scalp.

Principles:

- Sacrifice of spinal accessory nerve is debilitating. Get shoulder pain and droop with limited abduction. Modifications have been developed to preserve the spinal accessory nerve.

- Other modifications preserve other non-lymphatic structures. These operations preserve shoulder function, improve cosmesis, protect internal carotid artery and enable bilateral procedures.
- Bilateral node metastasis is not infrequent. Usually require staged bilateral radical neck dissection. Removing both IJVs can lead to death, blindness and permanent facial distortion.
- Selective neck dissection aims to remove nodes which are likely to be involved in N0 necks. This concept is not applicable if there is clinical metastasis. Sentinel node mapping is less predicable in the head and neck, but may improve selection.

Rules of neck dissection:

- Perform an elective neck dissection for large tumours (T3 and T4), in cases in which the primary lesion is easier to resect with the neck, in obese patients and in unreliable follow-up patients.
- Modified dissection is suitable for clinical N0 neck or possibly for micrometastasis.
- Bilateral dissection, either therapeutic or elective, is appropriate for lesions close to the midline and is usually staged.
- Multiple nodal involvement, a node more than 3 cm in size or extracapsular spread – give radiotherapy.
- Submandibular gland enlargement due to a blocked Warton's duct may give a false positive.
- Rarely are posterior triangle nodes involved in an N0 neck.
- Resect in continuity if possible, but not essential.

Indications:

- *Radical neck dissection* is performed for high-grade tumours with N2 neck, recurrent disease, invasive nodal disease.
- *Modified radical neck dissection* for T3, T4, N1 tumours, T2 tongue, in a thick neck.
- *Radiotherapy:* controversial. Usually if there is extracapsular spread, also some advise if there is positive histology following a neck dissection, others for N2 disease.

Operations:

- *Incisions:* McFee, utility, triradiate, visor.
- *Radical* or comprehensive – described by Crile in 1906:

○ Along with the cervical nodes (level I-V) are taken the SCM, omohyoid, internal jugular vein, cervical plexus, submandibular gland and tail of parotid gland. Usually used for bulky nodal metastasis.

○ Perform through Y incision or McFee particularly for bilateral disease Find lower end of SCM remove from clavicle.

○ Dissect out internal jugular vein and divide. Find anterior edge of trapezius – posterior boundary. Dissect posterior triangle from posterior. Identify accessory nerve and brachial plexus. Accessory nerve exits SCM in top half, enters trapezius 3 cm above clavicle.

○ Divide posterior belly of omohyoid. Preserve phrenic on scalenus anterior. Don't go lateral to vein as this will damage lymphatic ducts.

○ Elevate internal jugular vein and expose carotid and vagus. Medially take tissue up to strap muscle. Dissect up and over hypoglossal nerve.

○ Find central tendon of digastric.

○ Excise SCM from mastoid to expose posterior belly of digastric. Cut through lower pole of parotid, divide upper end of jugular. Preserve cervical and mandibular branches. Take submandibular gland, preserve lingual nerve.

Complications:

• *Intraoperative:* bleeding, _Air embolus_, pneumothorax, carotid artery injury, nerve injury – phrenic, X, brachial plexus, lingual, XII, IX.

• *Intermediate:* flap necrosis:
   ○ *carotid blow out:* often with salivary fistulas;
   ○ *chyle leak:* due to thoracic duct injury, milky drainage, reduce by fat-free diet, may need TPN.

• *Late:* scar contracture, neuroma, shoulder pain, facial oedema.

For intra-operative bleeding from IJV: Tell

the anaesthetist of the problem, control vein distally to prevent air embolus. Isolate bleeding with suction, dissection. Repair or plug defect. Can use segment of SCM to plug defect. See _Head and neck cancer_. See _Lymph node levels in head and neck cancer_.

Neck reconstruction
Local flaps:

• Vertical scarring may be helped with Z-plasties. Elevate flaps in deep subcutaneous planes.

• Bilobed flaps and cervicohumeral flaps can be used, but can leave ugly scars.

Musculocutaneous flaps:

• Including trapezius, pectoralis major and latissimus dorsi can be used, but has a thick muscular pedicle.

• The cervicodorsal fasciocutaneous flap fed by cutaneous branches of the superficial cervical vessels and posterior intercostal perforators arises in the posterior neck and can be raised as large as 30×7 cm.

• The cervicoscapular flap may include a vascular network of the circumflex scapular artery which can be as large as 32×12 cm.

SSG and splinting:

• The most frequently used reconstruction.
• Release the contractures deep.
• Orientated seams horizontally.
• Splint for at least 6 months, which gives less than 17% recurrence rate.

Tissue expansion:

• Placement in the unscarred supraclavicular region.
• Difficult to expand in the soft neck.

Microsurgical restoration of the neck unit:

• Radial forearm flap has been used, giving thin pliable skin but may be small, hairy with a poor donor site.

• The free scapular flap blends well. It may require debulking in fat patients. It may be pre-expanded.

• Other sources are the groin flap, thoracodorsal and TRAM.

Necrobiosis lipoidica

• Commonly associated with diabetes mellitus, but may occur in patients without diabetes and it may precede the clinical onset of diabetes mellitus.

• The lesion begins as a dusky red plaque, which progresses to atrophy of the skin followed by central ulceration.

• It is more common in the pretibial area.

• The lesion is progressive, despite control of the diabetes.

- Some patients present with the cosmetic problem of unsightly legs.
- Resection of the involved area and resurfacing with split-thickness skin grafts have been successful.

Necrotizing fasciitis

- A rapid aggressive and life threatening infection of soft tissues characterized by the spread of infection and necrosis through the fascia and subcutaneous fat.
- It may be:
  - *type 1:* polymicrobial;
  - *type 2:* pure group A strep infection.
- NF includes Fournier's gangrene, suppurative fasciitis and haemolytic strep gangrene – Meleney's ulcer.
- The term was coined by Wilson in 1954.
- With synergistic organisms one group may use up O_2 thus allowing anaerobes to grow. *Streptococcus* produces streptokinase. Exotoxins in clostridial infections produce multiple effects.
- Meleney's synergistic gangrene occurs over days or weeks. This may be an infection with *entamoeba histolytica*. There is a slow time course.
- Association of NSAIDs.

Clostridia: Present with severe pain out of proportion to the signs. Progression to skin necrosis with crepitus.

Fungal infections: Typically in diabetic, immunocompromised and elderly patients. Most infections are caused by *Zygomyces* and *Mucorales*. Usually presents as purple and indurated and mould may be seen at the wound edge. Most are superficial. Some may progress rapidly. Treat with amphotericin B 0.5 mg/kg/day up to a maximum of 50 mg/day.

Hyperbaric oxygen: May be a useful adjunct to radical debridement. with NF. NSAID slow polymorphs.

Neoplasm

Abnormal mass of tissue the growth of which exceeds and is unco-ordinated with that of normal tissue and which persists after the initial stimulus which provoked the change. A malignant neoplasm invades normal tissue and may metastasize.

Characterized by:
- *Initiation:* change in genome of cell.
- *Promotion:* change made permanent by cell division.
- *Progression:* further division to form an invasive tumour.

Neovascularization

- Free transfer of arteriovenous pedicles to another site can lead to neovascularization allowing the surrounding tissue to be raised on the new pedicle.
- For example, the radial arteriovenous pedicle of the radial forearm flap has been transferred to the neck and buried under the supraclavicular area and subsequently used to resurface a severely burned face.
- After 6 weeks the surrounding tissue can be raised.
- The crane principle has been used to implant the same pedicle in a second donor site.

Nerve conduction studies

- Neuropraxia leads to absent conduction over the site of the block, with normal conduction above and below.
- In compression get prolonged *latency* and decreased *amplitude.*
- First finding is increase in sensory latency. Sensory axons are larger than motor axons and are more sensitive to pressure changes. Normal value for latency is <2.2 ms at 8 cm distance. Later get prolonged motor distal latency. Increased latency means the velocity has decreased. This occurs in response to demyelination of nerve fibres, shorter internodal distances within segments of remyelinated nerve fibre or a conduction block due to ischaemia. Latency can be compared between ulnar and median nerve.
- Fibrillation and positive sharp waves are indicators of denervation when spontaneous muscle activity occurs. They appear 2–4 weeks after injury depending on the distance between site of injury and muscle.

Nerve graft

- The _Sural nerve_ can provide 30–40 cm of nerve graft. When a limited amount of graft material is required the medial or lateral antebrachial cutaneous nerve can be harvested from the injured upper extremity.

- The lateral antebrachial cutaneous nerve is found adjacent to the cephalic vein. 8 cm of nerve graft can be obtained and the loss of sensation is slight
- The medial antebrachial cutaneous (MABC) nerve, found in the groove between the triceps and biceps muscles adjacent to the basilic vein, has a posterior and an anterior division. Harvesting of the anterior branch is preferred because the posterior branch causes numbness over the elbow. 20 cm of graft can be obtained.
- In patients with median nerve sensory loss the third web space nerve can be harvested to reconstruct the median nerve defect, providing up to 24 cm of nerve graft.
- Also the dorsal branch of the ulnar nerve can be harvested to reconstruct the ulnar nerve.
- Posterior interosseous nerve – the terminal branch is useful for bridging small defects in small diameter nerves. It is located on the radial side of the base of the 4th extensor compartment at the wrist.

Nerve injury
Anatomy:
- Axons are surrounded by *Endoneurium*. Large axons are individually myelinated, smaller axons are grouped together and wrapped by Schwann cells. The greater the myelination the faster the conduction.
- Groups of axons are bundled together and surrounded by *Perineurium*.
- Fascicles are arranged in groups which are surrounded by the *Inner epineurium*.
- The periphery is encased in *Outer epineurium*.
- Peripheral nerves originate where the dorsal and ventral roots of spinal cord coalesce. Afferent (sensory) fibres originate in the dorsal spinal cord with cell bodies outside the spinal cord as the dorsal root ganglia. So brachial plexus lesions can be diagnosed as supraganglionic if there is sensory loss, but no Wallerian degeneration.
- The axon extends from spinal cord to the motor end plates and sensory receptors. Proteins are produced in the cell body and transported to where they are needed. If the cell body dies the entire cell dies.

Injury:
- Get Wallerian degeneration distally. Without the nucleus the axon degenerates along with the myelin sheath. Adjacent Schwann cells become phagocytic. Get a hollow endoneurial sheath, which collapses. Proximally get limited degeneration.
- Various cytokines such as NGF are released by Schwann cells stimulating axonal regeneration.
- The cell body produces structural proteins.
- Axons sprout both from the cut end and from the nodes of Ranvier, producing a growth cone. Tendriles called filopodia reach out from the growth cone until they find a favourable substrate. Then the axon grows into it within several days of injury. Once this is found the other sprouts degenerate.
- All the structures need to come from the cell body and this is the rate limiting step in nerve production.
- Nerves by preference grow towards other nerves, but this is dependent on a critical gap distance.

Repair:
- Affected by the amount of scar, the length of time particularly for motor nerves, age, the level of division with distal levels having better outcomes.
- Anatomical guides to fascicles can be used.
- Also electrical stimulation of the distal stump can be used to differentiate motor from sensory fibres (for 72 hours).
- Stimulation of sensory fibres gives a sharp pain, whereas stimulating a motor fibre results in a dull ache.

Prognosis:
- Young patient, distal lesion. Regeneration occurs at 1 mm per day with a 1/12 lag before recovery starts.
- Muscles can regain function up to 1 year after denervation. Get loss of up to 40% of sensory neuron population after nerve division. Neuron rescue has been attempted in animal models using neuroprotective substances, such as acetyl-L-carnitine.

See Seddon. See Sunderland.

Nerve repair
- Can be performed as epineural, perineural (fascicular) or group fascicular repair. No technique has been shown to be superior.

- If end-to-end repair is not possible then non-vascularized nerve grafting, vascularized grafting and nerve conduits can be used.
- No evidence that vascularized is better than non-vascularized, but it makes sense if the bed is poor.
- Conduits have been made out of vein or synthetic material.
- To ensure correct alignment, topographical maps can be referred to. Muscle can be stimulated directly for the first 72 hours. Histochemical techniques have been described to allow differentiation of motor from sensory nerves.

Nerve stimulator

Can be used to stimulate a nerve and observe muscle contraction. Useful in identifying the facial nerve and its branches. In a laceration, a motor nerve may continue to conduct impulses distal to the division resulting in muscle contraction up to 72 hours after division. When using the disposable stimulator, attach the earth to the muscle being stimulated otherwise the current may not be strong enough to detect a response.

Neurilemoma

- A benign tumour of nerve sheath.
- Also called Schwannoma as they originate from the Schwann cells of the neurilemoma. The tumour appears as a slightly elongated swelling along the course of a nerve, which may cause some pain or sensory change. Tapping may cause paraesthesia. They present when they are small. The tumour should be separated from normal fascicles. Recurrence is uncommon.

Neurocutaneous flap

Suprafascial paraneural vessels supply not only the nerve, but the skin that the nerve supplies via the formation of choke or true anastomosis between networks of fascial perforators. The major superficial venous channels serve as the outflow from the paraneural plexus, e.g. the sural flap includes the short saphenous vein. See *Fasciocutaneous flaps*.

Neurocutaneous melanosis

- The association of a large CMN with multiple small CMN ('satellites') with CNS involvement.

- CNS manifestations include hydrocephalus, seizures, focal deficits, or partial paresis usually occurring before 2 years of age.
- If neurological symptoms occur most patients will die from progression of melanosis or malignancy.

See *Congenital naevus*.

Neurofibroma

- Solitary tumour or multiple as part of Von Recklinghausen's disease.
- Plexiform neurofibromas are large with thickened nerves.
- Treatment may be required for cosmetic reasons or functional disturbance.
- Neurofibromas are difficult to resect from the nerve.
- Malignant degeneration can occur when the neurofibroma is associated with Von Recklinghausen's disease.
- Solitary lesions are seen in the first decade, multiple lesions after 30 years.

See *Mesodermal tumours*.

Neurofibromatosis

Autosomal dominant inherited syndrome with variable penetrance and high rate of spontaneous mutations.

Type I:

- Multiple neurofibromas, café au lait spots, axillary freckling, Lisch nodules on the iris (ocular neurofibromatosis) and other findings.
- Incidence 1:3000. Manifests in infancy with the café au lait spots. Also have freckling in the axilla. It progresses to affect skin, soft tissue, nerve and bone. Tumour progression is most aggressive at the time of puberty.
- The commonest presentation is with facial masses.

Type II:

- Presents with less skin lesions, but more meningiomas and acoustic neuromas (bilateral). Plexiform neurofibromas are large infiltrative lesions usually found in the head and neck region.

Head and neck neurofibromas

- Highly vascular lesion.
- Orbital lesions need to address the expanded orbit. Approach through lid incision or with a craniofacial approach. If there is no vision, removing the globe may give a better outcome.

- Cheek and lip reduction may need to be staged.
- Facial nerve will require dissection with resection of tissue superficial to it. Often there is a lot of bulk medially in the cheek which will require a wedge excision with suspension of lip.
- Also suspend tissue to bone using Mitek anchors. The slow insidious growth may undo any corrections achieved.

Neuroma
Present with pain and localized tenderness and dysaesthesia in the distribution of the nerve.

Types:
- *Neuroma-in-continuity:*
  - *spindle:* with chronic irritation in an intact nerve;
  - *lateral:* at site of partial nerve division;
  - following nerve repair.
- **End-neuroma:** following traumatic division and amputation.

Common upper limb neuromas:
- Palmar cutaneous branch of median nerve.
- Superficial branch of radial nerve.
- Radial digital nerves.
- Dorsal branch of ulnar nerve.

Palliation: desensitization, TENS, drugs such as carbamazepine.

Surgery:
- Resection and coagulation.
- Ligation, crushing or capping (with vein or histocryl glue).
- Multiple sectioning (may form multiple neuromas).
- Epineural repair over cut end.
- Bury nerve end in bone or muscle.
- Implantation into a nerve – another or the same nerve.

Neuropraxia
See <u>Seddon classification</u>.

Neurotmesis
See <u>Seddon classification</u>.

Nevus flammeus neonatorum
Salmon patch.

- The common fading macular stain that occurs in 50% of neonates.
- Commonly located on the glabella, eyelids, nose, upper lip ('angel kiss'), and nuchal area ('stork bite').

See <u>Port wine stain</u>.

Ninhydrin printing test
To test for sweating. The hand is cleaned with soap and alcohol. Place hand under a lamp and obtain an imprint. Spray with ninhydrin. Get a purple pattern with normal sweating.
See <u>Sympathetic function testing</u>.

Nipple

Nerve supply: Principally from the anterior branch of the 4th lateral intercostals nerve. It enters the breast at the chest wall 1.5 cm from the lateral edge of the breast.

Nipple inversion:
Classification:
- *I:* inverted, but everts easily and stays out. Try suction with nipplet or home-made nipplet using cut-off syringe.
- *II:* inverted. Able to evert, but retracts.
- *III:* inverted and will not evert.

Surgery: For II and III treat operatively. Evert nipple with skin hook. Using scalpel or nipple cut fibrous bands at the base of the nipple until it remains everted. Use purse string suture with clear prolene to maintain eversion.

Nipple reconstruction:
- Perform as second stage after breast reconstruction to get accurate positioning. Banking is usually not safe oncologically and gives a poor cosmetic result.

Nipple sharing: Can be used if there is an adequate size contralateral nipple, but will usually result in small nipples and a scar on the previously unaffected breast.

Local flap: The best way to produce nipple projection. Determined position of nipple by comparing with the opposite breast. Measure nipple to sternal notch and nipple to midline distance. Make small adjustments to fit nipple correctly on to the reconstructed breast mound. Nipple diameter should be the same as the opposite nipple, but projection should be at least twice as much.

Areola: Use tattooing – 4 months after the reconstruction, a tattoo should be darker as it fades within the first few weeks or FTSG from inner thigh. Can improve projection using cartilage graft. For nipple projection use one of a variety of flaps, e.g. skate flap, C–V flap, mushroom flap, Maltese cross (de-epithelialized areas), also Arrow flap, star technique.

No man's land

Zone II of flexor tendons: from distal palmar crease to middle of middle phalanx. Coined by Bunnell due to the poor results after attempted repair.

No reflow phenomenom

- Different tissues can tolerate different amounts of ischaemia. Skin and bone tolerate ischaemia well – up to 6 hours of warm ischaemia. Muscle shows irreversible damage after 4 hours.
- No-reflow describes the state of failure of perfusion once flow is re-established.
- The theories of no reflow are:
  o capillary leak increases haematocrit causing sludging;
  o endothelial swelling increases resistance;
  o capillaries are plugged by leucocytes;
  o interstitial oedema causes external compression on capillaries.
- Small capillary beds are occluded causing AV shunting. Treat with fibronolytic drugs, NSAIDs
See *Microsurgery*.

Nodular fasciitis

An uncommon lesion that must be distinguished from palmar fasciitis – part of Dupuytren's disease. It occurs more commonly in the forearm sometimes after a traumatic event. It presents as a small (<3 cm), tender, growing mass. It can be confused with a fibrosarcoma.

Noma

- Noma, also known as cancrum oris or necrotizing ulcerative stomatitis, is an orofacial gangrene which occurs in young children and untreated is usually lethal.
- Noma literally means wildfire. The condition results in extensive unilateral loss of the lips, oral commissure, nose, cheek and occasionally the lower eyelid. The bones of the maxilla, nose, zygoma, and mandible may be eroded and masticatory muscle involvement often causes trismus.

Non-ossifying fibroma

- Localized defects in the cortex of long bones.
- Seen in first decade of life.
- They form eccentric metaphyseal lesions.
- *Histology:* abundant immature fibroblasts.

Treatment: Observe. Most ossify at skeletal maturity.
See *Bone tumours*.

Notta's node

Nodule palpable in *Trigger finger*.

Nuss technique

Used for the treatment of *Pectus excavatum*. A preformed hooped bar inserted via a thoracoscope racked into position. Good results reported.

O Obesity to Ozone

Obesity

WHO weight classifications are based on the *Body Mass Index (BMI)*.

Underweight	<18.5
Normal range	18.5–24.9
Class I overweight	25–29.9
Class II obese	30–34.9
Class IIa obese	35–39.9
Class III obese	≥40

Oblique retinacular ligament (ORL) of Landsmeer
See *Landsmeer ligaments*.

Oedema
Impairs wound healing. In normal tissue each cells lies close to a capillary, and receives oxygen and nutrients by diffusion. Increase of extracellular fluid increases this distance. Also leads to protein deposition which can act as a barrier to diffusion. Growth factors and nutrients are also diluted.

Ohngren's line
Theoretic plane that joins the medial canthus of the eye with the angle of the mandible. Tumours below the line are considered infrastructure and carry a better prognosis than those above.
See *Maxilla/midface*.

Ollier's disease
- Multiple *Enchondromas*.
- Up to 25% of patients may get malignant degeneration of enchondroma to chondrosarcoma by the age of 40 years.

OMENS classification
For *Hemifacial microsomia*. Classifying the condition by the major affected structures:
- Orbit.
- Mandible.
- Ear.
- Facial nerve.
- Soft tissue.
OMENS plus is used to include the expanded spectrum: cardiac, skeletal, pulmonary, renal, gastrointestinal, and limb anomalies

Omentum
- Can be used pedicled, particularly for *Sternotomy wounds* and free, e.g. to provide soft tissue bulk in Rhomberg's disease.
- Upper midline incision. Lift omentum from colon. Free any adhesions. Isolate filmy attachments and divide. Clamp small vessels. Divide the short vessels between the gastroepiploic arcade and the greater curvature of the stomach. Now the omentum is attached by the left gastroepiploic (branch of splenic) and the right gastroepiploic.

- The omentum can usually reach the head and neck. It should fit loosely into the defect. Close the abdomen. Leave the upper wound open for 3–4 cm. Close skin and uncover chest. Either tunnel or lay open and skin graft. Potential complications include hernia, wound infection and bowel injury.

Omohyoid: anatomy

Origin: Inferior belly, tendon and superior belly. Inferior is from scapula and suprascapular ligament. It passes upward and forward across post. triangle. Passes under sternocleidomastoid to tendon held by loop of deep fascia slung to clavicle. Superior belly goes up in anterior triangle.

Insertion: Hyoid.

Nerve supply: Ansa cervicalis.

Action: Acts to depress hyoid.

Omphalocoele
- Developmental anomaly occurring in 1 in 3200–10 000 births.
- Often have sternal and diaphragmatic abnormalities, heart defects and bladder extrophy. Large defects have a high mortality rate.
- Results from failure of fusion at the umbilical ring.
- The sac of amnion and chorion commonly contains liver and midgut.
- The defect develops during the 6–12th week of gestation when the midgut passes out of the abdomen. Defects range from those around the umbilicus to those extending to the xiphoid and pubis. It is not a hernia.
See *Abdominal wall reconstruction*, *Gastroshisis*.

Oncogene
A gene that normally directs cell growth. If altered, an oncogene can promote or allow the uncontrolled growth of cancer. Alterations can be inherited or caused by an environmental exposure to carcinogens.

Onychomycosis
- 50% of patients with dystrophic nails have a nail bed fungal infection.

- Diagnosis is confirmed by microscopic visualization of hyphae on nail scrapings using a 20% KOH preparation.
- Other causes are psoriasis, lichen planus and trauma.
- More common in the foot.
- Treatment was previously problematic.
- Lamisil (terbinafine) is an effective antifungal. The dose is 250 mg per day for 6 weeks. LFTs are not required unless there is a history of liver disease. The dose is different for feet. 30% of patients will have a recurrence. An alternative is itraconazole.

Oppenheimer effect

Most implants in animals can induce tumours regardless of the material. Maximal tumirogenesis occurs with smooth surface. In rats the minimal size was 0.5 cm^2 and minimal time was 6 months with latent time of 300 days. There is not a strong association in humans. See _Alloplasts_.

Opponens pollicis

Origin: TCL deep to APB, ridge of trapezium and capsule of 1st CMC.

Insertion: radial border of 1st MC.

Nerve supply: motor branch of the median nerve.
See _Muscles_.

Opposition

- Thumb opposition is a composite motion through 3 joints to position the thumb pad opposite the distal phalanx of the middle finger.
- Abduction, pronation and flexion occur at the CMC joint, abduction and flexion at the MPJ and flexion or extension at the IPJ.
- Get 40° abduction at the CMCJ and 20° at the MPJ.
- Get 90° pronation.
- IP extension gives pulp-to-pulp grip and flexion for pinch.

Opposition thumb tendon transfers

- _Bunnell:_ FDS ring through pulley of FCU.
- _Camitz:_ PL with strip of palmar fascia to APB.

- _Burkhalter:_ EIP.
- _Huber:_ ADM.

Oral cancer

Risk factors:

- Tobacco products, alcohol. Also poor oral hygiene, mechanical from dental appliances, mouthwash, syphilis, Plummer–Wilson syndrome, candida, toxic irritants.
- _Leucoplakia_ and erythroplakia are premalignant – white and red lesions.

Cancers

- 30% of head and neck cancer.
- Tongue the most common – 30% of cases, most being in the anterior part, next is floor of mouth.
- 90% are SCC, next adenocarcinoma. SCCs can be differentiated, undifferentiated, adenoid squamous and verrucous.

Outcome: Determined by tumour size, thickness and nodes. Treatment based on TNM. Surgery mainstay of treatment, but also radiotherapy.
See _Head and neck cancer_.

Oral cavity reconstruction

Extend from vermilion to junction of hard and soft palate. Aim to maintain oral continuity, aid swallowing, prevent aspiration, preserve speech, provide wound healing.

Anatomy:

- _Lips:_ extend from skin vermilion to mucosa in contact with opposite lip.
- _Buccal mucosa:_ all the mucosa on the inner surface of cheek and lip up to alveolar ridge.
- _Lower alveolar ridge:_ formed by the alveolar process of the mandible and gingival mucosa.
- _The retromolar trigone_ is the mucosa overlying the ascending ramus of the mandible up to the maxillary tuberosity.
- _The upper alveolar ridge_ is the counterpart on the maxilla.
- _Hard palate_ extends over the palatine shelves.
- _Floor of mouth_ (FOM) extends from the gingiva of mandible to ventral tongue. The anterior tongue is from the tip to the V-shaped circumvallate papillae.

Specific sites:
- *Hard palate:* rare and should be biopsied first.
- *Alveolar ridge:* may get poorly fitting dentures. Metastasis unusual, but mandibular invasion is common.
- *Retromolar trigone:* easily invade adjacent structures up to skull base.
- *FOM:* become large before presenting. Often get occult bilateral neck metastasis.
- *Buccal mucosa:* aggressive metastatic potential.
- *Tongue:* invades easily and reaches a large size before presentation.
- *Lip:* tend to present early.

Surgical approach:
- Preserve tongue mobility.
- Small defects can be grafted or closed with local flaps or nasolabial flaps. Tongue flaps may be used.
- Radial forearm flap is the most commonly used flap for larger defects. Can be sensate with lateral antebrachial nerve to lingual nerve.
- Tongue can be reconstructed with a more bulky flap such as free rectus abdominus. Laryngeal suspension in a cephalad and anterior vector is important.

Oral cavity:
- *Small defects:* FOM defects may be able to be closed directly, but this may interfere with speaking and swallowing. Tongue and buccal mucosa can be closed directly. Tongue flaps can be useful and a posteriorly based lateral flap can fill a tongue defect but the tongue should not be tethered.
- *Large defects:* tongue, FOM and buccal mucosa defects can be reconstructed with a SSG using the quilting method. With anterior FOM defects coverage is important to prevent tongue tethering. It can be covered with nasolabial flaps. The pedicle is divided at 2 weeks. Bite blocks are required if there are teeth. Distant pedicle flaps have been used: forehead flaps, cervical apron flap, deltopectoral, pectoralis major, trapezius, lat dorsi, platysma and SCM flaps. The most frequently used flaps are the deltopectoral and pectoralis major. Bone can be carried with trapezius, lat dorsi, serratus anterior,

pectoralis major and SCM. Trapezius carrying spine of scapula is the most reliable.
- *Free tissue transfer – mucosa:* the best mucosa replacement are the radial forearm flap, ulnar forearm flap, scapular flap, lateral arm flap and dorsalis pedis flap. The radial and ulnar forearm flaps and the scapular flap are the most commonly used. Jejunal patches have been used but jejunal mucosa may be somewhat exuberant and may continue to produce mucus. Small doses of radiotherapy have been given to flatten the mucosa and reduce secretions.
- *Free tissue transfer:* mucosa and bone.
- *Replacement:* fibula flap, radial forearm flap, scapular flap, dorsalis pedis flap, and iliac flap based on the deep circumflex iliac vessels. The one most commonly used is the fibula flap.
- *Other reconstructive measures:* post-maxillectomy defects are skin-grafted and a dental prosthesis is placed in the defect.

Complications:
- Salivary fistula may occur and be difficult to deal with in the irradiated patient.
- The incidence of complications is increased when a simultaneous neck dissection is performed.
- *Carotid blowout:* particularly associated with a fistula and radiotherapy. Immediate cover with a muscle flap is advocated and may be performed prophylactically at the time of neck dissection.
- *Chyle leak:* may be repaired immediately if noticed, but usually become apparent once the patient is fed. Rarely require reoperation. Treat with fat free diet or TPN.
- Long-term complications include problems with the scar, shoulder pain and cosmesis.

Specific flaps:
- *Platysma flap.*
- *Temporalis muscle and fascia flap.*
- *Nasolabial flap.*
- *Lingual flap.*
- *Palatal flap.*
- *Forehead flap.*
- *Pectoralis muscle flap.*
- *Sternocleidomastoid flap.*
- *Trapezius muscle flap.*
- *Jejunal flap.*
See *Head and neck cancer.*

Orbicularis oculi

- Innervated by facial nerve.
- There are two portions, the orbital and palpebral.
- Orbital overlies orbital rims. It facilitates forceful eye closure.
- The palpebral portion is subdivided into pretarsal and preseptal. Continuous with SMAS in upper face:
  - ○ Pretarsal orbicularis is divided into superficial and deep components and is primarily responsible for involuntary eyelid blink.
  - ○ Preseptal orbicularis also has a superficial and deep component. Lacrimal pump intimately associated with muscle. Contraction of the pretarsal muscle shortens and closes the canaliculi, preseptal muscles pull on the diaphragm giving negative pressure in the sac. On relaxation tears are driven into the nasolacrimal duct. Also involved with voluntary eye closure. The orbital orbicularis acts as a medial brow depressor and performs forced eyelid closure. The muscle of Riolan is the smallest striated muscle in the body and is situated on the lid border.

See *Eyelid reconstruction*. See *Eyelid anatomy*.

Orbit

Anatomy:

- The orbit is comprised of 7 bones – frontal, zygoma, lesser and greater wing of sphenoid, ethmoid, lacrimal, palatine and maxilla.
- The optic foramen is situated medial to the superior orbital fissure.
- The anteromedial portion of orbital roof is the extension of frontal sinus. The rest is made of thin orbital plate of frontal bone and lesser wing of sphenoid. The roof is triangular in shape.
- The lacrimal gland sits in a concavity behind the rim. The optic canal is 8–12 mm in length. The floor is triangular. Most is made of the orbital plate of the maxilla. The palatine bone lies in the posterior aspect of the floor. Medially is the ethmoid.
- The infra-orbital nerve traverses the floor of the orbit in a groove.

- The sphenoid bone is the bone through which all neurovascular structures pass.
- Tenon's capsule is a fascial structure that divides the orbital cavity in two. The anterior half is filled with the globe and the posterior half with fat, muscles and neurovascular structures.

Orbital dystopia

Vertical or horizontal. With vertical dystopia the orbits do not lie on the same horizontal plane. In horizontal or transverse dystopia, the orbits are displaced laterally (orbital *Hypertelorism*) or medially (*Hypotelorism*). Orbital dystopia must be distinguished from ocular dystopia where the position of the globe is altered.

Causes: Vertical include craniosynostosis, torticollis, craniofacial microsomia and facial clefting. The most common cause of vertical orbital dystopia is a congenital condition. Surgery is beneficial.

Surgery: The box osteotomy moves the entire orbit. Frontal craniotomy allows movement of the orbital roof. The medial and lateral walls, floor of the orbit, zygoma, and maxillary osteotomies are performed. The procedure is performed through coronal, eyelid and gingivobuccal sulcus incisions. Diplopia may occur post-operatively, and more commonly with vertical repositioning.

See *Exorbitism*, *Exophthalmos*. *Enophthalmos*.

Orbital fractures

- Occur in conjunction with zygomatic fractures, naso-ethmoid fractures, high Le Fort fractures.
- Isolated orbital fractures result from pressure applied to the globe. The orbit fractures at its weakest point, the inferomedial floor known as the lamina papyracea (paper layer).
- The orbits can be divided into thirds. The orbital rim consists of thick bone, the middle third is thin then thickens in the posterior third. So the middle frequently breaks first followed by the anterior portions of the rim. This protects the important neurovascular structures posteriorly from severe displacement.

Symptoms and signs:
- Bruising and swelling.
- Subconjunctival haematoma with no posterior limit.
- Palpable steps in the orbital margin.
- _Enopthalmos:_ caused by increased volume of the orbit due to fracture, decreased volume of contents due to herniation, tethering at the fracture line. May occur late due to fat atrophy.

Diplopia:
- Caused by entrapment of fat, fascia or muscle within fracture, contusion of recti or oblique muscles. Usually on upward gaze due to fractures being tethered inferiorly.
- Visual field, globe pressure, fundoscopy. Assess lacrimal system. Examine for trapped muscle by the forced duction test. The insertion of a rectus muscle is grasped and the globe is moved.

Radiology: Plain XR – PA, Water's views – tear-drop sign may be present resulting from herniation of orbital contents through fracture line into maxillary sinus. CT and 3D CT.

Indications for surgery: Perform if there is diplopia, enopthalmos, evidence of orbital entrapment radiologically, large bony defects, or other fractures requiring fixation.

Fracture pathology:
- The commonest orbital fractures are zygomatio-orbital and malar fractures. The commonest infra-orbital fracture is the orbital floor. A blow-out fracture is due to a blow usually on the orbital rim causing an increased intra-orbital pressure resulting in a fracture to the thin inferior and medial wall. Orbital contents herniated through the fracture.
- Frequently get hypoaesthesia in the distribution of the infra-orbital nerve. The inferior oblique arises from the medial aspect of the orbital floor adjacent to the lacrimal groove behind the rim. Objects greater than 5 cm will increase intra-orbital pressure resulting in a pure blow-out fracture. Objects <5 cm diameter will cause globe rupture.

Fracture treatment:
- Aim.

- Release trapped structures and restore muscular function.
- Replace orbital contents into the orbit.
- Restore size.
- The orbital floor can be approached through a bicoronal incision, subciliary lower eyelid incision, midlid incision, transconjunctival incision, lateral brow incision, medial canthal and intra-oral incision.
- Fractures are fixed with interosseous wires or miniplates. The orbital floor is reconstructed with bone grafts or implants – rib, iliac crest anterior maxilla or split calvarial bone graft, titanium mesh, gore-tex, silicone or medpor.

See _Facial fractures_

Oropharyngeal tumours

Commonest sites in oropharynx are tonsils, tongue base, soft palate and pharyngeal wall.

Glottic and subglottic ca:
- The glottis is surrounded by ligamentous structures, which act as a barrier, and it is poorly supplied with blood vessels and lymphatics. Therefore the risk of cervical metastasis is low for T1 and T2 tumours – <10%.
- Supraglottic region is richly supplied with vessels and therefore the risk of cervical spread is much higher with 50% of T1 and T2 tumours having cervical metastasis.

Elective neck dissection: Supraomohyoid neck dissection is recommended for stage I and II tongue cancers as there is a high chance of occult metastasis – 30% for stage I and 50% for stage II. If two or more nodes present then also perform radiotherapy.

Surgery V radiotherapy:
- Stage I and II disease of the oropharynx is relatively uncommon, and often present with a neck mass. Either modality is effective for early disease.
- _Surgical complications:_ dysarthria, dysphagia, aspiration.
- _Radiotherapy complications:_ xerostomia, dysgeusia (distortion or absence of sense of taste), dysphagia, but symptoms after radiotherapy less than after surgery.

Surgery:

- Access is either transorally or through a pharyngotomy. For wide exposure perform a mandibulotomy with a mandibular swing. The lateral pharyngeal wall can be accessed through a lateral pharyngotomy.
- *Ca larynx:* laryngectomy has been the standard treatment. However, radiotherapy and combined radiotherapy and chemotherapy have been tried in an attempt to preserve the larynx and has given good results though the role of each is unclear.

Voice restoration.
See *Head and neck cancer*. See *Oral cancer*.

Orthodontics

For *Cleft* and craniofacial disorders. Dental development is usually slower than normal. Maxillary lateral incisors are often missing on the cleft side. Teeth are not removed unless they are causing problems. Maxillary central incisors are usually rotated.

Passive prosthetics (neonate):

- To fill the cleft palate.
- It is made from *Methylmethacrylate*.
- It aids breathing and feeding and placing the tongue in the correct position.
- It prevents medial collapse and promotes maxillary transverse growth.
- It must be adjusted every 6 weeks.
- Nasal moulding can be tried.

Presurgical orthopaedic correction (POC) (neonatal):

- To correct abnormal bony relationship and provide a better platform for repair. It can be passive or fixed devices.
- Passive devices are difficult to maintain, they are unpredictable and take a long time.
- Pinned retention using devices such as designed by Latham are more invasive, but quicker. A screw is turned regularly to realign segments which is usually complete within 3 months. POC may cause reduced maxillary growth

Orthopaedic management: primary dentition (3–6 years):

- Used to treat crossbite, narrow maxillary arch and openbite.

- The prostheses produce maxillary distraction and anterior repositioning.

Mixed dentition (age 7–11 years):

- By maxillary expansion, orthodontics, extractions and tooth straightening.
- Alveolar bone grafting occurs in this period.

Adolescent and adult dentition (age 12–17 years and over):

- Maxillary expansion may be used.
- The missing lateral incisor is replaced with a prosthetic tooth or by moving other teeth into position.

Orthognathic surgery

Corrects malposition of the dentofacial skeleton. Two most common conditions treated are mandibular and maxillary retrusion. Also maxillary vertical excess and mandibular prognathism. Most are developmental. Some are associated with congenital problems such as clefts.

Evaluation:

- Assess form and shape of face. Use aids such as the classic canons of vertical facial thirds. Also look at the AP relationship. The nose is the key to the central face and the lip-tooth-chin for the lower third.
- *Look at occlusion: Angle classification*, assess overbite and overjet. See *Teeth*. Assess the temporomandibular joints, looking for any dysfunction which may first require treatment. *Cephalometric analysis* is used.

Treatment plan:

- Aim to obtain a Class 1 occlusion after jaw repositioning. See *Le Fort*.
- *Maxillary vertical excess:* dissect subperiosteally to piriform rim and infra-orbital nerve. Osteotomy made at least 5 mm above the root apexes. Resect bone.
- *Vertical maxillary deficiency:* only one osteotomy cut is needed placed 5 mm above the apex of the roots. Intermaxillary fixation is performed with an acrylic wafer inserted to get correct position. Bone graft is inserted, cranial strips. Rigid internal fixation.
- *Maxillary retrusion:* often idiopathic. Also associated with cleft lip and palate. Get flattened or dished in midfacial region. Get Class III malocclusion. Get reduced SNA

angle and normal SNB angle. Perform a LeFort I osteotomy and rigidly fix. Relapse is high so some perform an overadvancement.

- *Mandibular retrusion:* most evident in the profile view. Get class II malocclusion. Get a decreased SNB angle. Prior to surgery, orthodontics corrects any flaring that will limit the amount of advancement. 3 types of osteotomies are performed:
  - o vertical and oblique ramus;
  - o inverted L;
  - o *sagittal split osteotomy:* may relapse, but less with rigid fixation, the most common problem is mental nerve dysfunction; this is common, but usually resolves, may get limited mandibular opening.
- *Mandibular prognathism:* often get mild mid-face flattening. Need set back. Use sagittal split for less than 1 cm and inverted L for larger osteotomies.

Chin deformities: can occur independent or together with other facial deformities. 7 types of deformity – macrogenia, microgenia, combination macroand microgenia, asymmetric chin, pseudomacro and pseudomicrogenia, witches' chin deformity (soft tissue ptosis).

Ortichochea flap

- Used for *Scalp reconstruction* with large scalp defects.
- Axial flaps, which allow the entire remaining scalp to be elevated.
- The 3-flap technique (banana peel) uses an anterior pedicle based on supratrochlear and supra-orbital vessels, a lateral flap on superficial temporal artery vessels, and a posterior flap incorporating occipital vessels. Good for frontal and occipital defects. Galeal scoring may allow as much as 20% increase to flap area.

Ortichochea sphincter pharyngoplasty

- For the treatment of *Velopharyngeal incompetence*.
- Aims to tighten the central orifice.
- Originally described by *Hynes* and modified by others, such as Ortichochea and Jackson. Involves the construction of palatopharyngeus myomucosal flaps from the posterior

tonsillar pillars, which are sutured to the posterior pharyngeal wall.

- The flaps are not sutured to the posterior pharyngeal wall laterally. There have been no studies validating its use. The height of insertion of the flaps appears to be critical for success.

Osborne's ligament

A tendinous arch formed by the two heads of *Flexor carpi ulnaris* under which ulnar nerve passes.

Osseointegration

- Direct anchorage of an implant by the formation of bony tissue around the implant without the growth of fibrous tissue at the bone–implant interface.
- Developed in the 1970s in oedentulous patients for the anchorage of dental prosthesis. Also used for fixation of hearing aids to the temporal bone and for small joint reconstruction in the hand and for the fitting of prosthesis in the hand and other sites.
- Titanium fixtures are used and the titanium oxide layer formed at the surface of the implant is probably important in this phenomenon.
- In thumb prosthesis there is a capacity for tactile stimulation – osseoperception. This may be based on the transfer of tactile stimuli from the thumb to the intra-osseous nerves via the osseointegrated implant.

Ossification of hand

Age of appearance of ossification centres:

- Capitate and hamate – 2/12.
- Thumb metacarpal – 1.6 year.
- Triquetral – 1.7 year.
- Thumb proximal phalanx – 1.7 year.
- MCP joint of fingers – 1.5 year.
- Distal phalanges – all by 2.5 year.
- Lunate – 2.6 year.
- Middle phalanges – all by 2 year.
- Scaphoid, trapezium, trapezoid – 4.1 year.

Ossifying fasciitis

- Rare benign tumour similar histologically to nodular fasciitis, composed of metaplastic bone with calcification.

- Rapidly growing lesion which may be mistaken for a malignancy. Usually found in the trunk and upper and lower limbs.
- Most common in women 20–30 years, may be associated with trauma (10%).
- Treatment is local excision.

Osteoarthritis

Can be secondary to gout, Wilson's disease, haemochromatosis, trauma, Kienbock's, infection, Ehler's–Danlos syndrome, haemophilia.

Osteoblastoma

See _Bone tumours._

- Similar histologically to osteoid osteoma, but a different XR appearance and clinical course.
- They are larger – usually over 2 cm.
- They occur in the cancellous bone of the posterior column of the spine.
- They are slightly more aggressive.
- They have plumper osteoblasts.
- Some are stage 3 with a high recurrence rate.

Osteochondroma

- The most common benign _Bone tumour_.
- Cartilage-capped bony exostosis near the epiphyseal cartilage plate.
- Usually painless.
- Growth often stops within 2 years of skeletal maturity.
- Most occur in the 20s.
- May get local pressure on adjacent structures.
- May be solitary or multiple.
- Multiple may be hereditary as autosomal dominant (20% have a negative family history).
- Most commonly in the radius and ulna and in the hand in the metacarpal and phalanges.
- Treat if becomes large and causing cosmetic or functional problem.
- Malignant transformation may occur though very rare – more likely with multiple osteochondromas.

Osteogenic sarcoma

- >80% occur in patients <30 years old.
- Present with pain unrelated to activity.
- Most common in the distal femur then the proximal tibia.

- In the upper limb the proximal humerus is the most common site followed by the distal radius. In the hand usually found in the metacarpals or phalanges.
- 90% are stage IIB on presentation.
- Secondary osteosarcomas with Paget's or after radiotherapy is very aggressive.

Histology: Consists of malignant proliferating spindle cell stroma producing osteoid bone.

_XR:_ See _Sclerotic expansile destructive lesion_. MRI shows widespread marrow involvement. With soft tissue extension with sunburst pattern.

Treatment: Aggressive radical excision with neoadjuvant and adjunctive chemotherapy. >90% can have limb salvage surgery. Survival is 50–70% 5-year without lung metastasis. See _Bone tumours._

Osteoid osteoma

- Benign osteoblastic lesion consisting of a well demarcated core (nidus) with surrounding zone of reactive bone.
- _XR:_ get area of sclerosis with central radiolucency. CT will differentiate from a Brodie abscess.
- 3 types are cortical, medullary and subperiosteal.
- They are reported in all bones, mainly in the lower limb. In the hand they are most common in the proximal phalanx.
- They present in the 20s and 30s.
- Patients complain of a dull aching pain with point tenderness.
- Treat with observation and NSAIDs until the disease burns out in 2–3 years.
- _Surgery for pain:_ complete excision of the nidus. Also radiotherapy has been used. See _Bone tumours._

Osteomyelitis

Most commonly caused by penetrating trauma and predisposing conditions such as DM. Direct trauma will most often lead to _S. aureus_ or streptococcal infection. Infections following ORIF are often _Staph. epidermidis._ Surgical debridement is required.

Classification: _Cierny and Mader classification_.

Ota: naevus of
- A blue naevus seen at birth or in adolescence.
- Mainly in Oriental women.
- Flat irregular grey-blue patch on the face in the distribution of 1st and 2nd trigeminal nerve may involve the eye. 5% are bilateral. Do not disappear spontaneously, and may hyperpigment.
- Benign, but associated melanoma has been reported.
- Q-switched ruby and argon lasers may be effective.

See Blue naevus, Naevus.

Ozone
- O_3, which occurs in the stratosphere due to the splitting of O_2 to O by *Ultraviolet radiation (UV)*, which then combines with O_2 to form O_3.
- Ozone is more effective in blocking UVA than UVB.
- 95% of radiation, which reaches the human skin is UVA. However, the minimal UVB causes the acute sunburn and malignant skin changes.
- Since 1969 there has been a 3–7% decrease in ozone. With each percentage decrease there is a 1% increase of melanoma.

P P53 to Pyogenic granuloma

P53
Tumour suppressor gene, mutated in the majority of cancers.

UV-related mutations have been linked to mutations of the p53 tumour suppressor gene.

Pacinian corpuscles
- Only found in the hand.
- Rapidly adapting myelinated A fibres mediating moving touch and vibration. They respond to the onset of mechanical stimulus.
- They are situated in connective tissue along nerve trunks. They are served by a single myelinated fibre.
- There are up to 120 on the palmar surface of each finger.

See Sensory receptors.

Paget's disease
- Eczematous lesion of the nipple and areola, which is also found in extramammary areas.
- Extramammary Paget's occurs in both sexes, more common in older women.
- Found primarily in the anogenital region, mainly the vulva.
- Biopsy is required. Microscopically large round Paget cells lie within the epidermis.

These have large nuclei and lots of pale staining cytoplasm. Mucin stains differentiate these cells from melanoma.
- Paget's disease of the breast without an underlying mass requires excision and has a good prognosis. If a lump is present this will require treatment and prognosis will depend on the nature of the lump.
- Extramammary Paget's requires wide and deep excision with a careful search for an underlying carcinoma. Paget's cells may be found outside the clinical limits of excision and wide excision will reduce chance of recurrence. Prognosis is poor if an underlying carcinoma is present.

Pairolero classification
For *Sternotomy* wound infections.

Palatal flap
Total palatal mucoperiosteal tissue can be raised on a single greater palatine artery. This can be transposed to cover defects in buccal mucosa, retromolar triangle, tonsillar and soft palate. Donor area left to granulate. Not pliable, contraindicated with previous RT.
See Oral cavity reconstruction.

Palate carcinoma

- More commonly in older men. Rare in the West.
- Due to tobacco and alcohol and in India a thermal element due to reverse smoking.
- Presentation may be with swelling, bleeding or pain. Bone invasion occurs late. Nodal involvement is seen in 16% of hard palate cancers and 37% of soft palate lesions.

Treatment:

- Resection through the mouth with underlying bone.
- Radiotherapy may cause bone exposure and necrosis.
- With more extensive lesions, a partial hemimaxillectomy is performed through a Weber-Fergusson incision, and reconstructed with a skin graft and a prosthesis.
- More extensive lesions require total hemimaxillectomy.
- As long as the inferior peri-orbitum is not breached, there is no change in position of the eye and no double vision. If the orbit is involved, the orbital contents must be removed; if the tumour extends into the ethmoid sinus, an intracranial approach is advised.
- Cervical node involvement requires neck dissection, which includes the parotid region.
- Radiotherapy is given for large tumours, for incompletely excised tumours, and after neck dissection.

Results: The 5-year survival rate is 31%.
See *Head and neck cancer*.

Palm infections

3 potential spaces deep to flexor tendons

- *Thenar space:* radial to oblique septum, which extends from palmar fascia to 3rd metacarpal. Flexor sheath infection of the index finger may rupture here. Incise in the-nar crease.
- *Mid-palmar space:* ulnar to oblique septum. Middle and ring sheath infections may rupture here.
- *Hypothenar space:* rarely involved. Incise on radial side to avoid a tender scar.

These are only potential spaces. Distinguish from the radial and ulnar bursae which are synovial sheaths enclosing the flexor tendons of the thumb and little finger, which communicate with the space of Parona. Infection can lead to a horseshoe abscess.
See *Infections*.

Palmar branch of the median nerve

Arises 5–6 cm proximal to the distal wrist crease between palmaris longus and flexor carpi radialis. It passes superficial to the radial margin of the flexor retinaculum to supply the skin of the palm. It is frequently injured during carpal tunnel release though it never runs ulnar to a line drawn from the ulnar side of the middle finger.

Palmar fascia

Longitudinal fibres extend into fingers. Natatory ligaments in web space. Cleland's (dorsal) and Grayson's (volar) ligaments extend to middle phalanges.
See *Retinacular system*.

Palmaris longus

Origin: flexor pronator origin. Muscle belly is small with a long thin tendon which runs superficial to TCL
Insertion: apex of palmar aponeurosis. Absent 10–15% people.
Nerve supply: median nerve.
Action: weak flexor of wrist. Used in tendon transfers or grafts.
See *Muscles*.

Papillomatosis

An increase in depth of corrugations at the junction between the epidermis and dermis.
See *Skin*.

Papineau technique

Staged bone grafting for infected non-union of a tibial fracture:

- *Stage 1:* excision of infected bone, external fixation, pack with antibiotic swabs.
- *Stage 2:* cancellous bone grafting with antibiotic swabs.
- *Stage 3:* flaps and skin grafts to achieve soft tissue cover.

See *Lower limb reconstruction*.

Parakeratosis
The presence of nucleated cells at the skin surface.
See _Skin_.

Parascapular flap
See _Scapular/parascapular flap_.

Paré
Ambroise Paré: 1517–1590, a military surgeon and a devoted Catholic. He was a great observer. Also surgeon to the king. He changed the practice of using oil to cauterize gunshot wounds (used as all such wounds were thought to be poisoned) when he had run out of oil and noted that wounds cleaned more gently healed better. He also revived the practice of vascular ligation. Above his chair was the motto 'I treated him but God healed him'.

Parkes–Weber syndrome
Now called fast flow _Complex combined vascular malformations_.

Parkland formula
- Fluid regime used in _Burns_ resuscitation.
- Also called the Baxter formula.
- Use Ringer's lactate.
- Fluid for first 24 hours = 4 ml × wt × % burn.
- Half given in first 8 hours, second half in next 16 hours.
- For children, also give maintenance fluid. Beware hypoglycaemia.
- Tends to overestimate fluid needs in adults with moderate-sized burns. Adjust based on the patient's response.

Parona: space of
Retrotendinous space in the distal forearm. The synovial sheath enclosing FPL can connect with that of the little finger through this space. This can give rise to a horseshoe-shaped abscess if all three spaces are involved in septic tenosynovitis.

Paronychia
- An infection in the nail fold along the perinychium. Cellulitus can be treated with antibiotics. Pus under the nail requires removal of part of the nail. If chronic, it may require marsupialization of the nail fold.
- Chronic paronychia may point to an underlying disease such as diabetes or scleroderma. Most commonly seen in middle-aged women. Many have _Candida albicans_.
- Treatment is difficult. Marsupialize eponychium. Remove nail and apply anti-fungals to nail bed.

Parotid duct: trauma
The duct travels from the anteromedial border of the parotid gland to the anterior border of masseter on a line between the tragus to the middle of the upper lip and exits in the mouth opposite the second maxillary molar (bicuspid). A vertical line drawn from the lateral canthus indicates where it divides intra-orally. Lacerations in this area may divides the duct. It lies very close to the buccal branch of the facial nerve so the two are likely to be injured at the same time. The duct can be cannulated and if divided should be repaired over a stent.

Parotid tumours
See _Salivary tumours_.

Parotidectomy
Superficial parotidectomy:
- Use no muscle relaxant to aid identification of the nerve.
- _Incision:_ upper anterior ear, down along pre-auricular crease and back over mastoid process then anteriorly towards the hyoid bone.
- Elevate skin flaps, preserving greater auricular nerve.
- Separate the tail of the parotid from the sternocleidomastoid and digastric muscles
- _Facial nerve:_ approach proximally or distally.
  - ○ Antegrade: visualize cartilaginous tragal pointer; facial nerve 1 cm deep to this point; use nerve stimulator; separate superficial lobe from the nerve.
  - ○ _Retrograde:_ identify distal branches at the following sites:
    - ■ cervical branch alongside retromandibular vein;

- marginal branch below lower border of mandible as it runs over the facial artery;
- buccal branches alongside parotid duct which can be cannulated to identify it.

Parry–Romberg's disease
See *Hemifascial atrophy*.

Parsonage–Turner syndrome
Pain around shoulder and upper arm is followed in a few hours by atrophic paralysis of anterior interosseous nerve. Pain can be bilateral though paralysis is unilateral. May have recent flu-like illness. Recovery occurs after 15–36 months. Treat conservatively.
See *Anterior interosseous syndrome*.

Passavant's ridge
This is the bulge on the posterior pharynx caused by the contraction of levator palatini and superior constrictors. May be seen in *Velopharyngeal incompetence* in an attempt to cause velopharyngeal closure.
See *Cleft palate*.

PDS
Polydiaxanone. Monofilament. Absorbed more slowly than the other absorbable sutures. It loses its strength at 3 months, absorbed by 6 months. Used as a dermal suture in areas prone to stretched scars.

Pectoralis major
Origin:
- *Clavicular head:* anterior surface of medial half of clavicle.
- *Sternocostal head:* sternum, upper 6 ribs, external oblique aponeurosis.

Insertion: Intertubercular groove of humerus.

Action: Adducts and medially rotates humerus. Clavicular head flexes and sternocostal head extends humerus.

Nerve supply: Lateral and medial pectoral nerves. Clavicular head C5 and C6, sternoclavicular head C7,C8,T1.

Arterial supply: Pectoral branch of thoracoacromial trunk.

Pectoralis major flap
- Described by Ariyan in 1979.
- Type 5 muscle supplied by thoraco-acromial artery and segmental perforators of IMA.
- Thoracoacromial artery starts from midpoint of clavicle and turns to run along line from acromion to xiphisternum. Accompanied by vein and lat pectoralis nerve.
- For a pedicled flap, the defect is measured and the skin island is drawn over the muscle. Skin is incised down to deep fascia. Muscle is exposed. Muscle is elevated and divided from attachments along sternum. The thoraco-acromial pedicle can be searched for. It arises just medial to the coracoid process of the scapula.
- Carry dissection toward the humeral insertion. Divide muscle, avoiding axillary neuromuscular structures. Divide clavicular attachments, working towards the pedicle. Transpose the flap into the defect. It can be used as a turnover flap.

Sternal reconstruction:

Oesophageal replacement:
- Paddle is outlined in a trapezoidal shape with the longer edge placed inferiorly and the short edge superiorly.
- The edges should equal in length the circumference of the oropharyngeal and oesophageal remnants.
- The paddle should lie entirely over pectoralis major muscle. Once the skin is incised down to fascia, the muscle is freed and the entire flap rotated to the neck.
- The flap is tubed and the long suture is placed laterally and the muscle overlies the skin tube. The pectoralis muscle is sutured to prevertebral fascia for support. Any exposed muscle is grafted.
See *Pharynx*.

Pectus carinatum
- *Pigeon breast:* protrusion deformity of anterior chest wall.
- The opposite of *Pectus excavatum*.
- Much less common.
- Can be chondrogladiolar (most prominent at xiphisternum) or chondromanubrial (most prominent at sternomanubrium).

Reconstruction: Similar to pectus excavatum. Resect abnormal costal cartilage. Reposition sternum. Support sternum with a substernal metallic strut. Secure strut with wires. Shave sternum and use shavings as on-lay for the hollows.
See *Chest wall reconstruction*.

Pectus excavatum

- Chest deformities occur in 1 in 300 births. M:F 2:1, may be familial.
- May be associated with Marfan's syndrome.
- Pectus excavatum (funnel chest) is the most common.
- The depression begins at the sternal angle and reaches the deepest point at the xiphoid. It may be so severe that the sternum contact the vertebral bodies. This results in cardiac displacement, rotation of the heart and reduction in lung space.
- Due to overgrowth of costal cartilages forcing it posteriorly or anteriorly (pectus carinatum). In a 5-year-old child a sterno-vertebral distance of <5 cm is severe, 5–7 cm is moderate and >7 cm is mild.

Reconstruction:
- Prosthesis can be inserted into the defect.
- *Ravitch technique.*
- *Sternum turnover procedure:* transection of ribs and intercostal muscles at costal arches. Transect sternum above deformity. Remove and turn over. Suture sternum with wires and heavy silk.
- *Nuss technique.*
See *Chest wall reconstruction*.

Pelvic wall reconstruction
Anatomy:
- Defined as the region above lower extremities and below abdomen. Bony landmarks are iliac crest, pubic symphysis, sacrum and greater trochanter.
- Major arteries are the common iliac, deep circumflex iliac and inferior epigastric artery. Internal iliac artery enters the true pelvis, and divides into anterior and posterior. Anterior divides into inferior gluteal, obturator, internal pudendal, umbilical, inferior vesical, middle rectal, uterine and vaginal arteries. The posterior divides into superior gluteal, iliolumbar and lateral sacral.

Operations: Local muscle flaps are often the first choice for small defects. Include gluteus maximus, *Rectus abdominus*, rectus femoris, vastus lateralis.

Anterior defects: Abdominoperineal hernias can be a problem and reconstruction should include fascia. Also mesh can be used covered with muscle flaps. TFL and rectus femoris can be used for inside and outside mesh cover.

Lateral defects:
- Local muscle flaps for smaller defects, including rectus abdominus, external oblique and rectus femoris.
- *Hemipelvectomy:* involves removal of the entire lower extremity and hemipelvis. If radical the bone is divided proximal to the sacroiliac joint. For a groin tumour choose a posterior flap. For a posterior tumour choose an anterior flap.
- *Posterior flap:* anteriorly start 5 cm proximal and 2 cm medial to ASIS. Follow inguinal ligament. Laterally from ASIS over anterior greater trochanter then distal to the gluteal groove. Divide iliac vessels, preserve sacral roots to bladder and rectum. Elevate myocutaneous flap.
- *Anterior flap:* uses a myocutaneous flap supplied by perforators of the external iliac and superficial femoral arteries.

Penile prosthesis
2 types available. A permanently stiff rod which keeps the penis firm, the other is inflated with a saline pump.
See *Peyronie's disease*.

Penis: anatomy
Root:
- Attached to perineal membrane.
- Bulb is the posterior end of corpora spongiosum.
- Lateral crura are the posterior ends of corpora cavernosa.
- Ischiocavernosus muscle moves the erect penis.
- Bulbospongiosus muscles empty the urethra of semen and urine.

Body: 3 erectile bodies, 2 corpora cavernosa and corpus spongiosum surrounding the urethra. The NVB contains the deep dorsal vein, dorsal artery, paired dorsal nerves.

Fascia:

- Tunica albuginea surrounds corpus cavernosa and spongiosum.
- This is surrounded by Buck's fascia deeply and Dartos fascia superficially.
- Between tunica albuginea and Buck's fascia lie the dorsal artery of penis, dorsal nerve of penis and deep dorsal vein of penis.
- The suspensory ligament attaches the penis to the symphysis pubis.

Urethra:

- *Posterior:* prostatic and membranous.
- *Anterior:* penile.
- The urethra is lined by transitional epithelia just proximal to the external urethral meatus and distally is lined by squamous epithelium.
- The cross-section is a horizontal slit changing to a vertical slit at the meatus causing urine to spiral.

Blood supply:

- The common penile artery comes from the internal pudendal artery.
- Its branches are the bulbourethral, dorsal and cavernosal artery.
- Venous drainage is by venae comitantes draining into the internal pudendal veins and the deep dorsal vein, which drains into the prostatic plexus. Superficial veins drain skin.

Lymphatic drainage:

- Lymphatics running with the superficial dorsal vein drain to superficial inguinal nodes.
- Lymphatics of the glans drain to deep inguinal nodes and internal iliac nodes.

Nerve supply: The dorsal nerve carries afferent sensory stimulation to the pudendal nerve. Erotic or tactile stimulation stimulates the cavernous nerve, which relaxes the cavernosal smooth muscle. Relaxation causes a decrease in arterial resistance and expansion in the lacunar spaces leading to an erection.

- *Erection:* parasympathetic, pelvic splanchnic nerves from the sacral plexus (S2,3,4).

- *Ejaculation:* sympathetic nerves (L1 root from sacral ganglia).
- *Skin:* posterior scrotal and dorsal branches of the internal pudendal nerves (S2,3,4).
- Muscles the perineal branch of the pudendal nerves.

Development:. See Embryology. See Hypospadias.

Penis reconstruction

Indications: Ambiguous genitalia, female to male gender reassignments and a number of acquired conditions of penile loss, such as trauma, cancer, burns, infection.

Goals:

- Normal appearance and adequate length for intercourse.
- Should contain the urethra and allow voiding while standing.
- Protective sensation to contain erectile prosthesis.
- Tactile and erogenous sensation.
- One stage. These are only possible with newer microvascular techniques.

Total penile reconstruction: Radial forearm flap is most commonly used.

- *Chinese method:* using radial forearm flap. centre over radial artery. Include two sensory nerves. 15 × 15 cm flap. Bone can be harvested or rib graft inserted or prosthesis. Ulnar skin which is less hairy is used to create the neourethra. So 3 cm width of urethra and 10 cm to tube around it. For transsexual the urethra will need to be longer.
- *Modified Chinese:* centre neourethra over radial artery to give best possible perfusion. Shaft either side of this. Cricket bat design places urethra over radius and shaft in tandem but with significant loss of penile length. As the ulnar border is less hirsute, it can be raised on the ulnar artery. Disadvantages of forearm flap:
  - hair causes problems in neourethra;
  - not much bulk;
  - extrusion of the prosthesis;
  - large graft;
  - cold intolerance.
- <u>Lateral arm flap:</u> extends from deltoid insertion to proximal 1/3 forearm. Proximal

forearm becomes glans and is innervated by posterior brachial and antebrachial nerves. The urethra is centred over the pedicle and a flap 18–20 cm wide is required. In a thin arm the urethra is prefabricated with a FTSG centred over the pedicle and sutured around a catheter. This is left 3–6 months. This ensures a good urethra is formed prior to lifting the flap and allows all available skin to be used for the phallus.

- *Others:* free sensate osseocutaneous flap. This requires a FTSG for urethra. Second toe dorsalis pedis flap has been used with jointed skeleton allowing rigidity and yet folding.
- *Recipient site:* T incision. Dissect out left and right erogenous branches of internal pudendal nerve from clitoris or penile remnant, also ilio inguinal or genitofemoral. Use inferior epigastric vessels, gaining 15 cm of length. For a prosthesis a pocket is made beneath the rectus abdominus.
- *Transfer:* for transsexuals, a neourethra is made from labia minora flaps. Perform neurorrhaphy first then anastomose vessels.

Subtotal reconstruction: Release any existing scar. Deglove corporal bodies down to base. Skin graft. Z-plasty to break up longitudinal scars. W flaps. Division of suspensory ligaments in the midline (avoid neurovascular structures). Silicon spacer can be inserted. Girth can be augmented by fat-dermal composite graft. Take from abdomen and include 5–10 mm of fat. Excise suprapubic fat. Penoscrotal webbing may need Z-plasty. New coronal sulcus can be created by undermining. Tattooing can be performed for colour mismatch.

Complications: Fistulae and strictures secondary to ischaemia. Making it stiff enough is the biggest problem. An inflatable prosthesis inside a sensate phallus gives the best chance of success.

Perforator flaps

Developed from *Fasciocutaneous flap* and *Musculocutaneous/muscle flaps* when it was realized that the muscle itself didn't need to be raised as long as the perforating vessels were preserved.

Perifolliculitis capitis abscedens et suffodiens

Also called dissecting cellulitis of the scalp.

- Occurs most often in black men.
- Disease of the scalp similar to *Hidradenitis suppurativa*.
- The scalp is involved with a perifolliculitis that results in burrowing, encysted epithelium-lined tracts with associated chronic infection and granulation tissue.
- The conservative management has been discouraging.
- The only effective treatment is excision of the scarred, infected areas and resurfacing with split-thickness skin grafts or skin flaps from the adjacent scalp if the disease is limited.

Periodontium

Or gums. Specialized dense fibrous tissue covered with mucous membrane that attaches to the cervical margin of the roots of the teeth and the alveoulus of the jaws. Long-term survival of the tooth is dependent on this periodontal attachment.

Permacol

D porcine collagen/elastin matrix. Permanent, non-allergenic, cell friendly, biocompatible, supports revascularization. Comes in sheets. Will also be as liquid.

Peyronie's disease

- Peyronie was a French barber surgeon who commanded the surgical corps of Louis XIV. He described scar tissue causing upward curvature of the penis.
- Connective tissue disorder affecting 1% of males.
- Get painful erections, curve, nodules.
- The plaque may be an inflammatory response to traumas to the penis.
- Associated with beta-blockers.
- Dupuytren's disease is seen in 10–30% of patients with Peyronie's disease.
- Curve is usually up and to the right.
- Condition usually progresses over 2 years and then stabilizes or improves.

Goals of treatment: Preserve or restore sexual function. Consider erectile dysfunction, penile pain.

Investigations: Penile ultrasound for vascular anatomy.

Medical: Vitamin E until plaque matures or curve stable.

Surgical:
- Various implants have been tried – dermis, Dacron, dura, tunica vaginalis, dexon, vein.
- Plication (Nesbit plication) or excision of plaque and dermal graft (from non-hair-bearing groin skin).
- Dermal graft gives straight erections in 85% of patients.
- Consider a penile prosthesis at the same time as surgery for plaque if there is erectile dysfunction.

See Penile prosthesis.

Pfeiffer's syndrome
See Craniosynostosis.
- Autosomal dominant.
- Similar craniofacial features to Apert's syndrome.
- Craniosynostosis – turribrachycephaly secondary to the coronal and occasional sagittal synostosis.
- Midface hypoplasia with shallow orbits and exorbitism.
- Hypertelorism and downslanting palpebral fissures.
- Nose is often downturned with a low nasal bridge.
- Intelligence is reported to be normal.
- Enlarged broad thumbs and toes.
- May have partial syndactyly of 2nd and 3rd digits.

Phalen's test
- Probably the most reliable test in *Carpal tunnel syndrome.*
- Hold the wrist in maximal palmar flexion. Test is positive when symptoms occur within 60 seconds.
- Reverse Phalen's test is similar with the hands and fingers dorsiflexed.

Pharynx
- A muscle line tubular continuation of the oral cavity. It regulates food entry into the oesophagus and is a modulator for speech.

- *Nasopharynx:* rigid mucosa-lined box-shaped structure with the posterior openings of the nasal cavity (choanae) anteriorly.
- *Oropharynx:* includes tonsils and tonsillar pillars, base of tongue and cephalad portion of middle constrictor.
- *Hypopharynx:* lies lateral and posterior to the larynx and is surrounded by cricopharyngeus.
- The oral cavity prepares food for swallowing. When ready, the tongue pushes it up and back, the middle constrictor relaxes, the larynx elevates and closes and the food moves into the oropharynx and hypopharynx. The bolus moves down into the oesophagus. As it passes, the larynx descends and airway is reopened.
- *Nerve supply:* sensation is primarily the internal laryngeal branch of the superior laryngeal nerve, from vagus. Also glossopharyngeal nerve. Motor supply to upper pharynx is from the external laryngeal branch of the vagus and the lower pharynx is from the recurrent laryngeal branch. High injury to the vagus gives severe functional disruption to the pharynx and larynx. Lower injury gives only motor problems.

Malignancy:
- Paediatric tumours such as rhabdomyosarcoma can be treated with CT and RT without surgery.
- SCC of the larynx and pharynx is treated with resection +/– neck dissection and RT.
- Oropharynx and hypopharynx carcinoma frequently spread to the nasopharynx with lateral spread to lymph nodes. Intrinsic larynx ca is less likely to spread. Ca of cervical oesophagus spreads to thoracic oesophagus and may require total oesophagectomy. Removal of tumour with a 2 cm margin frequently results in a circumferential defect.

Reconstruction:
- *Total oesophagectomy* for malignancy, stricture and motility disorders. Reconstruction is performed with a right, left or transverse colon as a pharyngogastric conduit in a subcutaneous or substernal position. To gain extra length an arcade can also be anastomosed in the neck.
- *Gastric pull-up* occasionally used.

- *Local flaps* for small defects. Tongue flap and islands of buccal mucosa and muscle can be transposed.
- *Deltopectoral flap:* in two stages.
- *Pectoralis major flap:* can carry a skin island, so it can be a one stage operation. Not so easy in women and the skin is rather thick. It can be used as an onlay patch for defects which are not circumferential.
- *Sternocleidomastoid flap:* with skin can be used for small defects.
- *Jejunum free flap:* good choice of vessel is the transverse cervical vessels. Usually perform the pharyngoenteric anastomosis first followed by the microvascular anastomosis followed by the distal anastomosis.
- *Other free flaps:* radial forearm, lateral arm and scapula flaps can be used. These have potential for sensory reinnervation. They are anastomosed to the lingual, alveolar or cervical lexus sensory nerves. It is not clear whether this improves swallowing.
- *Gastro-omental free flap:* useful when a long vascular pedicle is needed. The gastroepiploic vessels that supply the greater curvature of the stomach can reach the axillary vessels and can replace gullet with omentum to cover neck structures.

See *Voice restoration*.

Phenol peels

- Use as a *Chemical peel* produces profound long-lived results.
- It induces a controlled predictable partial thickness chemical burn.
- This results in a smoother more youthful-looking skin.
- Penetrates to the upper reticular dermis causing a new stratified collagen layer.
- Effective for fine and coarse wrinkling and irregular pigmentation.
- Prolonged recovery period and significant bleaching with demarcation line.

Mechanism of action:

- Chemical injury that extends to the superficial dermis.
- This is reconstructed with neocollagen.
- Healing proceeds from epithelial appendages.
- Initial marked inflammatory reaction with epidermal regeneration at 48 hours.

- Most of the healing is complete within 3 weeks.
- The new collagen is more rigid and compact.
- The changes can last as long as 20 years.
- After a peel the melanocytes remain, but they do not produce as much melanin.

Toxicology:

- Phenol ingestion causes injury to kidneys and liver.
- Only small volumes of phenol are absorbed topically.
- If applied in less than 30 minutes there is a higher incidence of cardiac arrhythmias which can be avoided by applying over an hour. All patients should be monitored.

Patient selection:

- Not beneficial for acne scarring, capillary haemangioma, facial telangiectasia or hyperpigmentation after skin grafting.
- It is good for fine and coarse wrinkles, and blotchy skin pigmentation.
- Severe epithelial dysplasia after actinic keratosis respond well to deep facial peel.
- Regional peeling works in fair-skinned patients, whereas in darker complexions and red-haired freckled patients full peel should be performed.
- Men don't do well as they don't use cosmetics and have thick skin.
- Use on the neck, thorax and limbs can lead to hypertrophic scarring.

Technique:

- Sedation is needed for full facial peels.
- *Baker formula:* 3 ml phenol (88%), 2 ml water, 8 drops of soap, 3 drops of croton oil. The croton oil is a vesicant.
- It is applied with an applicator over at least an hour.
- After each region of the face is completed it is covered with an occlusive dressing to increase the depth of phenol penetration.
- Burning sensation occurs 30 minutes after the tape is applied.
- Sedatives are required for the first 6 hours after which the burning subsides.
- The mask is removed after 24–48 hours. The wounds are washed.
- Re-epithelialization occurs 7–10 days after phenol application.

- Lubricate the skin. Sun exposure should be avoided after.

Phocomelia

Intercalated deficiency of the upper limb. See _Transverse arrest_.

Photodynamic therapy

- Used for treating BCCs, actinic keratosis and Bowen's disease.
- An inactive photosensitizer is administered and accumulates in the tissue.
- Light is delivered to the tumour, which photoactivates the sensitizer, which in turn converts molecular oxygen to free radicals that are tumouricidal.
- It may have a role for treating widespread disease.
- 5-aminolevulonic acid is highly selective for tumour cells. It is a prodrug which is metabolized by the haem biosynthetic pathway. The active metabolite is protoporphyrin IX. This is activated by illumination at 635nm[3].
- Cream is applied for 3 hours then illuminated for 9 minutes.

Piano keyboard sign

Seen with _Caput ulna_.

Pierre Robin sequence

- Pierre Robin (1867–1950) was a French dental surgeon.
- The sequence consists of airway obstruction in a child with micrognathia and glossoptosis. Most also have a cleft palate (60–90%). Infants also often have feeding difficulties.
- It may be associated with other syndromes, notably _Stickler syndrome_.
- The neonate may require intervention to assist the airway obstruction. The measures which can be taken are:
  - lie the child prone;
  - tongue stitch;
  - nasopharyngeal airway;
  - tongue–lip placation;
  - cricothyroidotomy/tracheostomy – last resort as morbidity is high from this procedure in a neonate;
  - mandibular advancement and distraction osteogenesis.

- Usually neuromuscular control improves in a few days to weeks and the above measures are temporary.

See _Cleft palate_.

Piezogenic pedal papules

- First described in 1991.
- Painful or asymptomatic papules of the feet and wrists, which result from herniation of fat through the dermis.
- They are common, non-hereditary and not related to a connective tissue defect. They are apparent when weight is applied to the heels and resolve when weight is removed. Usually bilateral.
- Histology reveals fragmentation of the dermal elastic tissue.
- There is no recommended medical or surgical treatment.

Pigmented villonodular tenovagino-synovitis

See _Giant cell tumour (PVNS)_.

Pilar cyst

Also called _Tricholemmal cyst_. See _Epithelial cysts_.

Pilomatrixoma

- A benign solitary tumour usually on the face and neck or upper extremities mainly in children or young adults but can occur at any age.
- Nondescript firm nodule 0.5 cm in diameter, rarely greater than 2 cm. Get foci of calcification or ossification.
- They are firmly fixed to the overlying skin and often have telangiectasia.
- Histologically there are sheets of epithelial cells with basophilic shadow cells arranged in irregular bands. Masses of keratin are found interspersed between cells with calcification.
- Treatment is excision.

Pincer deformity

Nail deformity. See _Nail_.

Pinch graft

Described by Reverdin.

Pisiform
Fracture:
- Uncommon, often overlooked as difficult to see and half associated with severe injuries. Most common mechanism of injury is a direct blow. Also repetitive trauma. Difficult to see on XR. May need supination oblique and carpal tunnel views.
- May get avascular necrosis. May get non-union or pisotriquetral arthritis.
- Examine by loading the subpisiform joint laterally as with the thumb CMC joint.
- If symptomatic treat by excision, which doesn't appear to affect wrist flexion.

Dislocation:
- For dislocation to occur there must be massive disruption of the FCU tendinous complex. Rarely reported.
- Due to violent contraction of the muscle with a flexed wrist. If the rupture is proximal to pisiform get distal dislocation. If the rupture is distal to the pisohamate and pisometacarpal ligaments get proximal dislocation. May be associated with avulsion of the hook of hamate.
- Treat either by tendon reattachment or excise pisiform and restore tendon continuity.

Pisotriquetral arthritis
- Characterized by pain over the palmar ulnar aspect of the wrist. Palpation elicits tenderness over the ulnar aspect of the pisotriquetral joint (PTJ).
- The pisiform is a sesamoid bone. Flexion of FCU relaxes the pisiform and allows side to side or radioulnar sliding. With compression this causes pain. It should be distinguished from lunotriquetral synovitis (see carpus *Instability*, and *FCU tenosynovitis*).
- XR: obtain a 30° supinated oblique view tangential to the pisiform. A standard carpal tunnel view further defines the joint. XR may reveal an osteochondral loose body emanating from the joint.
- Injection may help to localize the point of the pain. Osteophytes may cause ulnar nerve symptoms.

Operation: Pisiform excision is carried out through a longitudinal palmar incision that crosses the wrist joint obliquely. The incision is radial to the pisiform. Incise the periosteum and peel off the FCU tendon. Excise the pisiform. Mobilize after a week.

Pitanguy line
Identifies frontal nerve which runs from 0.5 cm below the tragus to 1.5 cm above the lateral eyebrow.
See Facial nerve.

Pitres–Testut sign
In *Ulnar nerve palsy*. Two signs. Inability to abduct in radial or ulna direction the middle finger. Also inability to cone the extended fingers.

Plantaris: anatomy and harvest
- Located anterior and medial to Achilles tendon.
- Absent in 7% of cadavers though clinically Harvey found it absent in 20% of limbs. Can be detected with CT scan or USS. Also unusable at times due to its insertions.
- Harvest with transverse incision just anterior to medial aspect of Achilles tendon. Divide and pass suture then stripper.
See Tendon reconstruction.

Platelet-derived growth factor
See Growth factors in cytokines and growth factors.

Platysma flap
Based on the submental branch of the facial artery and raised on a superior muscle pedicle. The skin island is designed on a transverse axis distally. Innervated so can be used to give motor function to the lip and provide sensation. It can be transposed to reconstruct defects of the floor of mouth and tongue.
See Oral cavity reconstruction.

Poirier: space of
A fenestration in the capitolunate articulation where a capsular tear occurs with a lunate dislocation.
See Carpus.

Poland's syndrome
- Described by Alfred Poland 1841 when he was an anatomy demonstrator at Guy's hospital.
- Aetiology may be hypoplasia of the subclavian artery.
- Usually sporadic occasionally genetic.
- 1:30 000, Rt > lt. M > F, but more females want reconstruction.

Chest wall: Congenital, partial or complete absence of pectoralis major and pectoralis minor. Hypoplastic musculoskeletal components. Get partial rib and sternal agenesis, mammary aplasia, absence of latissimus dorsi, serratus anterior and pectoralis major. Also hypoplastic scapula. If mild get breast hypoplasia and nipple displacement. There may be extensive deformities of the costochondral cartilages and sternum and absence of portions of the 2–4th ribs.

Upper limb deformities: Symbrachydactyly – short fused fingers. Usually central 3 digits. Short arm.

Other disorders: Scoliosis and renal disorders.

Reconstruction: In females need to address the breast asymmetry. Both male and female may require latissimus dorsi transfer to reconstruct the anterior axillary fold. Sternal prominence may need correction.
See Chest wall reconstruction.

Pollicization
- Thumb opposition allows for power grip and precision grip.
- Loss of a thumb is a similar disability to loss of an eye.
- Loss can be congenital and traumatic.
- With *Thumb hypoplasia* pollicization is required for Blauth type IIIB, IV and V. Pollicization using index finger is preferred for congenital absence.
- Pollicization is the only procedure that can restore the CMC joint. Damaged fingers may make useful pollicization as they only really need to function well at the CMC joint.

Aims:
- *Provide adequate length and position:* It must be shortened. Resect most of the metacarpal

so that the head with distal epiphysis acts as the new trapezium and PIPJ becomes MCPJ. Ablate epiphysis if no further growth is required. Rotate finger 120°. Fix the remaining metacarpal fragment on the scaphoid. This provides a radial abduction of 20° and a palmar abduction of 35°.
- *Provide good soft tissue cover:* The metacarpal resection leaves sufficient skin to obtain primary closure. Preserve dorsal veins and provide a wide web space.
- *Provide skin sensation:* Careful handling of the neurovascular pedicle. Vascular anomalies can occur with congenital cases.
- *Provide muscle balance:* The first dorsal interosseous is not present with thumb aplasia. Separate the index abductor to insert into the distal part of proximal phalanx to act as APB. FDP and FDS don't require shortening but extensors must be shortened. Stability is more important than mobility.
See Thumb reconstruction.

Pollock's sign
- Clinical test in *Ulnar nerve palsy*.
- Loss of FDP to ring and little with inability to flex distal phalanges.

Polydactyly
- *Extra digits:* pre-axial, central or postaxial.
- *Post-axial or ulnar sided most common:* worldwide it is the most common congenital malformation of extremities. 10 × more frequent in blacks. May be associated with syndactyly – polysyndactyly.

Surgery:
- If joints are involved preserve collateral ligament. If at the MCP level take care to preserve the physis. A closing wedge osteotomy may be required.
- Revisional surgery may be required if there is recurrence of clinodactyly.

Ulnar polydactyly:
- Also called post-axial polydacty.
- The most common single hand malformation. 8 × greater than other fingers. Often bilateral.

Classification: <u>*Stelling.*</u> Treat by simple excision

Central polydactyly:
• Usually with syndactyly, often bilateral.
• Treat by releasing the syndactyly, excising the excess tissue and soft tissue reconstruction.

Radial polydactyly:
• Also called pre-axial polydactyly.
• *See* <u>*Thumb duplication.*</u>
See <u>*Congenital hand anomalies.*</u>

Polyethylene
• Polyethylene refers to plastics from polymerization of ethylene gas.
• Ultra-high molecular weight polyethylene has a very low frictional coefficient against metal and ceramics and is used as a bearing surface for joint replacement prosthesis. Also wear resistance is low.
• <u>*Medpor*</u> is a high density porous polyethylene. *See* <u>*Alloplasts.*</u>

Polymethylmethacrylate
See <u>*Methylmethacrylate.*</u>

Polypropylene
Similar structure to <u>*Polyethylene.*</u> They differ by a methyl group instead of hydrogen in each unit of the chain. Marlex mesh has a high tensile strength and allows tissue ingrowth.
See Alloplasts.

Polytetrafluoroethylene
Examples are Proplast, Gore-tex and Teflon. Proplast HA contains hydroxyapatite. Can be used for onlay without biofunctional loading. It supports fibrovascular ingrowth. Gore-tex comes in sheets and can be used for <u>*Guided bone regeneration.*</u>
See <u>*Polyethylene.*</u>

Pontén flap
Bengt Pontén of Sweden reintroduced the concept of the fasciocutaneous flap. He found that undelayed lower leg flaps could have greater length to width ratio if deep fascia was included. His flaps were proximally based and

sensate so they would also have been neurocutaneous flaps. *See* <u>*Fasciocutaneous flaps.*</u>

Porokeratosis
• Autosomal dominant disorder of abnormal keratinization with malignant degeneration into <u>*Basal cell carcinoma*</u> and SCCs.
• The most common type is porokeratosis of Mibelli.

Port wine stain
Also called capillary malformation.
• Combined capillary <u>*Vascular malformations.*</u>
• Incidence 0.3%.
• An intradermal vascular malformation present at birth and persists through life with no regression.
• Developmental weakness of vessel wall.
• It can be localized or extensive.
• Differentiate from the fading macular stain (*Nevus flammeus neonatorum*).
• In distribution of trigeminal nerve.
• Deep red-purple.
• Grows with child.
• Later become nodular (cobblestoning).
• Some fade others darken.
• Associated with <u>*Sturge–Weber,*</u> <u>*Klippel–Trenaunay,*</u> <u>*Parks–Weber.*</u>
• *Treatment:* cosmetic camouflage, argon-pulsed dye laser. Significant lightening occurs in 70–80% of patients.

Positron emission tomography (PET)
• First developed and used in 1953.
• Used for the detection of micrometastasis based on abnormal cellular metabolic activity, rather than relying on structural changes.
• Non-invasive high resolution imaging.
• Used in oncology because malignant cells have a higher rate of utilization of glucose. Glucose accumulates in malignant cells as does 2-deoxyglucose. This can be labelled with ^{18}F (^{18}F-FDG).
• As this decays it emits a positron, which collides with an electron. These annihilate each other leading to formation of two photons emitted at 180° to each other. The PET scanner detects these and where they came from.

PET for melanoma:

- High positive predictive value but a negative value does not rule out the presence of disease.
- One study found a sensitivity of 85% and specificity of 92% for detecting involved nodes. Another study found it to be less sensitive or specific than sentinel node biopsy. Sentinel node biopsy is accurate, but PET also detects distant metastasis.
- PET similar in sensitivity and specificity to USS. USS more practical. PET more sensitive and specific than CT, but less accurate anatomical localization, so conventional imaging also required.
- Cost-effective once the machine is bought. Present role in melanoma uncertain. No data to suggest the use of PET at time of initial diagnosis and less specific than sentinel node biopsy.

Posterior interosseous artery flap

Anatomy:

- The posterior interosseous artery arises from the common interosseous artery or ulnar artery just distal to the antecubital fossa.
- It passes through the interosseous membrane under supinator and on the APL close to the PIN.
- At distal end of supinator it divides into descending and ascending recurrent branches. The ascending branch courses retrogradely to anastomose with the posterior radial collateral artery just distal to the elbow.
- The descending branch travels on the dorsal aspect of the forearm on APL within the intermuscular septum between ECU and EDM.
- It terminates at the wrist where it anastomoses with the dorsal branch of the carpus and perforating anterior interosseous artery.
- Multiple septocutaneous perforators supply the overlying skin. The largest arises just distal to supinator.

Operation:

- Draw a line from lateral epicondyle to DRUJ.
- A large perforator which should be included is found distal to the junction of posterior

$^1/_3$ and distal $^2/_3$, usually between 5–11 cm from the radial humeral condyle. Centre the skin island over the artery. It can be a width of 6–8 cm. Incise the radial side of the flap through fascia.
- Extend incision to wrist. At the wrist the anastomosis between the posterior interosseous artery and communicating perforators of anterior interosseous artery can be seen. Retract EDC and EDM to expose supinator. The artery is seen emerging from the distal edge of supinator with nerve. Perforating vessels to skin can be seen. Divide artery proximally. Dissect ulnar side of flap. Elevate proximal to distal. Inset flap into defect. It can be elevated as a osseocutaneous flap.

Posterior interosseous nerve

- Supplies all wrist extensors except ECRL. ECRB and supinator are supplied before entering the arcade of Frohse.
- Just proximal to the elbow, the radial nerve divides into superficial and deep. The superficial branch is sensory and the deep branch, the PIN is motor. It supplies ECRB then passes into the forearm entering the supinator muscle. After emerging from supinator, it supplies EDC, ECU, and EDM. Long motor branches supply APL, EPL, EPB and EIP. ECRL is innervated proximal to the PIN so some wrist extension is preserved with loss of PIN.

Posterior interosseous syndrome

Compression can be caused by:
- *Trauma:* dislocation of elbow, fracture of the radial head.
- *Inflammation:* RA of radiohumeral joint.
- *Swellings:* ganglia, lipoma.
- *Iatrogenic:* after tennis elbow injection.

Contusion of the dorsal proximal forearm can injure the PIN. In this situation, triceps and ECRL will be spared. Supinator is tested in extension, thumb adduction is weakened due to the loss of EPL.

Preiser's disease

Idiopathic avascular necrosis of the proximal pole of the _Scaphoid_.

Prelamination/prefabrication

- Involves manipulation of the flap prior to transfer.
- Involves creating a multilayered flap prior to transfer. Especially for head and neck reconstruction. Thus, the surgeon is not limited by natural flaps. For example, forehead flaps can be lined with cartilage and skin grafts before transferring for a total nasal reconstruction.
- It also includes _Neovascularization_.

Premaxilla

The alveolar segment of the maxilla which includes the nasal spine and 4 incisor teeth. It is located centrally anteriorly to the incisive foramen.
See Cleft lip.

Pressure sores

Definition: An ulcer resulting from unrelieved pressure. All of the other factors are secondary to the effects of pressure.

History:
- Charcot (1879) thought that nerve injury released a neurotrophic factor.
- Brown-Sequard (1853) believed that moisture and pressure were key.

Aetiology: As well as unrelieved pressure, other factors are altered sensory perception, incontinence, immobility, shear and friction, poor nutrition.

Pathophysiology:
- _Pressure_ is the single most important factor. Capillary pressure ranges from 12 mmHg at the venous end to 32 mmHg at the arterial end. External force exceeding these pressures will cause a reduced capillary perfusion. There is an inverse relationship between the amount of pressure and the length of time to ulceration. Studies confirming this also demonstrated that the initial changes occur in the muscle overlying the bone. Low pressure for long periods is more destructive than higher pressures for short periods and a rest of just 5 minutes can reverse damage.
- _Denervation:_ neurologically injured patients are more susceptible to ulceration than patients with cerebral palsy. Denervated flaps have a higher bacterial count than innervated flaps.
- _Infection:_ bacteria accumulate in areas of increased pressure. Proposed mechanisms include impaired lymphatic function, ischaemia, denervation and impaired immune function.
- _Oedema:_ once external pressures are greater than 12 mmHg, veins become engorged, and tissue pressure increases. Plasma extravasation occurs leading to oedema. Denervated tissues also lead to loss of sympathetic tone, vasodilatation and oedema. Lymphatic pump requires active skeletal muscle so denervation also exacerbates oedema by this indirect way. Also secondary to release of inflammatory mediators.
- _Shear:_ vertical shear occurs when patients are pulled up the bed. Shear is eliminated with an air mattress.

Preoperative care: All components of care must be optimized before surgery.
- _Nutrition:_ 25–35 cal/kg should be delivered daily. 1.5–3 g/kg of protein is required daily. _Vitamin C_ and Vitamin A. _Zinc_, _Iron_ and _Copper_. Supplemental feeds may be required. Consider TPN.
- _Infection:_ urinary sepsis, leading to bacteraemia. Pulmonary infections with high spinal lesions. Osteomyelitis within the pressure sore. May require a bone biopsy.
- _Relief of pressure:_ turning associated with _Mattress_ systems.
- _Spasms:_ develop in spinal cord injury due to the separation of spinal reflex arcs from higher control. Efferent fibres from muscles end directly on afferent fibres.
- _Treatment:_ drugs include diazepam (10–40 mg/day) and baclofen (15–100 mg/day). Also intrathecal phenol or alcohol. Severe case may require cordotomy or rhizotomy (sectioning of some of the sensory nerve fibres entering the spinal cord).

Risk factors: Immobility, incontinence, nutrition, altered level of consciousness. Braden, Norton and _Waterlow_ scales are risk assessment for pressure sores.

Staging system: National pressure advisory panel (1–4), also Shea and Yakony-Kirk.
- *Stage 1:* non-blanchable erythema of skin.
- *Stage 2:* partial thickness skin loss involving epidermis and dermis, superficial ulcer.
- *Stage 3:* full thickness skin loss extending down to fascia. Deep crater.
- *Stage 4:* full thickness skin loss with damage to muscle, bone and other structures.

Osteomyelitis: May need to perform bone biopsies, CRP, CT scan and treat with antibiotics for 6–8 weeks prior to reconstruction.

Surgical principles: Surgery may be required for grade 3 and 4, drain collections, debridement, excision of pseudobursa, ostectomy, haemostasis and suction, closure without tension using well-vascularized tissue. *Vastus lateralis flap*, *Rectus femoris flap*, gluteal thigh flap.

Ischial pressure sores:
- Plan a flap that will cover the ulcer, but allow the use of secondary flaps.
- The inferior gluteal musculocutaneous rotation flap uses the lower half of the gluteus maximus muscle.
- Also a superiorly based gluteal flap.
- The biceps femoris V–Y flap.
- The TFL flap.

Sacral pressure sore:
- Mostly musculocutaneous and fasciocutaneous flaps.
- Mainly based on the *Gluteus maximus*:, based superiorly or inferiorly, rotated, advanced or turned over.
- Also *Lumbosacral back flap*.
- Attempts have been made to place sensate skin in the back, but with limited success.

Trochanteric sores:
- Develop in patients who lay laterally for long.
- *TFL* is most commonly used.
- Sensation is from L1–3 so this is potentially a sensate flap in patients with a spinal cord lesion lower than L3.

Proflavine

Proflavine hemisulphate (proflavine 3,6-diamino-acridine sulphate dihydrate) is a quinolone antimicrobial. It is bacteriostatic against many Gram-positive bacteria, but less useful against Gram-negative organisms and ineffective against spores. Can get hypersensitivity. Used as it forms a malleable dressing.

Progeria
- Rare autosomal recessive disorder.
- Characterized by growth retardation, craniofacial disproportion, baldness, prominent ears, heart disease.
- Premature ageing in children.

See Werner's syndrome.

Pronator syndrome
- Compression neuropathy of the median nerve proximally in the forearm (4 sites), the most common being bands within pronator.
- Compression points.
- *Ligament of Struthers:* arises from lateral supracondylar process on lower 1/3 of humerus. Test by resisted elbow flexion.
- *Lacertus fibrosus:* arises from biceps. Test by resisted supination with flexed elbow.
- *Pronator teres:* test by resisted forearm pronation with the elbow extended. Pronator teres can be tender, firm or enlarged.
- *Arch of FDS:* test by resisted flexion of PIPJ of middle finger.
- Get forearm pain, as well as paraesthesia in the distribution of the median nerve. Palmar paraesthesia will be present from involvement in the palmar branch of the median nerve.
- May get weakness secondary to pain. Patients often perform repetitive tasks. Get pain on palpation of the median nerve. No weakness of muscles. Tinel's sign positive in the forearm. Muscle cramps can occur.

Treatment:
- Try immobilization with elbow at 90°. 50% respond to non-operative treatment.
- *Operative technique:* lazy S incision over the elbow. Find median nerve proximal to elbow. Excise ligament of Struthers if present. Incise bicipital aponeurosis, follow to superficial head of pronator teres. Incise fibrous band of pronator teres. If there is a variation in passage through pronator, the

deep head can be detached to expose the nerve. Next look at superficialis arcade. Incise superficialis arch. Relieve any site of compression. Pronator is reattached.

See *Anterior interosseous syndrome*.

Pronator teres

Origin: From medial epicondyle. It passes distally and radially.

Insertion: Through a flat tendon into radial aspect of mid-radius. It pronates the forearm, wrist and hand in extension. Valuable for wrist extension in radial nerve palsy.

Nerve supply: Median nerve.

Blood supply: Ulnar artery, anterior recurrent ulnar artery.

See *Muscles*.

Prosthetics: myoelectric

Utilize EMG potentials from residual neuromuscular systems to control the terminal device. The EMG potentials are obtained from skin surface electrodes over agonist/antagonist muscle groups. The main advantage is durability, reliability and function.

Proteus syndrome

• A sporadic vascular, skeletal, and soft tissue disorder.

• Asymmetric growth.

• Tumour-like lesions consist of connective tissue, adipose tissue, Schwann cell structures, and vascular tissue.

• More often in thorax and upper abdomen.

• The vascular anomalies are of the CM, LM, CVM, and CLVM type.

• Get macrocephaly (calvarial hyperostoses); asymmetry of the limbs; partial gigantism of the hands or feet, or both; plantar thickening ('moccasin' feet) can be present. Verrucous (linear) nevus also occurs.

• Proteus syndrome may be on a spectrum with *Epidermal nevus (Solomon) syndrome*.

• May result from a dominant lethal gene that survives by somatic mosaicism.

See *Complex combined vascular alformations.*

Proximal interphalangeal joint

Anatomy:

• Normal ROM 0–110°, lateral motion 8°. Hinge (ginglymus) joint.

• Two condyles on the proximal phalanx articulate with facets on the middle. A median ridge creates a tongue in groove preventing lateral movement. Get convergence of the fingertips on flexion due to the slight asymmetry of the finger joints. The condyles of each joint are of differing heights. In the coronal plane they angle away from the second web space. There is also some rotation occurring during flexion.

• *Ligaments* form a 3-sided box. The sides are the collaterals, the floor is the volar plate. Collaterals are proper (PCL) and accessory (ACL). PCL is thicker and provides most joint stability. It fans out from proximal to distal. It blends with volar plate at the critical corner. ACL is a suspensory ligament for *Volar plate* and flexor tendon sheath. ACL prevents tendon sheath from moving away from PIPJ in flexion.

• Dorsal stability is provided by central slip.

Hyperextension injuries:

• Injuries can occur dorsally, volarly or laterally, but are most common as hyperextension. Under a ring block stability can be assessed

Classification: *Dray and Eaton.*

Operations:

• If stable, provide extension block splint for 1–2/52. Buddy strap for 1/12. Treatment of unstable type III is more difficult and varied. 3 main treatments is open reduction, skeletal traction or volar plate arthroplasty.

• *Open reduction:* most successful with a single fragment. Approach through volar Bruner incision. Elevate flexor sheath between A2 and A4. Reduce joint. Apply dorsal blocking K wire (flex PIPJ and pass wire through head of proximal phalanx). Hold fragment with a small screw or K wire from volar side. Remove dorsal block at 4/52. Cerclage wire fixation can also be performed.

• *Volar plate arthroplasty:* if the fragments are multiple, they can be excised with the collateral ligaments. The volar plate is freed from collateral ligaments. The volar plate is attached to bone through a pull-out suture avoiding the lateral bands. Collateral ligaments are then reattached.

- *Dynamic traction:* traction with movement for 6 weeks.

Chronic fracture dislocation of PIPJ: Difficult problems with pain and stiffness. Can perform capsulotomy and reduction. Also pin in 30° of flexion and perform osteotomy to base of middle phalanx to tilt the volar lip. Bone graft may be required. Chronic hyperextension may require *FDS tenodesis*.

Collateral ligament injuries: Most can be treated with splinting. Instability is usually due to proximal rupture or avulsion fracture. Repair with suture, mitek or interosseous wire. Only a small group require operative treatment.

Volar dislocations: Much less common. May get rupture of the central slip with some collateral ligament involvement. With some rotation one of the collateral ligaments may tear. The ipsilateral proximal phalanx condyle slips through the extensor mechanism making it irreducible. Attempt closed reduction but may need open. If irreducible the prognosis is better as the extensor mechanism is intact.

Arthritis: It is not commonly involved in OA. Treat conservatively. Occasionally, an osteophyte requires excision. Implants are more indicated for ring and little finger as they are used to grasp. If conservative treatment fails, patients will require an *Arthroplasty* or *Arthrodesis*.
See Joints.

Proximal row carpectomy

- Motion preserving *Wrist* arthrodesis procedure.
- Excision of scaphoid, lunate and triquetrum, allowing the capitate to articulate with the radius.

Indication: Radiocarpal or intercarpal arthrosis, spastic wrist contractures, malalignment of proximal carpus – Kienböck's disease, SLAC, scaphoid non-union.

Requirement:

- Undamaged articular surface of the lunate fossa of distal radius and proximal pole of capitate.
- Also perform radial styloidectomy to prevent impingement against the trapezium.

Prozansky classification

(and Murry and Mulliken) *Mandibular hypoplasia* in *Hemifacial microsomia.*

- *Type 1:* all parts present though hypoplastic.
- *Type IIa:* condyle articulates as a hinge.
- *Type IIb:* no condyle.
- *Type III:* the mandibular ramus is absent.

Prune belly syndrome

Also called Eagle–Barrett syndrome.

- Seen in newborn boys.
- Get absent abdominal wall muscles, cryptorchism, and dilated urinary tract.
- The muscle deficiency may be limited to one area.
- The abdomen is wrinkled and with growth looks more like a pear.
- Surgery is required to correct urogenital problems and muscle deficiency may require muscle flaps.

See Abdominal reconstruction,.

Pseudo-epitheliomatous hyperplasia

Seen in long-standing chronic ulcers, often in pressure sores. Epidermal thickening may look like malignant change. Get downward proliferation of epidermal cells and micro abscesses. It may be difficult to differentiate from malignancy.
See Squamous cell carcinoma.

Pseudogout

- Calcium pyrophosphate dihydrate deposition.
- Calcification through the triangular fibrocartilage of the wrist is diagnostic.

See Gout.

Pseudohypertelorism

A normal interorbital distance but an increased intercanthal distance – measured between the medial canthal tendons.
See Hypertelorism.

Pseudosarcomatous lesions
- Several clinically benign localized fibromatous proliferative lesions may show cellular changes and numerous mitoses that easily lead to a mistaken diagnosis of fibrosarcoma.
- *Infantile digital fibromatosis* is a rare pseudosarcomatosis characterized by asymptomatic, firm, red, smooth nodules up to 1 cm in size on the dorsal and lateral aspects of the distal phalanges of the toes and fingers during infancy and childhood. Surgical excision is the recommended treatment, but recurrences are reported to be frequent.
- *Atypical fibroxanthoma*.
- *Nodular pseudosarcomatous fasciitis*.

Pseudoxanthoma elasticum
- Degenerative disorder of elastic fibres.
- Mainly affecting skin eyes and arteries.
- Autosomal recessive and dominant types.
- Get premature skin laxity looks like plucked chicken skin.
- Redundant skin around the neck, axilla, trunk and limbs.
- May benefit from plastic surgery, but severe arteriosclerosis commonly develops as early as the third decade of life.

Psoriasis
- Common, benign, chronic, erythematous, scaling skin disease.
- Surgery should be avoided when the disease is worsening:
  - may induce *Köbner's* phenomenon;
  - high skin colonization bacterial count may increase infection.
- Treatment range from topical therapy to phototherapy and systemic therapy.

Psoriatic arthritis
- Negative RhF.
- 5% of patients with psoriasis develop arthritis.
- 1/3 have a family history of psoriasis.
- 20% of patients can develop skin changes after the arthritis.
- Asymmetric.
- Classically affects DIPJ.
- Arthritis mutilans or telescoping occurs in psoriatic arthritis and severe seropositive arthritis.

- *Nails:* get pitting, leukonychia and crumbling.
- *XR:* osteolysis with bone destruction and widening of the joint spaces. Get pencil in cup changes.
- *Treatment:* usually osteotomy, arthrodesis or arthroplasty.

Psychology and plastic surgery
Aesthetic surgery is unique in being initiated by the patient not the doctor. It is therefore important for the surgeon to assess the psychological condition of the patient. Some conditions are contraindication to performing aesthetic surgery.
- *Schizoid personality disorder:* patients may be withdrawn and express vague reasons for wanting surgery. Patients avoid eye contact and show little emotion.
- *Paranoid personality disorder:* this refers to an unwarranted scepticism of others. It most commonly relates to the unmarried male.
- *Histrionic personality disorder:* patients are excessively emotional, seeking constant attention. They have shallow emotional responses. They are constantly worried about their external appearance.
- *Depressive personality disorder:* these patients do not desire cosmetic surgery, but seek it in the hope that they will feel better about themselves.
- *Body dysmorphic disorder*.
- *Male patients:* seek cosmetic surgery less commonly than females, but cause more problems. They lack a clear body concept and awareness of their physical appearance. SIMON – single, introverted male, overly narcissistic.

PTFE
See *Polytetrafluoroethylene*.

Ptosis: breast
See *Regnault's classification*.

Ptosis: eyelid
- Drooping of the upper lid.
- Differentiate from *Blepharophimosis*
- Aim of surgery is to correct ptosis by increasing the power of the lid.

- The 3 sources of power are levator, Müllers and frontalis muscle. Müllers muscle is sympathetically innervated with slow lifting effect. It adjusts lid level. Paralysis of Muller's muscle drops the lid by 2–3 mm. Paralysis of frontalis causes brow ptosis. Levator is not strongly fixed to the tarsal plate. Fixation is through fibrous bands. So in correcting ptosis, aponeurosis can be lifted off the tarsus and fixed more firmly. This is effective as the attachment is now more firm than the rather elastic attachment prior to fixation.

Aetiology:
- *Myogenic:*
  o congenital levator dystrophy;
  o blepharophimosis syndrome;
  o progressive external ophthalmoplegia;
  o myaesthenia gravis.
- *Neurogenic:*
  o 3rd nerve palsy;
  o Horner's syndrome;
  o Marcus Gunn jaw-winking, aberrant 3rd nerve regeneration.
- *Aponeurotic:* defects in levator aponeurosis.
- *Mechanical:*
  o dermatochalasis;
  o tumour;
  o scar;
  o anophthalmos.

Clinical tests:
- Determine the lid margin level and the amount of levator function. Normal lid covers 1–2 mm of the upper limbus.
- *Margin-reflex distance:* patient looks at torch held ½ m away. Measure distance of lid from corneal reflex.
- *Levator function:* fix brow with thumb and measure excursion of upper lid between upgaze and downgaze. Normal levator function is 12–15 mm.
- *Bell's phenomenon.*
- *Jaw-winking:* ask patient to move jaw to the side opposite to the ptotic upper lid or open the mouth wide. The lid will lift if jaw-winking present.
- Also measure aperture and distance from upper margin of iris to lid. Check visual acuity, extraocular muscle movements.

Classification of ptosis:
- Ptosis severity:
  o mild: 1–2 mm;
  o moderate: 3 mm;
  o severe: 4+ mm.
- Levator function:
  o good: >10 mm
  o fair: 4–10 mm
  o poor: <4 mm.

Summary of treatment:
- *Good levator mild ptosis:* Fasanella–Servat. Repair aponeurosis if defective.
- *Ptosis >4 mm, good levator function:* resect aponeurosis.
- Levator function <4 mm perform brow suspension.

Treatment:
- *Congenital:*
  o *severe:* frontalis sling;
  o *less severe:* levator advancement/ tarsectomy.
- *Senile ptosis:* disinsertion and reattachment of levator.
- *Post-traumatic:*
  o neurogenic use sling;
  o trauma – reinsert.
- *Myogenic:* treat disease then reinsert or plicate.
- *Neurogenic:*
  o such as stroke us a sling;
  o *Horner's:* Müllerectomy, reinsertion of aponeurosis or F–S op.
- *Mechanical:* remove the weight.

Operations:
- *Fasanella–Servat.*
- *Excision of segment of levator aponeurosis:* through posterior or anterior approach. Excise transverse segment of levator and resuture the incised edges to correct the ptosis.
- *Excision of segment of levator palpebrae superiosis:* through an anterior or posterior approach. The amount resected depends on the levator function and the degree of ptosis.
- *Frontalis sling:* harvest fascia lata. Place sling in U or W shape. Place stab incisions in the brow and upper eyelid. Pass a needle, pass a wire and snare the fascia. The placement of

fascia on the lid should be as close to the tarsus as possible and as distally as possible. This fibrous tissue will hold whereas a sling placed in orbicularis will relax with time.

- *Frontalis myofascial flap from eyebrow:* the frontalis originates from galea and ends in the skin at the eyebrow region. Some fibres interlace with orbicularis. A superiorly based flap can be isolated and advanced downwards and attached to the tarsal plate. Frontalis power is measured by marking the inferior margin of the eyebrow arch and measuring the elevation. The flap is elevated through an incision where the superior palpebral fold should be. The flap is fixed to the midtarsal level with silk.

Complications: The commonest technical error is in suturing the edge of Whitnall's ligament to the tarsal plate. Also under-and overcorrection, dry eyes, bleeding.

Pulleys

- Thickened areas within the _flexor sheath_ which enclose the Flexor tendons. In finger there is the palmar aponeurosis (PA), and 5 annular pulleys and 3 cruciform pulleys. PA pulley is the transverse fibres of palmar fascia. Annular pulleys – odd numbers are over joints.
- The pulleys keep the tendon close to the bone, preventing bowstring without restricting joint movement. They also help to distribute the flexor tendon excursion across the digital joints.

Annular pulleys:

- *A2 and A4* are the most critical pulleys to prevent bowstringing.
- *A1* is 10 mm long. It is attached to the volar plate and distally to the proximal phalanx.
- *A2* is the strongest and longest at 17 mm. It is attached to the proximal half of the proximal phalanx.
- *A3:* thin band 3 mm long over the PIPJ, attached to volar plate.
- *A4*: mid-portion of middle phalanx, 8 mm long.
- *A5*: very thin over DIPJ volar plate, often absent.

Cruciate pulleys:

- Enable the sheath to conform to the position of flexion.
- C1 and C3 are most frequently found. In the thumb there is one oblique pulley at the level of the shaft of the proximal phalanx. It is 11 mm in length. It extends obliquely in a distal radial direction.

Thumb: Have an A1 pulley overlying MCP joint and an A2 pulley overlying IPJ and an oblique pulley. The latter is considered the most important.

Pulvertaft weave

See _Flexor tendon_. See _Late reconstruction_.

Pyoderma gangrenosum

- Multiple skin abscesses with necrosis and undermining ulcerations.
- It is often associated with ulcerative colitis (50% of patients).
- Also other gastrointestinal disorders, such as diverticulosis, regional enteritis, peptic ulcer disease, hepatitis and carcinoid tumour.
- Associated with rheumatoid arthritis, pulmonary diseases and haematological disorders.
- No associations with 20% of the patients with pyoderma gangrenosum.
- No specific organism associated.
- The basic lesion may be a necrotizing cutaneous vasculitis.
- The course is protracted and in some instances fulminant.

Treatment:

- Systemic and topical antibiotic therapy.
- Conservative debridement of only the grossly necrotic tissues.
- Do not incise the adjacent intact tissues, to avoid extension of the disease beyond the operative debridement.
- Local and systemic steroid therapy immunosuppressives (e.g. azathioprine) and systemic sulfones have been helpful. local injections may cause local skin trauma, which may induce new pyoderma gangrenosum lesions.

Pyogenic granuloma

- A proliferation of capillaries often at a site of trauma.
- There may be an associated infection, but the condition is not an infective process.
- They rarely appear before the age of 6 months, frequently occur in children, but may occur at any age.

- They are rapidly growing in the early stages, later remaining unchanged. They have a pliable surface and bleed easily.
- Red or blue-black, haemorrhagic.
- Most commonly found on the face and distal extremities.
- They may be excised or destroyed with diathermy, laser or silver nitrate. They may recur. Vascular proliferation may be deep and therefore may require excision.

Q Q-switched laser to Quantitative microbiology

Q-switched laser

- Q-switching is when one of the resonating mirrors is non-reflective for an interval of pumping.
- Stored energy is emitted as a pulse of light 10 billionths of a second in length.
- 3 available – ruby (694 nm), YAG (1064 nm or 532 nm) and alexandrite (760 nm).

See *Tattoo, Laser*.

Quaba flap

A rotational flap based on the dorsal intermetacarpal skin perforator. It can be used to resurface proximal digits. The anatomy is most reliable on the radial side of the hand.
See *Maruyama flap*.

Quadriga syndrome

Diminished grip strength caused by tethering of FDP thus reducing power in remaining flexors. Derived from the Roman chariots with 4 horses on one rein and coined by Verdan.

See *Amputation*.

Quadrilateral space

Defined by the long head of triceps medially, teres major inferiorly, teres minor superiorly, humerus laterally. The posterior circumflex artery and axillary nerve pass through it.

Quantitative microbiology

- Measure bacterial contamination by weighing a specimen, converting to a liquid and culturing like urine cultures.
- The result is as the number of organisms per gram. With $<10^5$ organisms invasive infection will not occur and wounds will close. $>10^5$ organisms will cause infection and wound problems. Streptococci in lower numbers will cause problems. 10^8–10^9 organisms will cause pus.
- A dog's mouth has $<10^3$ organisms unless it has eaten meat in the last 8 hours when it can rise to 10^7.

R Radial artery to Ruben's flap

Radial artery

- Radial artery runs superficially in the forearm from the division with the brachial artery to its exit under APL.

- It first lies on pronator teres beneath brachioradialis then on the radial head of FDS and FPL. Gives branches to the fascial plexus and on to the skin, radius and muscles. Accompanied by 2 or more venae comitantes.

- Runs medial to APL and EPB.
- Passes deep to these to cross the anatomic snuff box.
- It enters the palm between two heads of the 1st dorsal interosseous muscle and is covered by AP.
- It gives off princeps pollicis which gives the two thumb digital arteries. It runs medially between interosseus and AP to become the main component of the deep palmar arch. A dorsal branch joins a branch from ulnar artery to become the dorsal carpal arch.

Radial club hand

- Congenital longitudinal radial ray deficiency.
- Affects all preaxial structures from shoulder to hand.
- Spectrum involving thumb. Index may be involved.
- Wrist unstable and hand radially deviated, flexed and pronated. ROM of fingers reduced.
- Often other syndromes.
- No known aetiology.
- 50% bilateral.

Classification: Bayne and Klug. Type IV most common – 50–90% of cases.

Prevalence:
- 1:55 000. 0.5–10% of congenital hands.
- Bilateral > unilateral. M:F 3:2. absence > partial absence.

Aetiology: May be sporadic, syndromic, or associated with thalidomide or valproic acid.

Associations: See *Fanconi's anaemia, TAR syndrome, Holt–Oram syndrome, VACTERL syndrome.*

Clinical features:
- Short forearm, bowed radially, hypoplastic or absent radius with anlage (fibrous band).
- Hand radially deviated. Skin deficient radially.
- Elbow stiff, maybe due to synostosis, elbow extended, but improves with age and determines when to operate.
- Hypoplasia of radial structures such as radial nerve.

- Reduced wrist movement. Check mobility. Carpus is deviated radially and displaced palmarly. The scaphoid and trapezium are usually absent in type III and IV.
- *Thumb hypoplastic or absent:* 60% absent in type IV with absent metacarpal in absent thumb. The 2nd metacarpal may be abnormal proximally.
- Muscles abnormal both extensors and flexors and relate to severity of the radial ray deficiency. Muscles most commonly affected are pectoralis major, brachioradialis. supinator, extensor carpi radialis, flexor carpi radialis, muscles of thumb. FDS is usually present but abnormaliy fused to FDP with absence of index tendon. EDC is usually present but fused with ECRL or EDM. Thumb extrinsics are usually absent.
- *Nerves:* ulna nerve normal, musculocutaneous nerve is missing. Median nerve supplies anterior compartment, radial nerve often terminates at elbow after supplying triceps. Sensation radially is supplied by median nerve with an anastomosis to ulnar nerve.
- *Ateries:* radial artery often absent or small. Interosseous arteries are well developed.

Treatment principles:
- *I:* do nothing or lengthen.
- *II:* lengthen.
- *III and IV:* centralize or radialize.

Treatment: Regular manipulation and splinting. Operate between 6–18 months of age.
- *Centralize* carpus on ulna by carpal excision and transfer radial wrist muscles to ulna side, closing wedge osteotomy. Stabilize with a pin through the 3rd metacarpal.
- *Radialize:* requires full passive correction. Place the scaphoid over the ulna and secure with a pin through 2nd metacarpal. Transfer FCR to ulnar side of carpus to reduce radial deviating force.
- *Pollicization*: release constricting radial soft tissue.
- Later may require ulnar osteotomy, distraction lengthening or fusion.

Operative technique:
- Bilobed flap to make use of redundant ulna skin. Preserve dorsal veins and sensory nerves.

Beware the radial-median nerve just under the skin on the radial side.

- Incise extensor retinaculum and identify radial extensors and flexors. They may be fused. If present detach BR, FCR, ECRL, ECRB. Protect and retract finger extensors, and find ECU, FCU and ulnar nerve and artery.
- Incise dorsal and palmar wrist capsule transversely to release ulno-carpal joint, but preserve ulnar collateral ligament. Dissect distal ulnar head avoiding damage to cartilage and epiphysis.
- Excise residual fibrotic tissue until hand is easy to move, attached only by skin, tendons and NVBs.
- Transpose with carpal bones over ulnar head and fix with pin passed retrogradely through ulna then into 2nd metacarpal.
- If ulna is markedly bowed or there is marked soft tissue contracture, perform wedge osteotomy of ulna.
- Suture back capsule. Radial tendons may be transposed, but may be atrophic. Shorten and tighten ECU. Close bilobed flap.
- Long arm plaster for 6–8 weeks, then removable splint until 6 year.

Complications: Recurrent deformity, premature distal ulnar epiphyseal closure.

Outcome: Determined by presence of thumb, wrist motion, digital motion and ulnar length. See Congenital hand anomalies.

Radial dysplasia
See Radial club hand.

Radial forearm flap

- First described in 1978 as a proximally based free flap. Distally based pedicled flap described in 1981.
- Based on the radial artery and venae comitantes. Skin and fascia on the volar forearm, as well as a portion of radius, PL, and superficial radial nerve.
- It can be fasciocutaneous, osseocutaneous or pure fascial.
- 12% of hand have the radial artery as dominant with 3% having an incomplete palmar arch.

- 9% of individuals have an ulnar artery, which lies superficial to the deep fascia so when raising a radial forearm flap, inclusion of all structures superficial to deep fascia would devascularize the hand.

Disadvantages: Donor site.

Anatomy: Radial artery.

Operative technique: Mark out flap to size of defect. Elevate skin off fascia around flap. Preserve superficial branch of radial nerve and prominent vein in case venae comitantes not suitable. Incise deep fascia and suture fascia to skin. Raise fascia off tendons taking care to preserve paratenon. As the FCR is reached from an ulnar direction, traction on FCR will reveal the artery. The same will occur from the radial side with traction on brachioradialis. Incise the lateral intermuscular septum parallel and deep to the radial artery. Dissect the pedicle distally and ligate. Through a proximal incision elevate the flap up to the bifurcation.

Radial nerve

- Radial nerve from posterior cord – C5–T1.
- Passes along the spiral groove beneath the lateral head of triceps.
- Through the lateral intermuscular septum 10–15 cm proximal to the lateral epicondyle.
- Continues between brachialis and biceps with brachioradialis and ECRL laterally. Motor branches to 3 muscles come off before the elbow. It divides at the elbow into superficial and deep (posterior interosseous.). PIN goes deep to supinator (arcade of Froshe).

Superficial radial nerve: Passes between tendons of brachioradialis and ECRL near the mid-forearm, and pierces the deep fascia to become subcutaneous. It runs towards the snuff box superficial to APL and EPB. It gives sensory branches to the dorsum of thumb to radial half of ring finger and hand.

Radial tunnel syndrome

- The most frequent site for radial tunnel compression is the arcade of Frohse.
- Sites of compression:
  - a fibrous band tethering nerve to the radiohumeral joint;

- the leash of Henry – radial recurrent vessels, which pass across the radial nerve;
- the tendinous margin of ECRB;
- the arcade of Frohse – a fibrous band on the surface of supinator.

Symptoms:
- Pain is the predominant symptom. It can be confused with tennis elbow. Motor and sensory disturbance is uncommon.
- Extension of middle finger is positive in radial tunnel syndrome. Nerve conduction studies are unreliable.

Treatment: Surgical decompression from posterior muscle splitting or anterior approach.
See *Radial tunnel syndrome, Posterior interosseous syndrome, Wartenberg's syndrome.*

Radiation

See *Healing. Acute effects* include erythema, inflammation, oedema, ulceration. *Late effects*: depigmentation, atrophy, fibrosis, necrosis, neoplasia.

Radiation injury: Caused by:
- DNA disruption that can cause a lethal injury or cell death from disruption of division.
- O_2 free radicals that are directly toxic.

Early and late effects:
- *Early:* inflammatory response with erythema and hyperpigmentation.
- *Late:* fibrosis, pigment changes.
  - endothelial cell, capillary and arteriole damage with loss of blood vessels in the affected area and hypoperfusion;
  - fibroblasts proliferate less and collagen is deficient;
  - lymphatics are damaged causing oedema and infection;
  - keratinocytes are injured; dry desquamation if there is enough cells to replace the dead ones; moist desquamation if the dermis is exposed in places and an ulcer if all epidermis and adnexal structures are destroyed.

Treatment: Local wound care, flaps from outside the radiated field, and hyperbaric oxygen.

Technique: Absorbed radiation is now measured in grays. 1 joule/kg = 1 Gy = 100 rads. The therapeutic dose for carcinoma is tissue dependent, but range from 45 to 80 Gy.
- *Fractionating irradiation* allows treatment of the cancer, while not exceeding tolerance of the surrounding normal tissue. The dose for tumour irradiation is indexed to tumour volume. Also only dividing cells will be killed so that fractionating will target more cells.
- *Altered fractionation* is external beam radiation outside the conventional treatment.
- *Hyperfractionation* is used for rapidly growing tumours – smaller doses every 6 hours.
- *Accelerated fractionation* is the same total dose over a shorter period.
- *Hypofractionation* is used as palliation of advanced tumours.

Principles: Ionizing radiation occurs as either electromagnetic waves or particulate forms. Electromagnetic radiation used therapeutically is as short wavelengths, such as X-rays and gamma rays. Also discrete energy packets called photons. Particulate irradiation consists of small energized particles such as electrons, neutrons, protons, alpha particles and others.

Delivery: By external beam e.g. linear accelerators or by *Brachytherapy.* External beam is applied in daily fraction of 200 cGy/day over a 5–6 weeks course. Brachytherapy allows continuous radiation. Photons are short pulses of high energy. Absorption depends on their energy level. High-energy megavoltage treatments pass through the skin and are therefore skin sparing. So low-energy photons are used for superficial lesions and high-energy photons are used for deep seated tumours.

Carcinogen: Ionizing radiation including electromagnetic (X-rays and gamma rays) and particulate radiation (electrons, protons, neutrons, α-particles) cause change by ionizing cell constituents. A single exposure may produce a tumour after a long latent period.

Tolerance dose: Of different tissues and organs has been established as the likelihood of treatment related complications in 5 years using conventional fractionation. So if 50% of complications will occur, it is expressed as TD 50/5. The dose likely to irradicate a tumour is for example TD5 = 5% of tumours will be eradicated. The sensitivity of normal tissues is the LD (lethal dose). So LD50 is the dose which will kill 50% of normal cells.

Hyperbaric oxygen.

Radiation treatment of head and neck cancer: See *Head and neck cancer.*

Indications: For small lesions RT may be as effective as surgery. For larger lesions both are required. When combined survival is not particularly improved. Pre-operative RT is thought to eradicate subclinical disease and prevent tumour implantation and possibly make more tumours operable. However, it interferes with healing. Post-operative RT is indicated for large tumours, nodes with extracapsular involvement and for vascular and perineural invasion. As healing has already occurred higher doses can be given.

Outcome: T1 or T2 tumours do well with either surgery or RT with 80% disease-free for 3 years. 30% survival for T3–4

Complications:
- *Acute:* mucositis, loss of taste, xerostomia, with dryness, which is permanent and progressive.
- *Chronic:* progressive. Dry uncomfortable mucous membranes. Atrophic skin with poor healing. Oral hygiene should be good to prevent loss of teeth. Osteoradionecrosis can be a serious problem requiring hemi-mandibulectomy. Carcinogenesis. Spontaneous fistulization, carotid blow out.

Radiotherapy for sarcomas:

Most *Sarcomas* are radiosensitive to varying degrees. Ewing's sarcomas are very radiosensitive. Liposarcomas are reasonably radiosensitive. Post-operative radiotherapy reduces the risk of local recurrence. Radiotherapy typically consists of 50 Gy delivered in 25 fractions over 5 weeks. Indications for post-operative radiotherapy include high-grade tumours, incompletely excised tumours, tumours >5 cm in diameter, deep head and neck sarcomas.

Radio-ulnar synostosis

Proximal forearm, 60% bilateralL
- Primary has no radial head and extensive synostosis.
- Secondary – radial head normal, but dislocated.
- Get fixed pronation, but hypermobile wrist.
- XR shows heavy bowed radius.
- Restoring rotation is unsuccessful:
  - mild or unilateral, no treatment;
  - severe do rotational osteotomy, synostosis may occur in metacarpal.

Ramirez component separation

- A technique used for the closure of *Incisional herniation*.
- Enable rectus with overlying anterior rectus sheath to move to midline by separating rectus from post-rectus sheath.
- Requires incision in midline at junction of post-rectus sheath with anterior rectus sheath.
- Rectus released by incising external oblique fascia laterally.
- Suture with interrupted mattress running transversely to alignment of fibres and only into fascia not muscle. Both recti should be opposing each other.

Ramsay–Hunt syndrome

Post-infective facial nerve palsy. See *Facial nerve re-animation*.

Random flaps

See *Flaps*. No directional blood supply. Not based on any known vessel. Include local flaps to the face. Length breadth ratio is 1:1 in the lower extremity, but up to 1:6 in the face.

Ravitch technique

- Operative technique for the correction of *Pectus excavatum:*.
- Elevate perichondrial flaps and resect involved costal cartilage (4–5 on each side, preserve costochondral junction).
- Divide xiphoid process to allow sternal elevation.
- Posterior transverse osteotomy of superior sternum and fracture sternum forwards.
- Bone wedge used to stabilize the sternum.
- Stabilize sternum with wires to ribs.
- Bilateral pectoralis flaps to cover sternum.

Raynaud's disease

- Vasospastic disease of small vessels of unknown aetiology with intermittent episodes of skin colour and temperature change.
- Raynaud's phenomenom has an underlying disorder such as scleroderma, RA or cryoglobulinaemia.

Investigations:

- *Bone scan:*
  - *phase 1:* within 2 minutes of injection shows nucleotide in the vascular system;
  - *phase 2:* 5–10 min, shows nucleotide diffusing into soft tissue;
  - *phase 3:* 2–3 hours, binding to skeletal structures;
  - in Raynaud's get decreased perfusion in phase 1 and 2, sympathetic block may help to establish the sympathetic contribution.

Conservative treatment:

- Stop smoking.
- Prevent cold exposure.
- Drugs – calcium channel blockers, serotonin receptor blocker (Ketanserin) topical nitroglycerin, and alpha adrenergic blockers such as reserpine. Reserpine has been the most valuable.

Surgery:

- Principally sympathectomy.
- Cervicothoracic sympathectomy only provides short-term improvement.
- Distal sympathectomy provides longer-term relief. The radial artery receives sympathetic nerves from the radial nerve and lateral cutaneous nerve. The ulnar artery receives 3 branches from the ulnar nerve and one from the medial cutaneous nerve of the forearm.
- *Digital sympathectomy:* the sympathetic fibres to the digital vessels ramify in the adventitia so adventitia stripping will provide effective sympathectomy. Results are best with pure vasospasm.

See <u>Vasospastic disorders</u>.

Reagan's test

- Test for lunotriquestral instability.
- Press the thumb on the lunate dorsally and the index finger on triquestrum volarly.
- Compare with <u>Masquelet's</u> test.

See <u>Carpal instability</u>.

Recall phenomenom

- Seen in <u>Extravasation injuries</u>.
- The extension of necrosis, which occurred at the time of extravasation following recommencement of administration of the toxic substance (mostly seen with doxorubicin).

Rectus abdominus flap

Anatomy: Origin from costal margin of 6–9 ribs, inserts to pubic tubercle. Blood supply is inferior and superior epigastric arteries.

Pedicled extended DIEP flap:

- Elevate through a midline incision, open anterior rectus sheath and divide superiorly.
- Mobilize rectus and divide proximally.
- Swing down and bring over anterior sheath to enter thigh or tunnel under.
- Close sheath, stitch sheath to arcuate line.

Rectus femoris flap

Anatomy:

- One of the quadriceps.
- Originates at the ASIS, inserts into patellar tendon.

Blood supply:

- The lateral femoral circumflex vessels, running from medial to lateral.
- 2–3 branches enter the muscle in the proximal third, 10 cm below ASIS.
- A secondary supply is located 2 cm below the primary supply.

Reconstruction:

- Elevate through a lateral thigh incision.
- After transposition, approximate vastus lateralis and medialis.
- Good for reconstructing the lower abdominal wall. The tip reaches between the xiphoid and umbilicus.
- The mutton chop flap is an extended rectus femoris myocutaneous flap.
- Get slight weakness of knee extension.

See <u>Abdominal wall reconstruction. See Pressure sores</u>.

Reflex sympathetic dystrophy

- Also called Complex Regional Pain Syndrome (CRPS).

- A complex unpredictable response producing pain out of proportion to the inciting event that is associated with inflammatory or sympathetic change leading to dystrophic change.
- The three basic criteria for diagnosis are disproportionate pain, interference with function, and autonomic type abnormality.
- The pain is characterized by _Hyperpathia_ and _Allodynia_.

Classification:

- Reflex sympathetic dystrophy (RSD) has been renamed CRPS.
- CRPS is subdivided into sympathetically maintained pain syndrome (SMPS) type I and II and sympathetically independent syndrome (SIPS) type III.
- _CRPS Type I:_
  - follows noxious event;
  - has continuous pain not limited to a nerve territory;
  - there is evidence of oedema, blood-flow abnormality, abnormal pseudomotor activity;
  - there is no other cause for the pain.
- _CRPS Type II:_
  - develops after nerve injury;
  - is usually confined to a nerve territory;
  - pain is limited to the area but may spread;
  - evidence of oedema or blood-flow abnormality;
  - no other cause for the pain.
- _CRPS Type III:_ as above, but not responsive to a sympathetic block.
- Lankford classified RSD by precipitating causes and is still used. These are:
  - _Minor causalgia_;
  - _Minor traumatic dystrophy_;
  - _Shoulder-hand syndrome_;
  - _Major traumatic dystrophy_;
  - _Major causalgia_.

Incidence:

- Variable incidence reported but probably around 5% of trauma.
- Most commonly in the upper and lower extremity, but has been reported in other areas.
- M = F, usually 30–60 years of age.
- It may occur in children where it usually has a shorter duration and a better prognosis.

Prognosis and outcome:

- Complete remission is rare. Great variations between different studies.
- Overall reviews suggest that with most treatment methods:
  - $1/3$ of patients receive excellent to good relief of symptoms;
  - $1/3$ some improvement;
  - $1/3$ no improvement or worse;
  - a study of sympathetic block suggests $2/3$ improvement.

Precipitating causes:

- Very varied from minor trauma to spinal cord injury. Non-traumatic causes include ovarian carcinoma, stroke, shingles.
- The most common causes are carpal tunnel release and colles fracture.

Clinical manifestations:

- _Characteristic pain:_ unremitting pain is the most distinguishing feature, particularly _Hyperpathia_, _Allodynia_ and _Hyperalgesia_. Usually constant and aggravated by motion, temperature change. Mirror image pain may occur in the opposite extremity. An emotional response is usually denied but may be present.
- Patients with RSD tend to be emotionally demanding and accusatory.
- Functional activity is often impaired by the pain. The clinical manifestation of RSD is similar to some CNS-related pain syndromes.
- _Physical findings:_ the patient avoids touch. A low-grade inflammatory activity is present. Oedema may be pitting or non-pitting. Redness or cyanosis, temperature change with warmness early and coolness later. Joint swelling may be seen. Get 3 stages of RSD – acute:
  - stage I with burning, subacute – lasts about 3 months;
  - stage II with burning and warm and chronic – lasts 9–12 months;
  - stage III with permanent dystrophy – pain remains intractable with fixed flexion contractures, depression and suicidal tendency.
- _Clinical forms:_
  - _Causalgia_;
  - _Shoulder-hand syndrome_;
  - Sudeck's osteoporosis;
  - _Myofascial dysfunction_.

Biological mechanisms: the mechansisms remain unclear.

- *Neurogenic inflammation, substance P:* when pain stimulates unmyelinated fibres there is an inflammatory response. This is modified by centrally produced neuropeptides. As the stimulus travels up the axon so backflow called axon reflux occurs with substances such as substance P (SP), calcitonin gene-related peptide (CGRP), bradykinin, serotonin, etc. These promote inflammation so the main provoking source of inflammation may be the afferent receptors. The afferent receptor mediates pain to the CNS and also supplies inflammatory neuropeptides to the periphery. SP is the most likely neuropeptide implicated in RSD as it causes profound inflammatory changes. Capsaicin depletes neurones of SP. Application appears to cause desensitization to inflammatory agents. CGRP causes intense vasodilatation. Many other substances have been implicated, such as cyclooxygenase which is produced in the midbrain, and proinflammatory cytokines. Dysregulation of the neuropeptide system could result in inappropriate quantity and length of the neuropeptide secretion.
- *Sympathetic nervous system:* most reports assume abnormal sympathetic activity. The proof is sympathetic block, which is very variable.

Aetiology:

- No unifying hypothesis explains the disproportionate pain with vasomotor, inflammatory and dystrophic changes.
- *Peripheral basis:* E phase theory suggests that artificial synapses occur at the injury site with efferent fibres directly activating afferent fibres. This leads to abnormal sensitization.
- *Spinal cord level:* suggests that peripheral nerves could activate internuncial neural pool in the spinal cord, which spreads to sympathetic neurons. Nociceptors are activated leading to excitation of wide-dynamic range (WDR) neurons. These then respond to all afferent stimulation. Sympathetic activity is increased. Also get failure of inhibitory mechanisms.

- *Psychophysiologic mechanisms:* there may be a predisposing psychological make-up of patients in some or all of the cases. Some studies have found significant differences in psychological make-up – a high % of patients have alexithymia ('lack of words for mood or emotion'). Patients are more emotionally unstable and have significantly greater depression.
- *Opioid pain-control system:* endorphins have an inhibitory effect on substance P production. They may have a role in the strong placebo effect in RSD.

Diagnostic techniques: usually markers of inflammation are normal.

- *Radiography:* may see osteopenia, patchy demineralization. Doesn't pick up early changes.
- *Radionuclide bone scan:* 3-phase technetium-labelled diphosphonate bone scanning. Get changes earlier, but a negative scan does not rule out RSD.
- *MRI:* changes are non-specific.
- *Thermography:* some consider this the most sensitive, but there is great variability in temperature change, and the temperature varies with the stage of the disease.
- *Response to sympathetic block:* many regard this the best criteria for diagnosis. However, it is variable.

Surgical treatment:

- Many established treatments have not been tested against a placebo and many patients with RSD have a strong placebo effect. Techniques such as phentolamine and guanethidine blocks have not been shown to be effective against a placebo.
- The best treatment is prevention. This requires an early diagnosis of RSD and close follow-up. Once established, it is difficult to gain the confidence of the patient.
- *Sympathectomy:* most effective with proximal nerve injury and less useful with slowly developing dystrophy from minor trauma. Patients most likely to benefit are those who get transient benefit from blocks. There is significant morbidity which is reduced by endoscopic procedure.
- *Transaxillary decompression of the subclavian vein:* in one study, similarities were noted

between RSD and thoracic outlet syndrome, and some benefit noted by decompression.

- *Surgical control of peripheral nerve irritants:* first control the symptoms before tackling problems, such as neuromas, as otherwise the syndrome may persist. Surgery may exacerbate symptoms.
- *Implanted electrical stimulation:* has been tried at various sites both centrally and peripherally with variable response.
- *Nerve blocks:* can be successful though may be just the placebo effect. Alternate long- and short-acting anaesthetics to confound the placebo effect. If the effect from sympathetic block is convincing, but short-lived, then consider surgical sympathectomy. Regional blocks may help therapy. Biers blocks can be used with guanethidine.
- *Sympatholytics:*
  - *Clonidine:* alpha-2-adrenergic agonist. Suppresses CNS noradrenergic activity. Use as a patch.
  - *Phentolamine:* post-synaptic alpha-1 antagonist and presynaptic alpha-2 antagonist. Oral use poorly tolerated.

Regnault's classification
Classification for the grading of breast ptosis:
- *1st degree minor:* nipple-areolar complex (NAC) at or slightly above inframammary fold.
- *2nd degree moderate:* NAC below the inframammary fold, but on the anterior projection of the breast mound.
- *3rd degree major:* NAC is in the dependent position. If very severe the nipple points downwards.
- *Pseudoptosis:* the NAC remains above the inframammary fold, but the breast mound descends below the inframammary fold with glandular hypoplasia.
- *Glandular ptosis:* the breast is normal except that the breast mound has descended below the inframammary fold.

See *Mastopexy*.

Rendu–Osler–Weber disease
Hereditary haemorrhagic telangiectasia (HHT)
- Occurs in 1–2 per 100 000 births.

- A group of autosomal disorders of similar phenotype caused by several genes. The homozygous form is lethal.
- Get multisystem vascular dysplasia and recurrent haemorrhage
- Spider-like bright-red maculopapules, 1–4 mm in diameter occur on the face, mucous membranes, fingers and nail beds. Also on internal mucosal surfaces.
- They usually present after puberty and increase in number with age.
- Epistaxis is the most common presenting symptom.
- Arteriovenous malformations may develop in the brain, spinal cord, liver and lungs.
- Septic emboli from pulmonary AVMs may cause brain abscesses.

See *Telangiectases*.

Replantation
- Single digit replants distal to FDS insertion give good results. Zone 2 replants have poorer functional results.
- *Multiple digit:* thumb and middle or ring finger have highest priority to give grasp and pinch.
- *Storage:* place part in damp normal saline gauze and place in sealed bag surrounded by ice-saline bath to maintain at 4ºC. Never place directly on ice.
- *Absolute indications:* for replantation. Thumb, multiple digits, paediatric, mid-carpal wrist or distal forearm.
- *Relative indications:* single digit distal to FDS, female, proximal limb in child.
- *Ischaemic time:* measure from time of amputation to replantation. Needs to be <6 hours if proximal to the wrist or <12 hours for fingers though survival after 42 hours of warm ischaemia has been reported.

Operation:
- Start by operating on the amputated part. Use 2 midlateral incisions and tag structures. Tag tendons and veins as well as the NVB. Insert two K wires.
- Temporary knobby plastic shunts can be used for proximal extremity to allow rapid reperfusion. Bleeding is allowed from muscle and veins to flush toxic products away.

Fasciotomy is required for proximal amputations.

- Veins grafts may be required if there is significant trauma to the vessels and these can be harvested from the wrist. Digital arteries can be transposed or a digital artery from an adjacent healthy finger can be used.
- If there is flow across the anastomosis but no perfusion then there may be spasm distally. Distal side branches should be tied off or diathermied as these may cause spasm. Heparin or 50–100 000 units of streptokinase or urokinase can be used.

Treatment of the failing replant:

- *Poor inflow:* reduce dressing and ensure there is no constriction. A marcaine block can be given at the wrist. Papaverine can be injected through the skin incision. If there is no improvement explore. Thrombosis should be resected and vein grafted. Heparinize.
- *Poor outflow:* leech therapy.

Retinacular system

There are 4 layers of fascia in the palm. The retinacular system has several important functions. The attachment of retaining ligaments to the skin enhances stability. It also provides fascial compartments for hand structures.

Palmar fascia:

- *Midpalmar fascia:* triangular in shape. Proximally it is attached to palmaris longus or transverse carpal ligament. It extends to the base of the fingers and has longitudinal, transverse and vertical fibres. Longitudinal fibres can be superficial or deep.
- *Longitudinal fibres:* superficial fibres are the pretendinous bands palmar to the flexor tendons and sheaths. They diverge as they approach the MCP joints. The central fibres run parallel to the flexor tendons. The band to index angles radially to the radial side of the MCPJ and the band to the little finger does the opposite. The bands are attached to skin. Most end at the palmar skin crease. Some bifurcate at the MCP level to contribute to the spiral bands of Gosset. The deep longitudinal fibres pass distally beneath the natatory ligament to insert into the lateral digital sheet.

- *Vertical fibres:* a deep system divides the midpalmar space into several compartments. The superficial vertical fibres pierce the palmar fat pad to anchor skin to the palmar aponeurosis. The septa of Legueu and Juvara originate from the palmar fascia at the level of the proximal edge of the flexor tendon sheath and pass dorsally between the lateral surfaces of the A1 pulleys and the digital neurovascular bundles. They attach to the deep transverse metacarpal ligament at the point of insertion of the volar plate of the MCPJ. There are less vertical fibres over the thenar and hypothenar eminence giving a relative laxity here.
- *Transverse fibres:* thin strong shiny fibres which run transversely deep to the pretendinous bands in the distal palm just proximal to the A1 pulley. The vertical fibres pass between the transverse fibres forming the A0 pulley. There is no connection and the transverse fibres are not involved in Dupuytren's contracture.
- <u>Natatory ligaments</u>.

Retaining ligaments of the digits:

- These stabilize the skin and the extensor mechanism and support the neurovascular bundles.
- <u>Grayson's ligament</u>.
- <u>Cleland's ligaments</u>.
- <u>Transverse retinacular ligament of Landsmeer</u>.
- <u>Oblique retinacular ligament of Landsmeer</u>.
- *The spiral band:* a fibrous condensation formed by the pretendinous band, natatory ligament, and vertical septa. Distal to the natatory ligament it progresses to the digit as the lateral digital sheet.

See <u>Dupuytren's contracture.</u>

Retromolar trigone carcinoma

- The retromolar trigone is a poorly defined area covered under the terms 'posterior floor of the mouth,' 'posterior alveolus,' and 'anterior tonsillar pillar.'
- The main points of significance about this region are that diagnosis may be delayed, the region is less accessible, and reconstruction is more difficult.

See <u>Head and neck cancer.</u>

Rhabdomyosarcoma

- Sarcoma that tends to occur in younger children.
- Often involves the orbit and usually doesn't metastasize.
- Surgery, irradiation and chemotherapy has improved the 5-year survival to 55%.
- Most failures are due to local recurrence, so wider excision will improve local control and obviate the need for RT.

Rheumatoid arthritis

- Affects 2% of the population. F:M 3:1. 90% have hand involvement, 10% have significant hand involvement. 15% get severe disease.
- *Aetiology:* autoimmune reaction to an unknown agent in synovial tissue. Antigen interacts with IgG and IgM antibodies to produce synovial inflammation. 70% RhF +ve (IgG or IgM abs in serum).
- *Criteria for diagnosis:* 4 of 7 required. Simplified version is:
  - morning stiffness;
  - 3 or more joints involved;
  - hand;
  - symmetric;
  - rheumatoid nodules;
  - seropositive;
  - radiography.

Classification:

- *Monoarthropathy:* 1 joint, pauciarthropathy 2–4 joints, polyarthropathy >4.
- *Clinical cause:* monocyclic one attack or polycyclic. Progressive if worsening.
- *3 phases:* proliferative, destructive and reparative.

Pathology: 5 stages

- macrophages in synovium ingest and present foreign antigens to T cells, which initiates B cells to produce antibodies.
- B cells proliferate. Angiogenesis occurs and synovial cells proliferate. Chronic inflammation is perpetuated. expansive hyperplasia within synovium forms a pannus.
- Patient becomes symptomatic with warm swollen joints.
- Synovial pannus invades cartilage, bone, ligaments and tendons.

- Damage produces joint destruction, contractures and tendon ruptures. Cartilage is destroyed. Subchondral bone is eroded. Synovium expands and joint capsule is stretched with ligament destruction. Joint instability and subluxation.

Non-articular manifestation:

- *Eyes:* iritis, scleritis, uveitis. Sjögren's syndrome.
- *Nervous system:* polyneuropathy, carpal tunnel syndrome.
- *Blood:* anaemia, Felty's syndrome (splenomegaly and neutropenia).
- *Heart:* pericarditis, myocarditis, pericardial effusions.
- *Lungs:* pleural effusions, rheumatoid nodules, Caplan's syndrome (nodular pulmonary fibrosis in RA exposed to industrial dusts).
- *Kidneys:* amyloidosis.
- *Skin:* vasculitic ulcers, rheumatoid nodules are present in 20% of patients.

Investigations:

- RhF.
- *XR:* note joint space narrowing, erosions, soft tissue swelling, cysts in bone and osteoporosis.

Non-surgical treatment:

- Diet, rest, exercise, splint and medication.
- NSAIDs counteract inflammation, steroids, azothiaprine, gold and hydrochloroquinone.
- More specific drugs aimed at switching off the immune response are being developed. Cytokines are pro or anti-inflammatory. TNFa antibodies (infliximan) bind to TNFa and reduce inflammation. STNFR (Enbrel) is anti-inflammatory.

Surgery:

- *Rheumatoid nodules.*
- *Tenosynovitis.*
- *Tendon rupture.*

Indications: For pain, function, prophylactic and for cosmetic improvement.

Wrist RA: Pannus occurs in the volar radiocarpal ligaments. Scaphoid becomes unstable. Get volar flexion of scaphoid, carpal collapse and distal ulna subluxation. Carpus supinates on radius with ulna translation.

- Synovectomy.
- *Darrach* procedure.
- Arthroplasty (not commonly performed).
- *Arthrodesis:* gives stability, but sacrifices wrist movement.
- *Limited carpal fusion:* may be possible as the midcarpal joint may be spared.

Dorsal tenosynovitis:

- Proliferative tenosynovitis leads to a swelling that may cause tendon rupture due to synovial infiltration, abrasion (*Vaughn–Jackson syndrome*).
- Perform dorsal synovectomy and place extensor retinaculum under the tendons.

Extensor tendon rupture:

- Starts from ulnar to radial.
- Repair by adjacent suturing, EIP transfer or FDS-4 transfer.

Flexor tenosynovitis:

- Present with pain on flexion and decreased movement with crepitus. Tendon rupture may occur.
- Treatment is by flexor synovectomy.

Flexor tendon rupture:

- FPL is the commonest to rupture (*Mannerfelt lesion*).
- Treat with direct repair, graft, and FDS transfer. FDP rupture in the palm – attach stump to adjacent tendon.
- For FDP rupture in the finger perform DIPJ stabilization.

MCP joint:

- Get ligament disruption by pannus. Cartilage and bone destruction remove stability. Wrist radial deviation alters balance of finger deviators. Radial sagittal band attenuation. Tightened ulna intrinsics.
- *Treatment:* synovectomy. Soft tissue alignment with intrinsic release, crossed intrinsic transfer and extensor tendon stabilization, *Arthroplasty.*

Swan neck deformity.

Boutonnière deformity.

Thumb deformities:

- *Classification: Nalebuff.*
- *Aetiology:*

○ Boutonnières occurs when the pannus affects the dorsal MCP joint structures leading to flexion and subluxation.
○ Hyperextension of IPJ caused by EPL.
○ Swan neck occurs when the CMC joint ligaments are destabilized with dorsal subluxation, adduction contracture and compensatory hyperextension of the MCP joint.
- *Treatment:* depends on the stage of disease.
○ with flexible Boutonnières treat by synovectomy and extensor reconstruction;
○ MCP joint arthrodesis;
○ Swan necks are treated with CMC arthroplasty.

Rheumatoid factor

IgM autoantibody to IgG immunoglobulin. Not specific to RA. Patients with RA who are negative tend to have a milder disease.

Rheumatoid nodules

- Collagenous matrix over bony prominence. Commonly over olecranon. Can appear on the dorsum of the fingers.
- Probably over areas of attrition with microvascular damage and complement cascade and chronic inflammation.
- Histologically get central fibrous tissue surrounded by macrophages which show pallisading. As it expands get central necrosis.
- More common in males.
- They occur in 25% of patients with RA and are associated with aggressive disease.
- Surgery is indicated for relief of symptoms and cosmesis. Recurrence is common.

Rhinophyma

A severe form of acne *Rosacea* affecting the nose. There are 4 stages of rosacea, the 4th being rhinophyma.

Pathology: Possibly the vascular instability leads to fluid in dermis with inflammation and fibrosis. Sebaceous ducts become plugged. Get a lymphocytic infiltrate

Epidemiology:

- Rosacea is common – 50–10%, with a higher incidence in women though rhinophyma is more common in men possibly due to the androgenic influence.

- More common in English and Irish descent with a familial component.
- Rosacea begins in the 30s, acne rosacea in the 40s and rhinophyma in the 50s.
- There may be a link with alcoholism. Skin tumours can easily be missed within rhinophyma or mimic rhinophyma.

Treatment:
- *Non-surgical:* rosacea is treated with topical and oral antibiotics and retinoids. None has been shown to halt progression to rhinophyma. Irradiation has been reported to be successful for rhinophyma.
- *Surgical:* the mainstay of treatment is surgical. There are many treatments such as dermabrasion, cryosurgery, shave excision and CO_2 laser therapy. No one method has been shown to give superior results. All skin should be sent for histology. Only graft for severe nodular rhinophyma or underlying malignancy.

Rhinoplasty
Challenging as the anatomy is variable, form and function must be corrected and it is highly visible.

Anatomy:
- The external nose consists of three parts – the osseocartilaginous vault, lobule/tip and base.
- The bony vault consists of nasal bones and frontal process of maxilla, which overlaps the cartilage – upper lateral and dorsal septum.
- Assess dorsum for height and width and base for width. Assess nasofacial angle – 34° with concavity in females, 36° and straight in males. The width is the same as the philtral columns and the tip defining points 6–8 mm for females and 8–10 mm for males.
- The lobule is the entire area covering cartilage, but the tip is just the area in the tip defining points.
- *Alar cartilages:* 3 crura – medial, middle and lateral with 2 junctions – columellar breakpoint and dome-defining point. Excising lateral crura will reduce tip volume and modifying the domal segment of middle crura will increase tip definition.
- *Base:* alar base, nostrils and columella.

- Assess septum, anterior nasal spine and pyriform maxilla.

Function:
- Assess airways. The five functions of the nose are respiration, filtration, humidification, temperature regulation and protection.
- 50% of airways resistance occurs in the nose. Resistance is determined by the internal valve which is defined by the valve angle – the relationship between the upper lateral cartilage and the septum, and the valve area – the circumference of the airway. The angle is 10–15° and closes with negative pressure. If this area is affected by septal deviation, mucosal disease etc., respiratory obstruction can occur.
- If lateral cheek traction will reduce obstruction (positive Cottle sign) then spreader grafts may be of benefit.
- The turbinates also increase resistance. Inferior turbinate hypertrophy may require reduction.

Assessment:
- Assess the internal nose, specifically:
  - *nostril/vestibule:* septal deviation, external valve collapse;
  - *internal valve:* look at angle and reduction by inferior turbinate;
  - *septum:* deviation and mucosal lining;
  - turbinates.
- Externally the commonest problems are with the nasal hump, width and tip projection.

Surgery:
Open approach:
- Transcolumellar and bilateral marginal incisions, which allow the nasal tip skin to be elevated. Incise the columellar in the middle at the narrow waist.
- The marginal incision is made going from dome out laterally, then back medially around the domal segment down to the level of the transcolumellar incision.
- Undermine the skin over the lateral crura and domes.
- Dissect along the cartilages to expose all the alar cartilages.
- Expose dorsum.
- Extramucosal tunnels are created beneath the dorsum.

- Perform dorsal reduction in two steps. First the bone then the cartilage. Rasps for the bone and scissors to detach upper lateral cartilages. Septum and cartilages are reduced.
- *Septum:* either straighten or resect. Preserve an L-shape strut of septal cartilage. Relocate septum by mobilizing the cartilage along the inferior border of the vomerine groove. Fixed deformities are often resected.
- *Osteotomies:* to narrow the bony width of the nose and close the open roof. For minimal movement produce a greenstick low to high osteotomy. Insert into a small cut made in the pyriform aperture and advance to the medial canthus. Pressure will achieve the narrowing. If major movement is required, make two osteotomies to completely mobilize the lateral wall. First a transverse osteotomy from above the medial canthus to the nasal dorsum then a low-to-low osteotomy. When they join the osteotome is rotated medially to cause major movement.
- *Grafts:* grafts can be carved. Spreader grafts are matchstick size and placed either side of the dorsal septum to restore natural width following reduction. They minimize collapse of the upper lateral cartilage. They are placed parallel to the dorsal septum.
- *Tip surgery:* mainly cartilage excision through a closed approach, suturing the alar cartilages and strut and tip graft.
- *Base:* the most common procedure is nostril sill excision to narrow the amount of nostril seen on anterior view.

Closed approach:
- It is simple, quick and without external incisions. It is limited though. Most patients on whom it is used have a bump, wide nose or minor tip problems.
- Transcartilaginous: involves a single intracartilaginous incision which penetrates the lateral crura 4–5 mm above the caudal margin which allows removal of excess cephalic lateral crura. The incision should mirror the external tip defining line.
- *Delivery method:* two incisions, a marginal incision at the caudal border of lateral crura and an intercartilaginous incision at the cephalic border of the lateral crura, where it meets the upper lateral cartilage. The lateral crura is exteriorized. This method may be better if some tip modification is required. Dorsal exposure is performed in close contact with the upper lateral cartilages. Extramucosal tunnels are formed. Septal surgery is performed and dorsal hump reduction. Osteotomies are made. Small tip grafts may be required.

- *Secondary rhinoplasty.*
- Delay operation for at least a year. Grafts will probably be required, but may need to come from concha. Deep temporal fascial grafts can augment soft tissue. The radix often needs to be reduced.

Rhomboid flap

Also Limberg flap.
- A combination of rotation and transposition that borrows adjacent loose skin for covering a rhombic defect.
- A rhombus is an equilateral parallelogram with 60° acute angles and 120° obtuse angles.
- The short diagonal equals the length of each side. Extend the short diagonal by an equal length and draw a line of equal length at 60° which will be parallel to side of rhombus.
- A large defect can be converted into a hexagon to facilitate closure using 6 rhomboid flaps.

See *Dufourmental flap*.

Rib graft

- Split rib grafts can be used for *Cranium reconstruction*.
- Ribs can regenerate as long as the periosteum is left intact.
- Don't take more than two ribs in continuity.
- Manage pleural puncture by lung expansion. The defect is then closed. Cut the ribs as long as possible and split with a fine chisel.
- They can be embedded in various ways.

Ribbon sign

- Curled up arteries lying proximally.
- May get faint red streaks on amputated digit (Chinese red lines).
- Suggest the arteries have been avulsed distally and are a poor prognostic sign.

Riche–Cannieu anastomosis

Anastomosis of motor fibres between the median nerve and ulnar nerve at the level of the palm causing ulnar muscles to be supplied by the median nerve.

Ricketts' aesthetic plane

• A line drawn from nose tip to chin.
• The lower lip lies on this plane, the upper lip 2 mm behind.
See *Cephalometrics*.

Rieger flap

Dorsal nasal flap.
• A rotation advancement of dorsal nasal skin.
• Initially described as a random pattern flap with a wide pedicle encompassing the whole side of the nose, it can be based on a branch of the angular artery that enters the skin of the nasal radix just below the medial canthal tendon.
• Elevating the flap on a narrow vascular pedicle gives greater mobility.
• The dorsal nasal flap provides good coverage for <2 cm defects in the nasal dorsum up to the tip defining points.
• If used for infratip defects, it pulls the nasal tip cephalad and causes alar notching.
• It provides a single unit of closely matching tissue while leaving scars that coincide with 'aesthetic unit' junctions.
See *Nasal reconstruction, Marchac dorsal nasal flap.*

Riley–Smith syndrome

Microcephaly, multiple vascular malformations and pseudopapilloedema, but no lipomas unlike *Bannayan syndrome*.

Ring avulsion injuries

Classification by Urbaniak.
See *Degloving injuries*.

Rintala flap

For nasal tip and columella, rectangular dorsal nasal flap based on nasion with Burow's triangles cut at canthal level.
See *Nasal reconstruction.*

Robin sequence

• Cleft palate, micrognathia and glossoptosis.
• Heterogenous aetiology but one of the most common causes is Stickler syndrome.
See *Pierre Robin sequence. See Craniofacial genetics*.

Rolando's fracture

Same place as a *Bennet's fracture*, but more bony fragments, with a Y- or T-shaped intra-articular component.

Romberg's disease

See *Hemifacial atrophy*.

Roo's test

• Clinical test in *Thoracic outlet syndrome*.
• 'I surrender position'.
• Patient seated. Arms abducted to 90°, elbows flexed to 90°.
• Hands closed into a fist and opened repetitively for 3 minutes. Each cycle lasts 2 seconds.
• May get colour change or neurological symptoms. Rarely carried out for 3 minutes.

Rosacea

4 stages of rosacea – a cutaneous vascular disorder.
• Facial flushing.
• Thickened skin and facial erythema.
• Some progress to acne rosacea with erythematous papules and pustules.
• *Rhinophyma* in some patients. The nose is usually the only structure affected. The nasal skin is erythematous with pits. Skin becomes chronically infected. May get nasal airway obstruction. The framework is unaffected.

Rotation flap

• Semicircular flap raised from the edge of a triangular defect which rotates about a pivot point into an adjacent area.
• The line of greatest tension is from the pivot point of the flap to the edge of the defect nearest to where the flap previously lay. If the tension is great, a backcut may be made from the pivot point along the base of the flap. Also a Burow's triangle can be excised from skin adjacent to the pivot point.

- Most commonly used for scalp and sacral defects.
- Another type of rotation flap is the bilobed flap.
See Transposition flap.

Ruben's flap
- Flap raised from the periiliac fat pad, which is seen in subjects of this artist.
- Based on the deep circumflex iliac vessels.
- Can be used for *Breast reconstruction*.

S Saethre–Chotzen syndrome to Systemic lupus erythematosus (SLE)

Saethre–Chotzen syndrome
- Autosomal dominant syndromic *Craniosynostosis*.
- Caused by a mutation in the *TWIST* gene, which codes for a transcription factor.
- Characterized by coronal synostosis, facial dysmorphology, brachydactyly and cutaneous syndactyly.
- Can be confused with Crouzon's if no limb abnormalities
- Get a low-set frontal hairline.
- Facial asymmetry.
- Ptosis of the eyelids.
- Maxillary hypoplasia with a narrow palate.
- Intelligence is usually normal.
- A partial syndactyly or brachydactyly involving the second and third digits.

Safe position of hand splintage
- *Metacarpalphalangeal joint* flexed, PIP joint extended, thumb abducted, wrist mild extension.
- The position from which it is easiest to regain mobility.
- MCP joint has variable tightness of collateral ligaments in flexion and extension. The head is ovoid in the sagittal plane with a palmar flare in the transverse plane so the collateral ligaments need to be longer in flexion. Lax ligaments tend to shorten leading to extension contracture.
- The interphalangeal joints are the same in flexion and extension, but the volar plate overlies cartilage, where it will readily become adherent. The extensors are stable in extension and stressed in flexion. In flexion they will easily become attenuated with disruption of the transverse retinacular ligaments, leading to volar slip of the lateral bands and a boutonniere deformity.

Sagittal band
- A passive stabilizer for the *Extensor tendons* over the MCP joint.
- The distal part is covered by transverse fibres of the interosseous hood.
- It attaches to volar plate.
- It also limits the proximal excursion of the extensor and it is the primary extensor of the MCPJ. As the extensor contracts, the sagittal band is pulled, which lifts the base of the proximal phalanx.

Subluxing tendons:
- Loss of integrity of sagittal band by trauma or attrition results in subluxation usually into the ulnar gutters.
- The tendons may centralize in extension but slip in flexion. Eventually active extension is lost though it can be maintained if positioned passively.
- Most commonly affects the ulna 3 digits.

Tear:
- Get swelling over the MCP joint, pain on extension, extensor lag and deviation of the finger (to intact side).
- Treatment controversial. Splint initially, but if this fails perform primary repair with centralization and stabilization of the extensor tendon.

Sagittal synostosis
- The most common form of *Craniosynostosis*.
- Scaphocephaly (boat-like) due to premature fusion of the sagittal suture.

- Skull has increased anteroposterior length and decreased width.
- Sporadic, 2% genetic or familial predisposition.
- Get enhanced growth at the coronal lambdoid and metopic sutures.
- The entire sagittal suture may not be involved so that deformity may be predominantly anterior, predominantly posterior or both.

Operative procedure: Treatment varies according to the age of the patient and severity.
- Young patients with mild sagittal synostosis require a simple sagittal strip synostectomy.
- To correct frontal bossing a Pi procedure can be performed with a coronal osteotomy and two parasagittal osteotomies, with the frontal bone being drawn back onto the central sagittal section.
- Total cranial reconstruction can be performed with a central strip left intact over the sagittal sinus, and the other bones being removed, barrel staved and replaced.
- Alternatively, the whole cranium can be removed using horizontal strips.

Salivary tumours
- 3% of head and neck malignancies.
- 80% in parotid.
- 80% parotid masses are benign.
- 50% salivary masses are benign.

Factors indicating malignancy: Pain, obstruction, nerve involvement, invasion, bleeding, rapid progression.

Classification:
- Benign or malignant.
- primary or secondary.
- Long list of possible tumours.
See WHO classification.

Benign parotid tumours:
- *Pleomorphic adenoma:* benign mixed tumour. The commonest benign tumour of the parotid. Classified by some as a low grade malignant tumour. Presents as a slowly growing mass. Invasion of facial nerve is rare. Simple enucleation leads to a high rate of recurrence. Treatment is by superficial parotidectomy.

- *Adenolymphoma:* Warthin's tumour. Located in the tail of the parotid in elderly males. 5–10% are bilateral. Most are treated by superficial parotidectomy.
- *Others:* oncocytoma, sebaceous adenoma, cystadenoma.

Malignant parotid tumours: Most arise in the body of the gland. Occasionally in the tail and rarely in the deep lobe. They can be primary or secondary. All malignant parotid tumours require adjuvant radiotherapy.
- *Mucoepidermoid carcinoma:* Most common malignancy, 30% of malignant parotid tumours. 3 histological grades.
  - well differentiated with limited local invasiveness;
  - intermediate, which behave like well differentiated SCCs;
  - poorly differentiated – local invasion and regional spread, treat high grade with total parotidectomy, but preserve nerve if functioning and if possible; give radiotherapy to all.
- *Adenoid cystic carcinoma:* most common non-parotid malignancy. 20% of malignant tumours. 3 grades – cibrose, tubular and solid. Skip lesions along the facial nerve are common and perineural invasion common. It may recur many years after presentation. If the follow-up is long enough few patients are cured.
- *Carcinoma ex pleomorphic adenoma:* malignant transformation may occur after 10 years.
- *Others:* adenocarcinoma, acinic cell tumour, sebaceous carcinoma, lymphoma.

FNA:
- FNA biopsy can be useful particularly if the patient is at a high risk or if it is thought to be a metastasis.
- Some controversy as to the value of tissue diagnosis, but it is argued that tissue diagnosis should always be obtained first with FNA and if this is negative, with ultrasound assisted core biopsy. This is to exclude a tumour, which doesn't require surgery, principally a lymphoma.

Facial nerve: Resect facial nerve if it is invaded with tumour or the tumour cannot otherwise be removed.

Neck dissection: The role in N0 tumours is unclear, usually perform RT.

Salmon patch
See _Nevus flammeus neonatorum_.

Saphenous flap
A _Venous flap_, based on the short saphenous vein and used to reconstruct defects around the knee.

Sarcoidosis
- May present with cutaneous lesions as reddish translucent, smooth papules on the eyelid and nasal margins or as plaques and nodules.
- Steroid treatment for generalized disease often improves cutaneous lesions.
- Large masses may be excised after failure of medical therapy.

Sarcoma
Incidence:
- 1% of malignant disease.
- 50% of deep sarcomas are in the lower limb and most are in the thigh.
- Most common types are:
  - liposarcoma;
  - malignant fibrohistiocytoma;
  - fibrosarcoma;
  - synovial sarcoma;
  - rhabdomyosarcoma.

Aetiology:
- Previous radiation. Most likely to develop on the edge of the radiation field where less devitalized tissue exists. It can happen even with low-dose treatments such as for keloid scars but there is a long latency period. With higher dose treatments the latency is 10–15 years. The most common sarcoma secondary to RT is osteogenic sarcoma and fibrosarcoma.
- Retinoblastoma and Wilm's tumours are associated with subsequent sarcoma formation, with a chromosomal anomaly on 13q responsible.

- Association with some benign conditions such as neurofibromatosis, fibrous dysplasia and Paget's disease.
- Some chemicals, such as polyvinyl chloride, arsenic and dioxin are sarcomagenic.
- AIDS is linked to Kaposi's sarcoma.

Classification: classify by:
- Tissue of origin:
  - smooth muscle: leiomyosarcoma;
  - striated muscle: _Rhabdomyosarcoma_;
  - fat: liposarcoma;
  - blood vessels: _Angiosarcoma_, Kaposi's sarcoma;
  - lymph channels: lymphangiosarcoma;
  - fibrous tissue: fibrosarcoma;
  - nerve: malignant Schwannoma;
  - synovial tissue: synovial sarcoma;
  - skin: _Dermatofibrosarcoma protuberans_, _Atypical fibroxanthoma_, _Malignant fibrous histiocytoma_.
- TNMG classification:
  - T1: tumours <5 cm;
  - T2: tumours >5 cm;
  - T3: invading bone, vessel, nerve;
  - N0: no nodes;
  - N1: nodes;
  - M0: no metastases;
  - M1: distant metastases;
  - G1: low grade;
  - G2: intermediate grade;
  - G3: high grade.
- Stage:
  - stage 1: T1 or 2, G1;
  - stage 2: T1 or 2, G2;
  - stage 3: T1 or 2, N1, G3;
  - stage 4: T3, M1.
- _Enneking classification._

Deep sarcomas present as enlarging mass, maybe with pressure effects and systemic symptoms.

Investigations:
- _MRI:_ gadolinum-enhanced to improve resolution.
- _CT:_ for bony involvement.
- _Angiography._
- _Radionuclide imaging:_ arterial, venous and osseous phase.
- _Biopsy:_ after imaging. With FNA, Tru-cut or open – site of incision planned to enable excision of the scar and tract.

Surgery:
- Get pseudocapsule, which may be infiltrated by tumour.
- May be intra- or extracompartmental. If intracompartmental there may be seedlings anywhere in the compartment. If extracompartmental there may be spread along fascial planes.
- Limb-sparing surgery is possible in 90% of patients.
- Surgery is determined by type of tumour and site.
- Wide local excision with 2–5 cm clearance with adjuvant therapy gives results similar to radical excision.
- Resect with one uninvolved anatomical plane in all directions.
- Functional compartmentectomy should be performed if possible (preserving at least one muscle in the compartment). Include both origin and insertion of the muscle in which the tumour occurs. If this is not possible at least 10 cm of muscle should be excised on either side of the tumour. Major nerves should be preserved unless directly infiltatred by tumour.
- Reconstruction is with SSGs, local flaps or free flaps. Free flaps are required to cover exposed neurovascular structures, bone or prostheses and permit the use of adjuvant therapy without delay. Brachytherapy can be started 1 week after free tissue transfer.

Radiotherapy

Salter–Harris classification
For epiphyseal injuries in children.
- *Salter–Harris I:* # through growth plate. Epiphysis separates from metaphysis with shear force. Good prognosis.
- *Salter–Harris II:* after age of 10, # through plate and metaphysis.
- *Salter–Harris III:* after age of 10, # in epiphysis.
- *Salter–Harris IV:* any age, rare in hand, # in epiphysis and metaphysic.
- *Salter–Harris V:* compression # of epiphyseal plate – rare in hand.

Sauvé–Kapandji procedure
Fusion of distal ulna to radial sigmoid notch with removal of a section of ulna proximal to fusion.
See DRUJ.

Scalenus muscles
Scalenus anterior:
Origin: Transverse process of 3–6 cervical vertebra.

Insertion: Tubercle of first rib.

Nerve: Anterior rami of C5 and C6.

Action: Stabilizes the first rib or rotates and flexes the neck if the first rib is fixed.

Scalenus medius:
Origin: Posterior tubercle of transverse process of C2–7.

Insertion: Superior aspect of neck of first rib.

Nerve: Posterior branches of anterior ramus of C3–8.

Action: Flexes and rotates cervical vertebra, raises first rib. When acting bilaterally flexes the neck.

Scalp anatomy
S: Skin.
C: Subcutaneous.
A: Aponeurosis (galea) connects frontalis with occipitalis.
L: Loose connective tissue.
P: Pericranium.
- *Skin:* the thickest in the body, up to 8 mm thick. It is attached by fibrous septa.
- *Subcutaneous layer:* of dense connective tissue and fat binds the skin to the underlying galea. It contains the principal arteries and veins of the scalp, as well as the sensory nerves and lymphatics.
- *Galea aponeurotica:* the tough fibrous layer of the scalp. It is extensive in its attachments and is a part of the subcutaneous musculoaponeurotic system (SMAS) of the face. It connects the occipitalis muscle posteriorly with the frontalis muscle anteriorly and the temporoparietal fascia (superficial temporal fascia) in one temporal region with the

same layer on the contralateral side. The frontalis muscles originate from the galea aponeurotica and insert into the dermis at the level of the supraciliary arches.

- *Loose areolar plane:* beneath the galea, composed of thin, avascular connective tissue. It is the layer most often involved in avulsion injuries. The laxity within this layer provides for the mobility of the scalp. Haematoma and infection spread easily through it, and thrombosis of the emissary veins may extend to the dural sinuses.
- *Pericranium:* densely adherent to the outer table of the skull, it has a good blood supply.
- *Arterial supply:* supra-orbital, supratrochlear, superficial temporal, occipital and postauricular. The main supply is from the occipital and superficial temporal arteries with the latter being the longest and largest.
- *Nerve supply:* V cranial nerve – supra-orbital and supratrochlear. The lesser occipital nerve supplies the posterior scalp.
- *Lymphatics:* forehead and frontoparietal drain to the superficial parotid gland and retromandibular node, posterior drainage is to the occipital and posterior triangle nodes.

Scalp reconstruction
Indications:
- *Congenital: Aplasia cutis congenita,* haemangiomas, AVM, extravasation injuries, *Craniopagus.*
- *Acquired:* trauma, burns, tumours.

Goals of reconstruction:
- Reconstruct with hair-bearing skin if possible, debridement should be limited as there is an excellent blood supply.
- Prevent desiccation of bone with bone necrosis. If bone exposed need immediate cover.
- Galea can be scored. Skin graft can be used on a vascularized surface – bone can be drilled or decorticated.
- Management of scalp wounds with radiotherapy may require a flap.

Surgery:
- *Local flaps.*

- *Regional flaps* or free flaps will be required if >30% of the scalp is involved. Examples include *Ortichochea flap,* Juri flap, *Trapezius flap.*
- *Replantation:* avulsed scalp can be replanted – use vessels outside zone of injury, which may require vein grafts. *See Cranium reconstruction.*
- *Free flaps:* free flaps allow a one-stage procedure to cover exposed bone or brain. The most commonly used flaps are omentum, latissimus dorsi with or without serratus anterior and radial forearm. The radial forearm gives good cover with pliable tissue though it may need pre-expansion. Free flaps however are often bulky and non-hairbearing. Superficial temporal vessels can be used or preferably use vessels in the neck – occipital or facial vessels.
- *Tissue expansion:* the preferred method for secondary scalp reconstruction as it enables hair-bearing skin to be used to cover the defect. The main disadvantage is the long duration of treatment. May develop skull deformation following prolonged expansion in children. Up to 50% of scalp can be replaced with expansion. Place multiple crescentic expanders adjacent to the defect. The risks are infection, extrusion and device failure.

Scalping flap
- The most reliable way to deliver a large amount of skin from the forehead to the nose.
- Originally described by Converse in 1942. Useful particularly in the older patient.
- Elevate through a coronal incision behind the superficial temporal artery, extending to a skin paddle on the contralateral forehead.
- The frontalis muscle is not carried in the distal end of the flap, but the remainder of the pedicle is dissected in the subgaleal plane.
- The donor site on the forehead is closed with a FTSG.
- The temporary defect on the scalp is covered with a non-desiccating dressing.
- After the skin paddle is completely revascularized on the nose, the pedicle is divided and the anterior scalp is replaced.

- The advantages of the scalping flap technique are the rich vascular supply of the broad skin paddle and the lack of incisions on the central forehead.

See *Nasal reconstruction.*

Scaphoid fracture

- The commonest carpal bone to be fractured.
- Most fractures are either transverse or horizontal oblique, which tend to be stable. Vertical oblique are more prone to displacement and non-union.
- Earlier treatment with fixation leads to earlier bony union though no long-term difference.

Blood supply:

- From branches of radial artery through ligamentous and capsular attachments to the dorsal ridge. Orientation of blood flow is predominantly distal to proximal.
- The superficial palmar branch of the radial artery gives a volar supply to the distal scaphoid.
- The dorsal carpal branch gives a dorsal supply to the distal scaphoid. The proximal pole is therefore poorly supplied.
- Minimal intraosseous anastomosis so the blood supply to the proximal fragment may be disrupted following fracture leading to avascular necrosis (*Preiser's disease*).
- The scaphoid functions as a link between the distal and proximal carpal rows. 80% of fractures occur at the waist. Proximal $1/3$ fracture don't heal well.

Treatment:

- If undisplaced by cast. A long arm cast may reduce time of healing, so have a long arm cast for 6 weeks and a short cast until radiological healing.
- Displaced fractures require fixation.
- k wires are simple with high union rates but no compression.
- Herbert screws and Herbert–Whipple screws provide compression by differential pitch concept.

Non-union: Occurs in 30% of waste fractures and 100% of proximal pole fractures. Ligamentous injury leading to a *DISI will* increase instability.

Classification: of non-unions can be simplified to stable and unstable.

- *Stable non-unions* have a firm fibrous non-union, which prevent deformity of the length and shape of the scaphoid. OA is minimal. Stable may become unstable with time.
- *Unstable pseudoarthrosis* are nearly always associated with some degree of carpal collapse deformity. Get sclerosis, cysts and synovial erosion. May develop scaphoid non-union advanced collapse.

Treatment:

- *Internal fixation:* compression screw provides the best fixation for routine non-unions. Approach volar or dorsal. Volar disrupts ligaments, dorsal may disrupt blood supply. Vascularity is assessed but most will also require bone grafting.
- *Bone grafting:* dorsal inlay, volar inlay and peg grafts have been used. Russe describes a bicortical bone graft through a volar incision. If collapsed then perform a volar wedge graft.
- *Vascularized bone grafting:* avascular necrosis is a serious late complication of scaphoid fractures. Patients develop increasing pain and stiffness. Reconstruction is by vascularized bone graft with or without bone stimulation. This produces faster incorporation and increased viability. The dorsal aspect of the distal radius is supplied by four vessels, two superficial to the retinaculum and two deep. Distally these anastomose with the dorsal intercarpal arch. A bone graft harvested here may be pedicled to reach the scaphoid. Zaidenberg graft relies on a septal pedicle between the 1st and 2nd dorsal extensor compartments The benefit is the vascular reliability and the simplicity with a single incision. Volar grafting is based on the palmar carpal artery, the anterior interosseous and a branch of the ulnar. The pronator quadratus is usually transferred to maintain the blood supply. The flap has a limited reach.
- *Bone stimulation:* with electrical stimulation by external devices. Electromagnetic fields may upregulate mRNA of TGFα and BMP. One study showed 69% of non-unions

healed with casting and electrodes. There is controversy regarding efficacy.

Salvage procedures: May be required for persistent non-union with carpal collapse.

- *Conservative treatment:* wrist support and change of activity. Neurectomy for pain, usually of the posterior interosseous nerve. Also the anterior interosseous nerve can be cut. Limited radial styloid incision can relieve impingement. Partial scaphoid excision can be helpful if the distal scapholunate ligament is preserved. The retaining palmar ligaments must be preserved.
- *Limited intercarpal and midcarpal fusion:* the most used are the capitolunate, scaphocapitolunate and scaphotrapeziotrapezoid arthrodeses. The various midcarpal fusions allow correction of midcarpal joint subluxation while preserving radiolunate joint motion.
- *Proximal row carpectomy versus scaphoid excision:* proximal row carpectomy is standard procedure for SLAC, involving removal of scaphoid, lunate and triquetrum. Scaphoid excision and four corner arthrodesis is more demanding with longer immobilization. They seem to have similar outcomes.
- *Total wrist fusion:* this gives pain relief at the expense of motion. The AO plate fixation uses bone graft and a plate to align 3rd metacarpal with radius with dorsal angulation of 0–20°.

See Carpal instability.

Scapholunate instability
See Carpal instability.

Scapular/parascapular flap
Blood supply:
- Based on cutaneous branch of circumflex scapular artery.
- Arises from subscapular artery and passes between teres major and teres minor on axillary border of scapula.
- Divides into scapular art (horizontal) and parascapular (longitudinal).
- The position of the pedicle can be found by $D = (L - 2) \div 2$, where D is distance between the spine of scapula and pedicle, and L is

distance from spine of scapular to inferior angle of bone.

Anatomic landmarks:
- Scapular flap is based on a horizontal line from *Triangular space* (2 cm above posterior axillary crease) to vertebra. The medial end lies midway between the medial border of the scapular and the midline.
- The parascapular flap is centred on a vertical line from triangular space to posterior iliac crest. The distal line lies midway between the tip of the scapular and the iliac crest.

Uses: Good for cheek and hemifacial restoration. The thickness allows for sculpting and the colour match is reasonable. It does not atrophy and is good for Romberg's disease.

Technique: Raise medial to lateral just above the deep fascia. As the lateral border of scapula is approached, carry the dissection beneath deep fascia. Identify the triangular space. Up to 10 cm of bone can be obtained from the lateral margin by identifying the distal branch of the circumflex scapular artery. Separate skin and bone paddles can be obtained.
See Trunk reconstruction.

Schirmer's test
- To assess the function of the greater petrosal nerve by measuring tear secretion.
- *Schirmer 1:* place a strip of filter paper in the lower conjunctiva for 5 minutes <10 m of wetting is abnormal.
- *Schirmer 2:* LA can be added to block reflex tear secretion (Schirmer's test 2).
See Facial re-animation.

Schuchardt flap
- Used in *Lip reconstruction.*
- The defect is excised as a rectangular defect and the incision is extended around the labiomental fold to the submental region on each side to allow lip to slide into the defect.
- It requires the excision of triangles in the submental region unless a compensating crescentic excision along the fold can be made instead.

Schwannoma
See Neurilemoma.

Schweckendiek technique

- Protocol for the repair of _Cleft lip and palate_.
- Lip and soft palate are repaired before the child is 1 year of age.
- Hard palate is repaired at 8 years of age.
- Reportedly excellent midfacial growth due to reduced disturbance of the important growth centres around the palate, but poor speech due to palatal incompetence.

Scleroderma

Hard skin.

- Chronic autoimmune disease mainly affecting women aged 30–60.
- Get thickening of skin, but also affects arteries, joints, lungs and kidneys.
- Sclerodactyly designates the characteristic hand changes, consisting of atrophic skin of the fingers held in partial flexion with limitation of motion in both flexion and extension.
- Wound healing is poor and ulcers should be treated like ischaemic ulcers.

See CREST.

Scleroderma circumscriptum

- Band-like lesions.
- They often follow a dermatome pattern on the trunk or an extremity.
- They may appear in the paramedian region of the forehead – scleroderma en coup de sabre – associated with _Hemifaical atrophy_.
- Severely deforming atrophy of skin, subcutaneous tissues, muscle, and bone may result from scleroderma.
- The eventual extent of the disease is unpredictable in its early stages and spontaneous resolution occurs in some cases.
- The treatment is conservative so long as active disease is present. When activity has ceased soft-tissue may require augmentation possibly by microvascular transfer.

Scurvy

See Vitamin C.

Sebaceous adenoma

- Non-descript solitary lesion.

- Histologically the lesion is an incompletely differentiated sebaceous lobule with irregular shape and size.
- Adenoma sebaceum, associated with _Tuberous sclerosis_ is an angiofibromatous proliferation and not a true sebaceous adenoma.
- Multiple sebaceous tumours of the face, scalp and trunk with keratoacanthomas may be associated with internal malignancies in _Torre's_ syndrome.

Sebaceous cell carcinoma

- A rare tumour, but accounts for 2% of _Eyelid tumours_.
- They arise from meibomian glands or pilosebaceous glands.
- Usually slow growing and arise in the upper eyelid in patients over 60 years old.
- Delay in treatment significantly increases mortality.
- There is a 5-year survival of 60–70%.
- Diagnose by excision biopsy.
- Management is by wide local excision and orbital extension will require exenteration. Neck dissection may be required. Radiotherapy is controversial and is reserved for palliative therapy.

Sebaceous cyst

See Epithelial cysts.

Sebaceous epitheliomas

- Resemble basal cell epitheliomas as pale or yellow papules with central ulceration.
- Usually a solitary lesion on the face or scalp.
- Treatment is by either excision, electrocoagulation and curettage, or carbon dioxide laser vaporization, depending on their size and location.
- Biopsy may be required to differentiate it from sebaceous carcinoma.

Sebaceous glands

- Holocrine glands that drain into the pilosebaceous unit.
- They are called meibomian glands when they drain directly onto skin.
- More frequent on the forehead, nose and cheek.

- They are not the sole cause of sebaceous cysts which are of epidermal origin.

Sebaceous hyperplasia

- 2–4 mm papules on the face of middle-aged adults.
- Pale yellow with central umbilication and telangiectasia.
- Histologically the lesions are collections of sebaceous glands with enlarged lobules located around a central enlarged sebaceous duct.

See *Fordyce's spots*.

Sebaceous tumours

See *Naevus sebaceous of Jadassohn, Senile sebaceous hyperplasia, Sebaceous epitheliomas*.

Seborrhoeic keratosis

Also seborrhoeic wart, senile keratosis, basal cell papilloma.

- Occurs in males and females from 5th decade onwards.
- Related to sun exposure.
- Covered with greasy scale.
- Familial variant autosomal dominant.
- A variant called *Dermatosis papulosa nigra* is seen in black people.
- Get accumulation of immature keratinocytes between the basal and keratinizing layers.
- Treat by curettage, excision or cryotherapy.

Seddon classification of nerve injury

Described in 1943.

- *Neuropraxia:* local conduction block, no Wallerian degeneration.
- *Axonotmesis:* axonal damage with wallerian degeneration.
- *Neurotmesis:* Nerve division.

Semmes–Weinstein monofilament testing

- Technique of *Sensation testing* to evaluate light touch and deep pressure.
- Uses 20 nylon monofilaments with a constant length, but increasing diameter.
- They are applied perpendicular and the patient responds when feeling sensation.
- The figures range from 1.56 to 6.65 with 2.44–2.83 being normal for a finger.

Senile keratosis

See *Actinic keratosis*.

Sensation testing

- *Four main types of testing:* threshold, functional, objective and sudomotor:
  - ○ *Threshold:* temperature, pressure, touch, vibration, sharp stimulus.
  - ○ *Functional:* 2PD, stereognosis.
  - ○ *Objective:* object manipulation.
- *Light touch and pressure:* <u>Semmes-Weinstein</u> monofilament testing. <u>2PD</u> is a reliable way to test the quality of sensibility in the fingers.
- *Pain:* with a pin prick.
- *Vibration:* tuning forks of varying cycles.
- *Temperature:* tested with temperature specific probes.
- *Moberg pick-up test*

Classification: *Highet's*.

Sensory receptors

- 3 types in the hands, thermoreceptors, mechanoreceptors and nociceptors.
- They are either encapsulated or present as free nerve endings.
- Free nerve endings are either myelinated or non-myelinated and lie between epidermal cells. Free endings are usually nociceptors or thermoreceptors.

Mechanoreceptors:

- Rapidly and slowly adapting fibres.
- Rapidly adapting are myelinated A fibres. They include *Pacinian* and *Meissner* corpuscles, which mediate moving, touch and vibration.
- *Slowly adapting:* <u>Merkel cell.</u>
- Corpuscles of Ruffini and Krause are poorly understood mechanoreceptors found in the deep dermis. Ruffini are slowly adapting and Krause rapidly adapting mechanoreceptors.

Sentinel lymph node biopsy

- First described in 1991 by Wong.
- The sentinel lymph node is that which first receives the lymphatic drainage from the involved area. It is therefore the first to receive tumour cells. If this node is tumour-free then the others in the chain will also be. So sentinel node biopsy will spare patients

with tumour negative nodes the morbidity of lymphadenectomy. The sentinel node can be examined more extensively.

- SLNB is a staging procedure in _Head and neck_ cancer and in _Melanoma_.
- The node is identified using vital blue dye and also a radioactive tracer. A scan pre-operatively can help to identify where the sentinel node is.
- Routine histology identifies 1 positive cell in 10 000. Serial sectioning and staining increases this to 100 000.
- There is presently little evidence that sentinel node biopsy improves prognosis.

Serratus anterior

Origin: Outer surface of upper 8–9 ribs.

Insertion: Costal surface of vertebral border of scapula.

Nerve supply: Long thoracic nerve.

Vascular supply: Lateral thoracic artery.

Action: Abducts scapula at the scapulothoracic joint, raises ribs when scapula is fixed.

As a free flap: To avoid winging of the scapula use the middle and lower 4–5 digitations of the muscle.

Sex differentiation defects
- _Klinefelter's syndrome_.
- _Turner syndrome_.
- _Hermaphrodites_.
See _Ambiguous genitalia_, _Embryology_.

SGAP and IGAP
Superior and Inferior Gluteal Artery Perforator Flap
- Used in _Breast reconstruction_.
- The vessels tend to be short and the internal thoracic vessels are used as recipient vessels.

Shoulder-hand syndrome
- A subtype of _RSD_ involving the upper limb.
- Usually caused by a proximal trauma or painful visceral lesion with manifestation in the shoulder and eventually involving the whole of the upper extremity.
- Examples include neck injury, stroke and Pancoast's tumour, but any distal RSD in the

hand may progress to the shoulder with limited shoulder movement.

Shprintzen's syndrome
See _Velocardiofacial syndrome_.

Sick cell syndrome
Carbon monoxide binds to cytochromes, as well as haemoglobin. Cytochrome-bound CO is washed out after 24 hours causing a secondary rise in serum COHb and possibly post-intoxication encephalopathy.

Sickle cell disease
- Caused by substitution of glutamic acid by valine on the haemoglobin β chain.
- Inherited as an autosomal gene. Heterozygotes have both normal and abnormal haemoglobin.
- Sickle cell trait gives a relative resistance against malaria.
- Most common in West Africa, central India and also in Mediterranean populations.
- Distorted red blood cells increase blood viscosity with capillary and venous thrombosis, and organ infarction.
- Races at risk should be screened by electrophoresis.
- For surgery, patient should be well hydrated. Keep well oxygenated with O_2 concentrations of 40–50%. Keep warm. Tourniquets should be avoided if possible but can be safe if other factors optimal.

Sickle flap
See _Hatchet flap_.

Silicone
- Silicon is an element. Silica is silicone oxide. Silicone is interlinked silicon and oxygen with methyl, vinyl or phenol side groups. Polydimethylsiloxane (PDMS) has a repeating chain of -Si-O- units with methyl groups attached to the silicone atoms.
- Consistency can be changed by varying the length and cross-linking of the PDMS chains. Fluids are short straight chains, gels are lightly cross-linked and elastomers are longer chains with cross-links.
- Silicone is highly biocompatible, non-toxic, non-allogenic and non-biodegradable.

- Get a mild foreign body reaction. Capsular contracture is the most common complication. Get synovitis in joint arthroplasty.
- *Disadvantage as implant:* rubbers tear or fail when stressed (Swanson finger joints). Gel foam is difficult to remove following rupture. Bone resorption can occur. Smooth implants are more prone to extrusion. Rubbers are permeable so proteins and lipids may be absorbed altering the physical property.
- *Uses:* in plastic surgery silicone is used for breast reconstruction, facial reconstruction, orbital floor, tissue expanders, penile devices and finger joint replacements.

See *Alloplasts*.

Silicone controversy

- *1962:* first implant inserted.
- *1982:* Van Nunen linked implants to connective tissue disease (CTD).
- *1992:* cosmetic implants were banned in USA, France and Spain.
- *1994:* a class action settlement of $4.25 billion for any of 10 CTD developed within 30 years.

Findings of UK independent review group: Controversy over whether implants cause some autoimmune diseases or an increased risk of cancer. In 1998 the report concluded that:

- They are not associated with greater risk than other implants.
- No evidence of abnormal immune response.
- No association with connective tissue diseases.
- Local complications occur.
- National registry advised.

Findings of IMNAS in USA: Institute of Medicine of the National Academy of Science reported in 1999 that

- No evidence that silicone implants are responsible for any major diseases.
- No evidence that recurrent breast cancer is more prevalent with implants.
- Silicone augmentation is not a contraindication to breast feeding and milk formulas have a higher level of silica than breast milk with implants.

See *Breast implants*. See *Breast augmentation*.

Silver nitrate

- Used in *Burns* dressings.
- 0.5% concentration.
- It is broad spectrum and resistance to the silver ion is rare. There is minimal absorption so toxicity is rare.
- It is very hypotonic so its use can lead to loss of Na, K from the burn wound.
- Some organisms can reduce nitrate to nitrite and this can rarely lead to methaemoglobinuria.
- It stains everything brown or black, and this is the principle reason it is not used routinely.

Silver sulphadiazine

- Used in *Burns* dressings.
- This is the most frequently used topical agent.
- It has a water-soluble base at a concentration of 1%.
- This will inhibit the growth of most sensitive organisms.
- It is applied every 12–24 hours and is active against Gram –ve and +ve organisms, *Candida* and herpes. It is not painful and is non-staining. It makes burn depth more difficult to assess.
- Toxicity is rare though leucopenia often occurs after 2–3 days of treatment.
- Clinical trials suggest that silver sulphadiazine reduces bacterial density and delays colonization with Gram –ve bacteria.

Simian crease

Seen in 1% of the normal population. 50% of Down's syndrome and trisomy 21 have a simian crease. They also have brachymesophalangia and syndactyly.

Simon's classification

Grading for *Gynaecomastia*.

- *1:* small enlargement no skin redundancy.
- *2A:* moderate enlargement no skin redundancy.
- *2B:* moderate enlargement, skin redundancy.
- *3:* marked enlargement, marked skin redundancy.

Simonart's band

- A *Cleft lip* is often bridged by a band of lip tissue – the Simonart's band.

- This may be partial formation, healing or the remains after the fusion has separated.
- If the band occupies less than $1/3$ of the vertical height, the deformity is classified as a complete cleft lip. If more than $1/3$ it is an incomplete cleft lip.
- It is unclear who Simonart was.

Sjögren's syndrome

Triad of dry eyes (keratoconjunctivitis sicca), dry mouth (xerostomia) and *Rheumatoid arthritis*.

Skew flap below knee amputation

- A technique of below knee amputation with well-vascularized flaps and a well-contoured stump.
- Stump length should be 10–15 cm below tibial plateau. Too short gives insufficient lever, too long requires a wide unsightly prosthesis. Skin blood flow at this level is predominantly from saphenous and sural nerve artery.
- Mark level of amputation and measure circumference with tape. Mark point 2.5 cm lateral to tibial crest and mark half circumference from this. Divide tape into quarters to mark midline of each flap and also the inferior point.
- A 2-cm proximal extension anteriorly allows access for bone section.
- Elevate flaps with fascia. Divide saphenous and sural nerves. Preserve arteries as long as possible.
- Divide anterior compartment muscles transversely. Divide interosseous membrane. Raise periosteum. Divide fibula high. Divide tibia in curved fashion. Hold lower leg to expose tibialis posterior which is cut transversely to reveal posterior and peroneal NVBs.
- Separate gastrocnemius/soleus from tibia. Divide vessels and divide gastrocnemius/soleus 15 cm distal to bone section. Ligate vessels and divide nerves under tension. Thin muscle tapering to aponeurosis. Remove muscle medially and laterally. Under-run soleal sinuses.
- Suction drain. Smooth bone ends. Secure posterior muscle flap to anterior tibial fascia

with continuous suture. Suture skin under no tension.

Skier's thumb

See *Ulnar collateral ligament*.

Skin

Anatomy:
Epidermis:

- Stratified squamous epithelium 0.05–1.5 mm thick. Goal of skin is to maintain the waterproof *stratum corneum*. Cells migrate from the basal layer to the environment in 40 days.
- Comprised of basal cells, keratinocytes, melanocytes, *Merkel cells* and Langerhan's cells.
- *Stratum germinativum:* comprised of *Basal cells* are the innermost layer. Columnar. BCCs arise from basal cells. These divide to form *keratinocytes*, which provide a barrier. These are attached by *desmosomes*. They are attached to basal lamina. They make keratin and cytokines. Also contains melanocytes.
- *Stratum spinosum:* 5–12 cells thick. Also called prickle layer. They are joined to each other by tonofibrils (prickles). SCC arise from these cells. They are polygonal and they flatten to become stratum granulosum.
- *Stratum granulosum:* with granules of keratohyalin in them. These dehydrate and flatten further to form stratum lucidum.
- *Stratum lucidum:* only present in the thick skin of palms and feet.
- *Stratum corneum:* keratinocytes die leaving keratin as a barrier. As the cells move through stratum corneum they become disorganized.

Dermis:

- Represents 90% of skin thickness. Provides a collagen matrix, holds dermal appendages and provides nutrients. The boundary is undulating. Basal cells are attached to basal lamina which attaches to dermis – this is the basement membrane. Acts as a barrier.
- *Papillary dermis* is superficial and contains more cells and finer collagen.
- *Reticular dermis* is deeper and contains fewer cells and courser collagen.

Extracellular matrix:
- <u>*Collagen*</u>: thin outer layer of dermis is called the papillary layer. Collagen is randomly arranged and thin. Under this is the reticular layer with elastic fibres and thick aligned collagen. Type 1:3 ratio 5:1
- *Elastin:* also produced by fibroblasts. They can reversibly stretch to twice the resting length.
- *Ground substance:* fills the remaining dermal space. Provide aqueous environment for cell migration. Mucopolysaccharide can hold 1000 times its own volume of water. Produced by fibroblasts. Consists of glycosaminoglycans (GAGs), hyaluronic acid, dermatan sulphate and chondroitin sulphate.
- *Histiocytes and mast cells:* also in the dermis. Histiocytes are mobile macrophages, mast cells release histamine and heparin.

Sensory nerves: Tactile sensation is detected by Meissner's (palm and sole only) and pressure by Pacinian corpuscles (mainly in palms and soles). Pain, itch and temperature is detected by unmyelinated nerve endings.

<u>*Hair follicles:*</u> Develop from epithelial germ cells. Type of melanin gives hair its colour. Arrector pili smooth muscle is attached at the base of the hair. Innervated by adrenergic sympathetic supply. Action is to raise the hair and secrete sebum.

<u>*Sweat*</u> *and sebaceous glands:*
- *Apocrine* sweat glands are stimulated by adrenergic sympathetic fibres. Found in axillae and anogenital region and become active after puberty. The odour is from bacterial decomposition. The glands open into a pilosebaceous follicle.
- *Eccrine* sweat glands are supplied by cholinergic sympathetic fibres. Found in palms, soles, axillae, forehead mainly, but over most of the skin. Control body temperature. Sebaceous glands are appendages of hair follicles. They are under endocrine control. Found everywhere except palms and soles. They produce sebum, a mixture of fatty acids. Also lubricate hair.

Blood vessels: Adrenergic sympathetic fibres innervate blood vessels. Flow is also mediated by histamine. Get plexus at dermal-subcutaneous junction and at papillary dermis. Glomus bodies are AV shunts which can greatly increase blood flow and control body temperature.

Function: Protect from trauma. Resident bacteria is reduced by sebum. It is flexible, elastic and tough. It regulates fluid and temperature. Normal daily loss of 500–800 ml.

Physical properties: Collagen is convoluted, allowing stretching up to a certain point, after which there is sudden resistance. Return is by elastin fibres. If a load is prolonged, get irreversible extension. This viscoelasticity gives rise to <u>*Creep*</u>. During creep get a change in collagen fibre bonding. May be due to displacement of water from the ground substance.

Clinical implications:
- Resting tension is high over shoulders and sternum and may partly explain hypertrophy.
- *Wrinkles:* due to repetitive mechanical forces and reduced mass of collagen, and changing elastin. Muscle contraction and gravity pull collagen, which remodels.
- *Chronic ageing skin:* fibroblasts have reduced function, collagen cross-links increase. Skin is stiffer and thinner. Collagen is less convoluted. Dermis and epidermis thins. Ground substance which is responsible for skin turgidity is reduced.
- *Photo-ageing skin:* divided into 6 types. *See* <u>*Ultraviolet radiation*</u>. Most DNA damage is repaired except in <u>*Xeroderma pigmentosa*</u>. Long-term changes are irreversible. In epidermis get thickened heterogenous basal layer. In the dermis get tangled masses of elastin and collagen. Get reduced total collagen.
- *Racial differences:* Black skin has more layers of stratum corneum though it is the same thickness. Get 2.5 times increase in desquamation. Blacks have a greater water loss. Black skin is 4 times more photoprotective. Numbers of melanosomes per unit area is the same, but in black skin they are more dispersed.

<u>*Langer's lines.*</u>
<u>*Healing.*</u>

Histological terms: <u>*Acanthosis*</u>, <u>*Papillomatosis*</u>, <u>*Hyperkeratosis*</u>, parakeratosis.

Blister formation: Pathological extracellular fluid in the skin. They can be intraepidermal or dermal-epidermal and further subdivided.

Skin creases: hand

- In the finger: at the DIP joint there is one crease just proximal to the DIPJ. There are 2 creases at the PIP joint and another at the distal palmar digital junction mid-proximal phalanx. The crease ends at mid-axial level. There is no fat at the level of crease and minor injury can easily penetrate the tendon sheath.
- The distal and proximal palmar creases run obliquely over the palm. A1 pulley lies under them.
- The crease at the base of the thenar eminence merges with the proximal palmar crease. The radial digital nerve to index follows this line.
- The second longitudinal crease runs from the base of the long finger to the radial edge of the hypothenar eminence.

Skin grafts

History:

- First described in Hindu texts 2500 years ago.
- Astley Cooper performed a skin graft in 1817, taking the skin of an amputated thumb to cover the stump.
- Reverdin, 1869 used pinch grafts to improve healing.
- Ollier, 1872 used skin grafts to treat ectropion.
- Wolfe used grafts for a fresh surgical wound.
- Blair and Barrett Brown, 1929 used split skin grafts.

Type:

- *Split-thickness skin grafts (SSG):* consist of epidermis and a portion of dermis, average thickness 0.3–0.4 mm. A method for harvesting them was developed by Thiersch in 1886.
- *Full-thickness grafts (FTSG):* include the entire thickness of skin, epidermis and dermis.

Properties:

- *SSG:* take well, but shrink, thinner, more fragile and abnormal pigmentation.

- *FTSG:* thicker and more robust, but require well-vascularized bed and limited by size.

Healing: Initially white, then pink after a few days with capillary refill. By 2–3 weeks the graft surface thickens. Collagen replacement is complete by 6th week. Remodelling takes many months. Lymphatics are established by 5–6th day.

Graft take: 4 phases.

- *Adherence:* fibrin bonds form immediately. There are two phases of graft adherence. The first begins with placement of the graft on the recipient bed, to which the graft adheres because of fibrin deposition. This lasts approximately 72 hours. The second phase involves ingrowth of fibrous tissue and vessels into the graft.
- *Plasmatic imbibition:* during the first 48 hours allows the graft to survive. Diffusion of exudates allows access to nutrition and disposal of waste.
- *Revascularization:* by inosculation occurs next with anastomotic connections between graft and host.
- *Capillary ingrowth:* occurs at the same time with new vessels. Four theories have been proposed for graft revascularization:
  ○ neovascularization of the graft in which new vessels from the recipient bed invade the graft to form the definitive vascular structure of the graft;
  ○ communication occurs between existing graft vessels and those in the recipient site;
  ○ there is a combination of ingrowth of new vessels and re-establishment of flow into existing vessels;
  ○ the vasculature of the skin graft is made up, primarily, from its original vessels before transfer.
- *Remodelling:* architecture returns to normal.

Graft failure: Due to haematoma, infection, seroma, shear and bed vascularity.

Pigmentation: Varies with graft site. Grafts from thighs tend to darken and palms lighten with time. SSGs tend to become darker than FTSGs from the same site. Sunshine may affect pigmentation and should be avoided for

6 months. Pigmentation may be treated with dermabrasion.

Donor sites: The epidermis regenerates from adnexal structures, but dermis never regenerates. Therefore, donor sites can be recropped, but how many times is dependent on the thickness of the dermis and the thickness of the SSG.

Skin tag
See *Acrochordon*.

Skull base surgery
Tumours:
- *Malignant extracranial*, such as squamous cell carcinoma, adenoid cystic carcinoma.
- *Malignant intracranial*, such as malignant Schwannoma.
- *Malignant primary basicranial*, such as chondrosarcoma and osteogenic sarcoma.
- *Benign extracranial*, e.g. pleomorphic adenoma.
- *Benign intracranial*, e.g. primary adenoma.
- *Benign primary basicranial*, e.g. fibrous dysplasia.

Clinical findings: Symptoms may be vague. Benign tumours present with signs of compression. Malignant tumours present with headaches, fits and cranial nerve paralysis.

Imaging:
- *CT scan with contrast* provide information of bone involvement.
- *MRI with T1- and T2-weighted images* for soft tissue information.
- *Angiography and naso-endoscopy.*

Surgical exposures:
- The transfacial approach allows safe access to a difficult area. Facial units are separated. Wide exposure is actually safer with clearer visualization of tumour and vital structures. 6 levels. The first 3 are intracranial and the latter 3 extracranial providing exposure to the midline skull base.
- *Level I Transfrontal approach:* to access tumours of the anterior cranial fossa. Performed through bicoronal scalp incisions. A bicoronal craniotomy is performed. A supra-orbital bar is removed.

- *Level II Transfrontal nasal approach*: to access anterior cranial fossa and tumours growing anteriorly. A bicoronal incision is performed and the supra-orbital bar including the nasal complex is removed.
- *Level III Transfrontal naso-orbital approach:* the approach is the same as level II but includes the lateral orbital wall, so that the superior orbital roof can be included to enable lateral globe retraction.
- *Level IV Transnasomaxillary approach:* for wide exposure of midline skull base. Through Weber–Ferguson incision. Le Fort II osteotomy performed.
- *Level V Transmaxillary approach:* for small clival lesions. through an intra-oral approach, a Le Fort I osteotomy is performed.
- *Level VI transpalatal approach:* for lower clival and upper cervical. The palate is incised, mucoperiosteal flaps are raised and an osteotomy is performed in the hard palate.

SLAC
Scapholunate advanced collapse. The most common form of wrist OA. Also SNAC – scaphoid non-union with collapse.

Pathology:
- Rotary subluxation of the scaphoid following either acute rupture or chronic attenuation of the scapholunate ligament. The scaphoid palmar flexes with decreased surface area, but increase in joint contact forces between radius and scaphoid. Get carpal collapse with destruction of the capitolunate and lunohamate joints. In SLAC the radiolunate joint is preserved.
- Four stages:
  - *I:* stylocarpal arthritis.
  - *II:* scaphoid fossa involvement.
  - *III:* capitolunate arthrosis.
  - *IV:* diffuse wrist arthritis.

Surgery:
- Depends on the state of the proximal capitate and radiolunate articular surfaces. Two most common procedures are:
  - *scaphoidectomy* with 4-corner arthrodesis (capitate-lunate-hamate-triquetrum);

○ *proximal row carpectomy (PRC):* If the lunate fossa and proximal capitate are well preserved, PRC is better than arthrodesis.
* *Arthrodesis:* perform wrist if both articular surfaces are damaged.

SMAS

Superficial Musculo-Aponeurotic System.
* Layer of facial fascia. Contiguous with frontalis muscle, galea, temporoparietal fascia (superficial temporal fascia), platysma. It is tightly adherent to the zygomatic arch.
* In the parotid-masseteric area it is thick and attached to the parotid sheath. It becomes thin in the cheek region. The SMAS invests and extends into the external part of the superficial facial muscles, involving fibres of risorius, frontalis, platysma and peripheral part of orbicularis oculi.
* In the mandibular area the SMAS is in close contact with the superficial plane of platysma. The mandibular branch runs deep to platysma.
* Over the mastoid, SMAS is attached to dermis and fibrous tissue around the insertion of the sternoclavicular muscles.
* *Nasolabial fold:* SMAS is deep and thin here. Here it ends as a distinct layer.
* Sensory nerves are superficial and motor branches are deep to SMAS. The facial artery and vein lie deep to SMAS. Their perforating branches go through it.
* SMAS acts as a distributor of facial muscle contractions to the skin through its attachments to the dermis.
See Face lift.

Smoking

* Get a thrombogenic state due to effects on dermal microvasculature and blood constituents.
* Nicotine increases vasoconstricting prostaglandins such as thromboxane A2. Carbon monoxide leads to tissue hypoxia and increased platelet adhesiveness.
* Smoking adversely affects procedures with extensive undermining, such as facelifts. There has been no proven adverse affect in free tissue transfer.
* Smoking one cigarette leads to a 42% reduction in blood flow velocity to the hand, which may adversely affect replants.

Snap test

For assessment of lower Eyelid. Pull the lower eyelid downward and assess how long it takes to return to the normal position. A return of less than 1 second is normal.

Snodgras repair

* Operative technique for the correction of distal shaft and mid-shaft Hypospadias.
* Use when urethral groove is wide and deep. Tubularize urethral plate *in situ.*
* To address the problem of inadequate width the plate is incised in the midline so the plate can be hinged. A subcutaneous flap of preputce covers the urethroplasty. Glans wings close over the urethroplasty in the midline.

Snuffbox: anatomic

Hollow on radial side of wrist. Contents of first dorsal compartment border the palmar side, EPL is dorsal, radial styloid proximal, and the base of thumb metacarpal distal. The radial artery traverses snuff box. Scaphoid in floor of snuffbox.

Snuffbox: ulnar

Depression immediately beyond ulnar styloid. Bordered by ECU and FCU tendons. Floor formed by triquestrum in radial deviation, and joint of triquestrum and hamate in ulnar deviation.

Sodium bicarbonate

* Sometimes added to local anaesthetics.
* Local anaesthetics are in a balanced solution between ionized and non-ionized forms. The non-ionized form goes into the nerve more rapidly.
* Alkalization of the solution changes the concentration of the non-ionized form and increases the rapidity of onset.
* Dose to give are 1 mEq/10 ml lignocaine and 0.1 mEq/20 ml bupivicaine.

Soft tissue tumours: upper limb

Most are benign. Foreign body granulomas and inclusion cysts are frequent. Most common benign lesion is a lipoma.

Location: often most useful sign. Ganglia – dorsal or volar wrist. Mucous cyst DIPJ,

Retinacular cyst over volar aspect of finger at MPJ. Palmar fibromas are found in the palm.
Epidermoid inclusion cyst.
Fibroma.
Ganglion.
Giant cell tumour.
Granular cell tumour.
Mason's haemangioma.
Vascular leiomyoma.
Sarcoma.

Solar keratosis
See Actinic keratosis.

Sonic hedgehog
Implicated in limb development in the AP plane. Sonic hedgehog (*Shh*) is a segment polarity gene. It is expressed in the posterior mesenchyme of limb buds. It patterns the AP limb axis. It may maintain the progress zone of the AER while acting as a positional signal along the AP axis.
See Embryology.

Speech
- Need normal resonance, effort and consistency for intelligible speech. Some patient's speech deteriorates when tired. For proper speech the palate needs to be opened and closed in quick succession, e.g. in 'small'.
- Velopharyngeal closure is required for all consonants except m,n,ng. The others are in two groups, the plosives (b,p,t) and the continuants or fricatives (s,sh,z). Divide also into whether the vocal cord is used – voiced (b) or unvoiced (p). Unvoiced fricatives are sibilants.
- *Velopharyngeal insufficiency* (VPI) gives hypernasal speech. Obstruction gives hyponasal speech.
- Nasal escape is a sniffing or snorting sound heard during a sound that should be directed through the mouth.
See Cleft palate.

Speech restoration
See Voice restoration.

Spilled tea-cup sign
- Seen in volar lunate dislocation.

- Lunate displaced out of the fossa and into the carpal tunnel region.

Spina bifida
Failure of fusion of the neural groove.

Incidence: Commonest CNS defect. 1:200–1000. Related to folate deficiency. If a child is affected the risk is 5% if two then 10%. Inheritance is multifactorial.

Classification: 4 types:
- *Meningocoele:* meninges in herniation with no neurological defect.
- *Meningomyelocoele:* most common. Meninges and neural elements with neurological deficits.
- *Syringomyelocoele:* rare. Similar to meningomyelocoele, but with dilatation of the central canal of the cord.
- *Myelocoele:* rare. Exposed neural elements with no covering.

Clinical presentation:
- Spina bifida occulta presents with anomaly over the skin, such as a dimple, hair tuft, naevus or lipoma. XR shows a defect in the spinous processes and vertebra. A tethered cord may cause progressive neurological defect with growth.
- *Meningocoele:* usually lumbosacral bulge with poor or ulcerated skin. Bulge increases with crying.

Natural history: 90% survive, 25% have learning difficulties mostly due to infections, 85% walk with aids, 80% can become continent.

Treatment:
- Aim to close with 24–72 hours if cord exposed.
- 75% will close with wide relaxing incisions. Otherwise use bipedicled flaps, rhomboid flaps, latissimus dorsi or gluteus maximus. V–Y flaps based on paravertebral perforators.
See Trunk reconstruction.

Spitz naevus
- Also spindle cell nevus or benign juvenile melanoma.
- Mainly in children.
- Were thought to be melanoma, but is a compound naevus variant.

- Colour ranges from pink to purplish-red and a few are pigmented. Surface may be warty. Elevated firm nodules up to 2 cm in size. Vascular and may bleed.
- Often-rapid initial growth over 3–6 months.
- Close histopathological resemblance to melanoma.
- Occur before puberty and may be present at birth.
- Most frequently found on the face.
- The incidence of melanoma transformation is no different than any other compound *Naevus*.
- Excise with narrow margins. If not excised completely they may recur.

Sporothrix schenkii

Occurs in nurserymen. Infection with subcutaneous erythematous nodules with centripetal pattern along the course of lymphatic drainage. Isolate on Sabouraud agar at 30°. *See Infection*.

Spurling's test

- Clinical test for cervical disc involvement. Tends to affect upper plexus.
- Seat patient, extend neck and apply pressure to vertex of scalp down cervical spine then flex head to affected side to narrow intervertebral foramen. Flex away from affected side to open up foramen, but applying traction to the brachial plexus indicating brachial plexopathy.

See Thoracic outlet syndrome.

Squamous cell carcinoma

Incidence:
- 25% of that of BCCs.
- Related to sun exposure, radiation, chemicals, chronic ulcers.

Sites: Occur in areas of abnormal skin with sun damage, keratin horns, leucoplakia, chronic scar, *Solar keratosis*, *Bowen's disease*, *Pseudoepitheliomatous hyperplasia*.

Histology:
- SCCs arise from the keratinizing or malpighian (spindle) cell layer (stratum spinosum) of the epithelium. Dysplastic epidermal keratinocytes extend through the basement membrane into the dermis. The presence of keratin pearls is characteristic.
- They may be well, moderate or poorly differentiated.
- Bad prognostic indicators are increased depth of invasion, vascular invasion, perineural invasion and lymphocytic infiltration.
- Initially smooth, verrucous or ulcerative then becomes inflamed and ulcerated. Verrucous may be deeply locally invasive, but less likely to metastasize, whereas nodular have rapid growth and early ulceration. They are locally invasive and more likely to metastasize.
- SCCs >4 mm thick gives 35% metastatic rate.

Recurrence:
- Associated with degree of differentiation. 7% recurrence for well-differentiated, 28% for poorly differentiated.
- Overall risk of metastases at the time of presentation is 2–3% Higher tendency with *Marjolin's ulcer* and *Xeroderma pigmentosa*.

Treatment:
- Local excision. 0.5–1 cm excision margin recommended.

See Basal cell carcinoma.

Stahl classification

For XR changes in *Kienbock's Disease*.
- *I:* compression fracture.
- *II:* sclerosis.
- *III:* sclerosis and mild collapse, IIIa without fixed scaphoid rotation, IIIb with fixed scaphoid rotation.
- *IV:* sclerosis, collapse, fragmentation.
- *V:* sclerosis, DJD changes.

Stahl's ear

Congenital anomaly of the ear, which has a third crus.

Stainless steel

- A large group of iron–chromium–nickel alloys.
- They have a high degree of corrosion and implant failure.
- Galvanic current occurring between the screws and plates can result in corrosion.

Vitallium and titanium corrode less due to protective oxide layer on their surface.
See *Alloplasts*.

Steatoblepharon

Peri-orbital fat which is either excessive or protruding through a lax septum.
See *Blepharoplasty*.

Steele's classification

For base of phalanges intra-articular fractures.
- *Type 1:* non-displaced marginal fracture.
- *Type 2:* comminuted impaction fracture.
- *Type 3:* displaced intra-articular fracture.

Stelling classification

Classification of *Polydactyly*.
- *Type 1:* extra digit attached by skin bridge only.
- *Type 2:* extra digit articulating with metacarpal or phalanx.
- *Type 3:* extra digit articulating with extra metacarpal.

Stener lesion

Ulnar collateral ligament attaches deep to adductor aponeurosis. With complete disruption the adductor is interposed between UCL and proximal phalanx giving a Stener lesion.

Stensen's duct

Excretory duct of the parotid gland. 7 cm long, runs over the masseter muscle and buccal fat pad then bends medially to pierce buccinator muscle ending intra-orally at the level of the second maxillary molar.
See *Parotic duct*.

Stepladder technique

- Used in *Lip reconstruction*.
- Use for defects up to ²/₃s of the lower lip. It retains relatively good sensation and muscle continuity.
- The horizontal component measures one half the width of the defect, so 2–4 steps required. The vertical dimension of each step is 8–10 mm.

Sternal cleft

- Rare and often dramatic presentation of central chest defect.

- Fusion from mesodermal plates occurs from above, so defects usually involve the lower or entire sternum.
- Deformities range from sternal clefts only, *Ectopia cordis* and Cantrell's pentalogy with multiple deformities of chest, heart, diaphragm and abdomen.
- Most sternal defects can be reapproximated and secured with wires.
See *Chest wall reconstruction*.

Sternocleidomastoid

Origin: Sternum and medial half of clavicle.

Insertion: Lateral surface of mastoid process.

Blood supply:
- *Superior:* branches of occipital artery.
- *Middle:* branches of the superior thyroid artery.
- *Inferiorly:* branches of the thyrocervical trunk.

Innervation: Spinal accessory nerve.

Sternocleidomastoid flap

- Can be raised on inferior or superior pedicle.
- The skin island is outlined over the inframastoid area. The skin paddle is not very reliable. The 11th cranial nerve is usually sacrificed.
- It can be used in a functional neck dissection for intra-oral reconstruction proximally based on superior thyroid and occipital vessels.
See *Oral cavity reconstruction*.

Sternotomy wounds

- 0.4–5% of median sternotomies get infected with a mortality of 5–10%.
- Related to internal mammary artery (IMA) use – Cosgrove reported no infection with saphenous vein, 0.3% with unilateral IMA and 2.4% with bilateral. Other associated factors are diabetes, smoking, hypertension.

Classification: by Pairolero.
- *Type 1:* infection in first 3 days. Serosanguinous with negative culture. Need minimal debridement and rewiring.
- *Type 2:* first 2–3 weeks. Purulent mediastinitis.

- *Type 3:* present months to years after with sinus tracts from chronic osteomyelitis. Require debridement and reconstruction.
- Can also be classified by anatomical site which can help in deciding the reconstruction into type A – upper half requiring pec major reconstruction and Type B (lower half) and type C (whole sternum) requiring a combined pec major and rectus abdominus bipedicled flap.

Reconstruction:
- Single stage debridement with muscle flap successful in 95% of cases.
- *Pectoralis major:* harvest through sternotomy wound. Detach muscle from ribs and sternum. Find pedicle and divide humeral attachment. Dissect from clavicle and advance medially. Bilateral flaps can be used for large defects. If the IMA is intact a turnover flap can be used. Ligate thoracoacromial pedicle and elevate from lateral to medial, preserving medial 2–3 cm of muscle.
- *Rectus abdominus:* use with pectoralis or if pectoralis not available. Based on the deep superior epigastric artery, a terminal branch of the IMA. Type III muscle (dual dominant supply). Midline incision, incise anterior rectus sheath, divide muscle inferiorly, separate from posterior sheath and transpose. It can be used if the IMA has been harvested based on the 8th intercostal vessel, but vascularity is more tenuous.
- Combined pec major and rectus abdominus bipedicled flap. Blood supply from the thoracoacromial artery superiorly and the deep inferior epigastric artery inferiorly. First a skin flap is raised then the plane deep to pec major is developed. Rectus abdominus is elevated from the posterior rectus sheath. Lateral rectus and pec major are divided.
- *Omentum:* used alone or with other flaps.
- Latissimus dorsi and external oblique (based on intercostals perforators) are used as back-up flaps.

See *Chest wall reconstruction.*

Stereognosis
The ability to recognize objects based on touch.
See *Moberg pick-up test.*

Steroid

Hypertrophic scar: Blunt the inflammatory response by stabilization of lysosomal membranes thus preventing the secretion of enzymes and cytokines. This leads to impaired capillary budding, inhibition of fibroblast proliferation, decreased protein synthesis and diminished epithelialization. Vitamin A counteracts the effects of steroids. Response rate of 30–100% with intralesional steroids but side-effects include atrophy, depigmentation, and telangiectasia

Haemangiomas:
- *Action:* augments the sensitivity of the terminal vascular bed to catecholamines and inhibit fibroplasia.
- Dose is 2–3 mg/kg/day of prednisolone given systemically or orally over a 2–3-week period.
- Haemangiomas will respond within 7–10 days. After getting a response, lower the dose to 0.75 mg/kg/day. If they respond slowly, treat with a 4–6 week course then rest for 3–4 weeks, then another course. May see a rebound phenomena. If so, treat with 2–3-week cycles with reducing doses. $^1/_3$ respond quickly, $^1/_3$ equivocal, $^1/_3$ no response.
- Triamcinolone at a dose of 3–5 mg/kg can be used intralesionally. Usually require 3–5 injections at 6–8-week intervals.

See *Wound healing.*

Stewart–Treves syndrome
See *Lymphangiosarcoma.*

Striae
Caused by disruption of dermis with loss of continuity of elastic fibres.

Stickler syndrome
- One of the most commonly reported syndromes resulting in cleft palate.
- Get myopia, retinal detachment, clefts and arthropathy.
- At least one form is due to a defect of collagen type II gene.
- It is autosomal dominant.
- Patients should be screened for vision.

See *Craniofacial genetics.*

Stork bite
See Nevus flammeus neonatorum.

Stranc and Robertson

***Classification** of Nasal fractures:* 3 groups.
- *Plane 1:* disruption of the cartilagenous septum. The nasal bones are unaffected.
- *Plane 2:* disruption of the bony septum and nasal bones.
- *Plane 3:* these injuries extend beyond the nasal skeleton into the piriform aperture and medial orbital rim. They represent mild naso-ethmoidal fractures.

Strawberry naevus
See Haemangioma.

Streptokinase
- It is the least expensive fibrinolytic agent, but highly antigenic with a high incidence of untoward reactions. It is produced by beta-haemolytic streptococci.
- It binds with free-circulating plasminogen or plasmin, which forms a complex that can convert additional plasminogen to plasmin. The active half life is about 20 minutes. It can cause febrile reactions.
- It cannot be used safely a second time within 6 months.
- It is useful for breaking up clots in failing free tissue transfers.
- Use 5000 units/ml and infuse 25–50 000 units, which will be effective locally, but not problematic systemically.

Struthers: ligament of
- One of four sites of potential compression of the *Median nerve* in the forearm along with lacertus fibrosis, pronator teres and arch of FDS.
- The ligament may originate from a supracondylar process.
- It forms an accessory origin for pronator teres.

Sturge–Weber
- *Port-wine stain* with congenital glaucoma or ipsilateral leptomeningeal angiomatosis.

- Occurs in the distribution of the trigeminal nerve V1, V2 and V3 involvement (not V2 alone).
- There is a low risk of brain involvement.
- It can be associated with seizures, contralateral hemiplegia, and variable developmental delay of motor and cognitive skills.

Succinylcholine in burns
- Succinylcholine is an acetylcholine agonist, which may cause a massive sometimes fatal release of potassium in burn patients.
- It has been documented as long as 18 months after a burn so its use is not recommended up to 2 years after a burn.
- Burn victims have an increased number of muscle receptor sites for acetylcholine.
- Non-depolarizing relaxants such as D-tubocurarine, pancuronium Atracurium and Vencuronium are recommended, although burn patients have variable resistance with these.

Sudeck's osteoporosis
Seen in association with reflex sympathetic dystrophy (RSD). Diagnosed because of the apparent skeletal involvement. It frequently responds to intramuscular calcitonin treatment. Apart from the radiographic pattern it is indistinguishable from other forms of RSD. The demineralization is similar to disuse, but more rapid than can be explained by disuse.

Sulphuric acid
- A strong acid and oxidizing agent.
- It is used in car batteries and electroplating.
- Strong thermal reaction occurs on contact with water.
- The skin is leathery and becomes red-brown, then grey. No systemic toxicity occurs. Upper and lower airway injury may occur.
See Chemical injuries.

Sunderland classification of nerve injury
Classification of *Nerve injury*
- *I:* conduction block – neuropraxia, recovery <4/12.
- *II:* axonal damage – axontmesis, recovery 4–18/12.
- *III:* endoneurial damage – recovery mixed.

- *IV:* epineurium intact – neuroma in continuity recovery mixed.
- *V:* division epineurial – neurotmesis, needs repair.
- *VI:* mixed – recovery depends on damage.
See Seddon classification of nerve injury.

Supercharging

A method of augmenting the blood supply to a large pedicled flap by performing a microvascular anastomosis to a secondary pedicle of the flap. It is most often used for unipedicled TRAM flaps.

Superficial palmar arch

- Lies distal to the transverse carpal ligament (TCL) in a line from the base of the extended thumb to the hook of the hamate.
- Formed by the anastomosis of ulnar artery to superficial branch of radial artery.
- It gives off the common digital arteries, which divide at the base of the fingers to give off the digital arteries.

Superficial temporal artery

- Terminal branch of external carotid artery. Supplies the lateral aspect of the scalp and is the longest and largest of the scalp vessels.
- It arises from beneath the parotid anterior to the tragus. It travels along the temporoparietal fascia and bifurcates into an anterior and posterior branch 2 cm above the zygomatic arch. The main continuation is the posterior branch.
See Scalp reconstruction.

Superior pedicle breast reduction

Operative technique: Mark as for inferior pedicle with 90–100° angle. Limbs 8 cm and horizontal lines a little shorter. De-epithelialize around nipple/areolar complex. Cut nipple on pedicle 0.5 cm thick. Score inferior line and cut through dermis obliquely to the chest wall. Mobilize whole breast off pectoralis. Stabilize the breast and cut medial limb then vertical and lateral limb. Suture breast in two layers. Suture vertical limb to horizontal limb, which will rotate the breast tissue upward under the nipple to create projection. De-epithelialize the new areolar position and suture in the nipple.

Supra-orbital nerve

- V1, exits from the supra-orbital foramen and supplies sensation to upper lid, conjunctiva, forehead and scalp up to the lambdoid suture.
- Block by inserting the needle under the midportion of the eyebrow while palpating the foramen.

Supratrochlear nerve

- Supratrochlear nerve comes from the medial aspect of the supra-orbital rim to supply the medial aspect of the forehead, upper eyelid, skin of upper nose and conjunctiva.
- Block by injecting medial portion of orbital rim lateral to the root of the nose.

Sural nerve

- *S1–2:* supplies skin of the lateral arch and lateral aspect of the heel.
- For nerve grafting, harvest through longitudinal or through stab incisions on the posterolateral aspect of the leg posterior to the lateral maleolus.

Sushruta

Circa 700 BC. Wrote in the Samhita (encyclopaedia). First to describe a facial (forehead) flap for the reconstruction of a nose.

Sutures

Absorbable:

- *Catgut:* from submucosal layer of sheep intestine. Hydrolysed by proteolytic enzymes within 60 days. Tensile strength lost within 10 days. Prolonged by chromatization.
- *Vicryl/Dexon:* synthetic. Minimal tissue reaction. Tensile strength lost in 1 month completely absorbed in 3 months. Both are braided sutures which can potentiate infection.
- *Polydiaxone (PDS):* synthetic absorbable monofilament. Minimally reactive. Retains tensile strength at 3 months, absorption complete by 6 months. Can spit out.
- *Maxon/monocryl:* absorbable monofilaments, similar to PDS, but retain tensile strength for only 3–4 weeks. Absorption complete by 3 and 4 months.

- So vicryl, dexon, monocryl, maxon, lose strength by 3 weeks, absorbed by 3 months. PDS loses strength by 3 months absorbed by 6 months.

Non-absorbable:
- Monofilament sutures (ethilon, prolene) have minimal inflammatory reaction, slide well, can easily be removed and retain tensile strength. Prolene keeps tensile strength better than ethilon.
- Braided sutures (ethibond, ticron, silk) give an inflammatory reaction.

See _Alloplasts_.

Swan neck deformity
Hyperextension of the PIP joint with flexion of the DIP joint.

Causes of swan neck:
- _PIP:_ volar plate deficiency.
- _Flexor:_ rupture of FDS.
- _Intrinsics:_ intrinsic muscle contractures.
- _Extrinsics:_ chronic mallet finger, extensor tension, e.g. wrist deformity.

In RA: Functional loss relates to loss of motion of PIP joint. 4 types determined by motion and joint space.

Classification:
- I – PIPJ flexible.
- II – flexion limited on MPJ extension (intrinsic tightness).
- III – limited in all positions.
- IV – stiff with XR charges.

Type 1 – PIP flexible in all positions:
- Full passive motion of PIP joint.
- Deformity may originate in DIP or PIP joint.
- May start with stretching or rupture of terminal extensor tendon attachment giving a mallet deformity. This can be presumed when the DIP deformity is greater than the PIP deformity.
- In others the PIP joint is the cause of the problem when synovitis stretches the volar capsule or flexor rupture. Then DIP flexion is secondary.
- Treat by preventing PIP joint hyperextension and restoring DIP extension.
  - _Splint_ around PIP joint;
  - DIP joint can be surgically fused;

  - dermadesis (take ellipse of skin from volar aspect of PIP 5 mm wide);
  - flexor tendon tenodesis (section one insertion of FDS proximally, pass through slit in A2 pulley and re-attach to itself);
  - retinacular ligament reconstruction (ulnar lateral band free from extensor mechanism proximally, but left attached distally; passed volar to Cleland's fibres and suture to fibrous tendon sheath. See _ORL_.

Type II – PIPJ flexion limited in certain positions:
- PIP joint flexion is influenced by position of MCP joint. When the MCP joint is extended, passive PIP joint movement is limited. Though initially the limitation is only on MCP joint extension, eventually the PIP joint will become stiff.
- Need to relieve intrinsic tightness and correct any MCP joint problem such as subluxation.
- _Intrinsic release:_ perform through dorso-ulnar longitudinal incision over proximal phalanx. Can be combined with DIP joint fusion or volar dermadesis.

Type III – limited PIPJ flexion in all positions:
- Significant loss of hand function. Often well-preserved joint spaces. Structures restricting movement are extensor mechanisms, collateral ligaments, and skin.
- Need to first restore passive motion.
- _PIP joint manipulation:_ may be possible with an MUA, usually with intrinsic release or Swanson arthroplasty. Splint in flexion. May need K wire fixation initially.
- _Skin release:_ oblique incision which is left open – graft not needed. Perform just distal to joint.
- _Lateral band mobilization:_ in established deformity lateral bands are displaced dorsally. Freeing them from the extensor tendon using two parallel incisions allows movement.
- _Flexor tenosynovitis:_ tendon adherence and tenosynovitis can lead to stiff PIP joints.

Type IV – stiff PIPJ and poor XR appearance:
- Require fusion or arthroplasty. Tend to fuse index for stability.

Swanson MCP joint arthroplasty: operative technique

• Transverse incision over dorsum over MCP joints. Expose extensor tendons, preserving all structures in between.

• Release intrinsics on ulnar side and reflect extensor tendon radially – usually requiring sagittal band division. Crossed intrinsic transfer – preserve intrinsic divided distally. Identify intrinsic on radial side and suture ulnar intrinsic to radial side of adjacent finger. Can be performed on middle, index and little finger.

• Try to preserve capsule, incise and reflect. Perform synovectomy. Put Mitchell trimmer and Howarth around metacarpal head and excise head with oscillating saw just around the metacarpal flare. Hold head with towel clip and excise preserving collateral ligaments. Perform thorough synovectomy with rongeurs cleaning off volar plate and under metacarpal, but being careful not to injure NVBs. Put traction on finger to increase space.

• Now prepare bones for prosthesis. Start with broach then move to reamers. Ream metacarpal square, but angle proximal phalanx slightly to recreate normal arc of hand. When reaming phalanx hold finger to enable accurate gauging of position of reamer. Use sizers to determine prosthesis. Drill hole in distal radial side of metacarpal and stitch radial collateral with ticron, pass through hole and clip. Retract all soft tissue out of the way and using a no touch technique insert the prosthesis – long end proximally. Ensure a snug fit and tie collateral.

• Suture capsule with PDS and reef extensor if necessary. Place Swanson drain transversely and suture skin. Put in volar backslab in slight MPJ flexion. After 1/52 put in outrigger.

Swanson classification
See _Congenital hand anomalies_.

Sweat glands
Two types.

• _Apocrine:_ in axilla and groin. Start to function in puberty and give an odour due to bacterial decomposition. Sympathetic adrenergic.

• _Eccrine_ glands are found throughout the body except lips and external genitalia. They are found more frequently in the eyelids, palms, feet and axilla. The eccrine glands on the sole of the foot and palm of hand differ from the rest of the body. Sympathetic cholinergic. The sweating of a graft follows that of the recipient site. Transplanted skin lacks lubrication until it is reinnervated.

Sweat gland tumours
• _Eccrine hidrocystomas._
• _Syringomas._
• _Cylindroma._
• _Eccrine spiradenoma._
• _Eccrine poroma._

Symblepharon
Fusion of the eyelids to the globe. It is sometimes caused by chemical burns. Localized areas may be corrected with Z-plasty, but the best method for correction is wide release of adhesions and conjunctival grafting. Larger areas will require mucosal grafts.

Symbrachydactyly
• Means short coalesced digits. Deficient bony framework leaves soft tissues unsupported. Get finger buds with nail appendages.

• Arises sporadically with mesodermal deficit in skeletal framework of fingers.

• There is a failure of formation and failure of differentiation in a longitudinal and transverse direction. Longitudinal deficiency centres around the middle phalanx, transverse affects index, middle, ring, little then thumb.

• Usually unilateral with no other abnormalities. 25–39% associated with ipsilateral pectoral or thoracic deficits.

• Short finger type is the most common. Usually the thumb is spared, but may get adduction of 1st web space. Categorize according to number of remaining phalanges (absence progresses from middle phalanx). All fingers affected but radial more severe. Some similarities in Apert's and constriction ring. It is the most common of the 4 types – 33–59%.

Classification: <u>Blauth and Gekeler</u>.

Treatment:
- If skin envelope is present, composite grafts can be inserted.
- May perform a reverse pollicization – transferring the index ray to the 3rd MC.
- Thumb reconstruction can be performed in a number of ways. Can use skin from cleft to widen 1st web space. Rotation osteotomy of border digits.

See <u>Congenital hand anomalies</u>.

Sympathetic function testing
- The sympathetic nervous system controls vasomotor response, sweating and pilomotor activity. These 3 can be assessed along with trophic changes.
- *Trophic changes:* get atrophy and tapering of the fingers – 'pencil-pointing effect'. Skin is smooth and finger prints disappear.
- *Vasomotor:* change in skin colour and temperature. May be blue or pink as heat regulatory capacity is lost. <u>Ninhydrin printing test</u> is the most accurate assessment. Wrinkle test assesses wrinkling after placing hand in water.

See <u>Sensation testing</u>.

Symphalangism
- Originally described absent PIPJ with normal length of phalanges. Also used to describe stiffness of MCPJ and DIPJ and also includes shortened digits.
- Rare autosomal dominant inherited condition due to failure of differentiation. Can be seen in drug-induced anomalies and other non-inheritable anomalies such as Poland's and Apert's. Most common in Caucasians, rare in blacks.
- Clinically no discernable finer creases, get square articular surfaces.

Classification:
- *3 types:* true (single or multiple), symbrachydactyly and symphalangism assoc with other anomalies.
- *Cushing:* fusion of PIPJs most common.
- *Drey:* involvement of DIPJs of all fingers with hypoplastic nails.

- *Kermisson:* index to little finger severely malformed, absent nails and distal phalanges, short middle phalanges, fused PIPJs.
- *Fuhrman:* radiohumeral synostosis, carpal and tarsal fusion.
- *WL symphalangism:* brachydactyly syndrome. Autosomal dominant with conductive hearing loss, broad nose, pes excavatum.

Treatment:
- Arthroplasties have been tried, but none are successful in producing a mobile joint.
- Vascularized 2nd toe transfer. Operate at age 10 as exercise is very important.
- Alternatively perform osteotomies when the epiphysis are fused. Do it at 20°, 30°, 40°, 50° for D2, 3, 4 and 5, respectively.

Syndactyly
Two or more partially or completely fused digits. Arise because of failure of apoptosis (programmed cell death).

Epidemiology:
- 1:2000 births. 20% have a positive family history. M:F 2:1. Autosomal dominant with incomplete penetrance. Common in Caucasians.
- It may be associated with syndromes such as Apert's and Poland's. Linked to FGF receptor deficiency.
- Middle-ring web in 54% of cases, ring-little in 30%, middle-index in 15%, thumb-index 1%.

Classification:
- Complete up to the tips of the fingers or incomplete.
- *Simple:* only soft tissue, complex with bone or acrosyndactyly with bone fusion distally.

Treatment
- Surgical release not usually before 1 year though earlier if 1st or 4th web involved due to the length discrepancy. Also complex and acrosyndactyly are released earlier as the bony connections will affect growth.
- Only operate on one side of a finger at a time.
- Do border digits first.
- Straight line scars may cause more contractures. Important to bring a large dorsal flap to palmar surface to create the web space

and prevent web creep (Bauer design). Use interdigitating flaps volar and dorsal. Grafts are required for the defects. Use interdigitating flaps from the hyponychium to reconstruct the lateral nail fold.

Synostosis

- Abnormal fusion of two bones which may be partial, permitting reduced motion or complete, with no motion.
- It can occur at any site in the upper limb where two bones are adjacent.
- Synostosis in the phalanges occur in complex _Syndactyly_.
- Forearm synostosis may require rotational osteotomy.

Synovectomy

See _Rheumatoid arthritis_.

Syringocystadenoma papilliferum

- Usually a verrucous lesion that occurs most commonly on or near the scalp.
- A hamartomatous growth often in association with naevus sebaceous type.
- It begins to develop during childhood and may be bulbous.
- Basal cell epithelioma occur in about 10% of the lesions.
- Treat with excision of the lesion and any surrounding sebaceous nevus.

Syringomas

- Occur in adult women on the lower eyelids and upper cheeks, and also the trunk, neck, and extremities.
- Pink or yellow papules, usually 2–3 mm in diameter.
- They are often confused with trichoepitheliomas, xanthelasma or basal cell epithelioma.
- Removal for diagnosis and cosmesis with excision, cautery or laser.

Systemic lupus erythematosus (SLE)

- Usually young women (15–25 year). Female: male 9:1.
- Varies from a mild to a fatal disease.
- When active get leucopoenia, anaemia, raised ESR, positive anti-nuclear factor and low serum complement with vasculitis.
- Hand deformities can resemble RA with volar subluxation and ulnar drift. XR show deformity with no erosive changes or joint space narrowing. Hand deformities are passively correctable as the ligaments are lax. Therefore, position can usually be maintained by splints though arthroplasty or arthrodesis maybe required.
- Skin grafts and flaps are not contraindicated in SLE patients and the benefits of steroid therapy in suppressing vasculitis outweigh the drawbacks.

T Tagliacozzi to **Two-point discrimination**

Tagliacozzi

- _Gaspar Tagliacozzi:_ 16th century Italian surgeon from Bologna who defined the ideals of plastic surgery.
- 'We restore, repair and make whole those parts of the face which Nature has given but which fortune has taken away, not so much that they may delight the eye but that they may buoy up the spirit and help the mind of the afflicted.'
- He learnt and further developed the pedicled flap from arm for nasal reconstruction.

Tagliacozzi flap

- Used for _Nasal reconstruction_. The original Tagliacozzi flap was based distally and required _Delay_ with a cotton lint being placed under the flap to prevent reattachment.
- A more recent modification uses a proximally based flap that encompasses the axial vessel to the medial arm skin. A delay procedure is not necessary.
- After transfer, the upper extremity is immobilized for approximately 3 weeks until the pedicle is divided.

- Good quality skin is supplied but there is often a significant difference in quality from normal nasal skin and better options are usually available.

Tanzer classification

For congenital ear anomalies.
- *Type I:* anotia.
- *Type II:* microtia.
  ○ *A:* microtia with atresia of external auditory meatus;
  ○ *B:* microtia without atresia.
- *Type III:* hypoplasia of the middle third of the ear.
- *Type IV:*
  ○ *A:* constricted ear;
  ○ *B:* crptotia;
  ○ *C:* hypoplasia of the upper third.
- *Type V:* prominent ear.
See *Ear*.

Tanzini

1906: performed a latissimus dorsi flap for breast reconstruction.

TAR syndrome

Thrombocytopenia Absent Radius. Usually get correction of the thrombocytopenia after 1 year with good prognosis.
See *Radial club hand*.

Tarsal tunnel syndrome

- Results from compression of the posterior tibial nerve within the fibrous tunnel. Usually get a burning pain in the medial part of the foot. Worsened by activity and at night. Tinel's sign. Sensation is decreased.
- May be confirmed by nerve conduction studies with prolonged latency and abnormal potentials.
- Treat by releasing the tunnel.
See *Lower limb reconstruction*.

Tarsorraphy

- Surgical closure of the eyelids indicated when any part of the cornea remains exposed when the eye is closed.
- A medial or lateral tarsorraphy can be performed. Pinch the eyelid to determine which side is best. A medial tarsorraphy keeps the

punctae in touch with the globe. It is better cosmetically, but more difficult as the punctae and canaliculi need to be avoided.
- *Margaret Brand procedure:* pinch the lids together. Mark the correct length. Add amethocaine and LA. Incise along the grey line (behind the lash follicles). Make another incision parallel to the first 1–2 mm thick. Dissect this strip of tissue. Repeat on the upper lid. Suture together over bolsters. Ensure no lashes project inwards. Remove sutures after 2/52. Give chloramphenicol drops.
- *McLaughlin procedure:* incise lower lid margin along intermarginal line (the line where the lids touch anteriorly) medially from the lateral canthus for 5–6 mm. Remove a piece of anterior lamella of lower lid. Split the intermarginal line of the upper lid and remove a similar sector of tarsus and conjunctiva. Evert upper lid and suture with a bolster.

Tattoo

- A foreign material entered into the dermis leaving an indelible mark. Depth varies. Professional tattoos are superficial and uniform and therefore more readily removable but have more ink than home-made tattoos. Tattoos were present in ancient Egypt. Polynesians had tattoos and this started the naval tradition.
- Medical tattoos are useful for vitiligo, nipple reconstruction, grafts. Also eyebrows and eyelids. Retattooing can cover up the offensive portion of a tattoo.

Safety:
- Dyes are generally safe. Patients can become sensitized to the pigment in a tattoo particularly the red from cinnabar. Usually it is a delayed hypersensitivity with itchy glaucomatous lesions. Some are photoallergic.
- Using Q-switched laser with an allergy may worsen the allergy as the dye is broken up. There is a risk of transmission of infectious diseases.

Treatment:
- *Excision:* may be the best option, particularly if there is an allergy to the dye.

May require serial excision, tissue expansion or a flap.

- *Laser:* short pulses disrupt tattoo material. Because the energy is high and the duration short, the pigment can be eliminated without injuring adjacent dermis. Match wavelength to colour. All work well with black and India ink:
  - ○ ruby not effective with red, but good for green pigment;
  - ○ YAG good for red poor with green;
  - ○ alexandrite good for blue-black and green, poor for orange and yellow;
  - ○ may develop scarring and hypopigmentation, response may be extremely variable; the most difficult to treat are the newer brightly coloured tattoos, whereas the easiest are the home-made as the load of ink is less.
- *Salabrasion:* skin is abraded and salt left on the wound allowing some pigment to leach out.
- *Tanic/oxalic acid:* use after abrasion to induce inflammation.
- *Dermabrasion:* the epidermis and superficial dermis is abraded. A dressing is changed daily allowing dye to leach onto the dressing. The problems are scarring and partial response. Also chemical peel and dermaplaning has been used.

Taylor classification
Nerve supply to muscles.
- *Type 1:* single unbranched nerve.
- *Type 2:* single nerve which branches.
- *Type 3:* multiple branches from same nerve.
- *Type 4:* multiple branches from different trunks.

See Musculocutaneous/muscle flaps.

Teeth
Classification:
- *Universal system* of notation of teeth. Maxillary teeth 1–16 from upper right third molar. Mandible numbered 17–32 from lower left third molar. The primary teeth are similarly counted using A–J for upper and T–K for lower.
- *Teeth names:* the 32 permanent teeth are divided into 4 quadrants. Each has a central incisor, lateral incisor, canine (cuspid), first premolar (bicuspid), second premolar (bicuspid) and first second and third molars. The 20 primary teeth are also divided into four each having a central and lateral incisor, canine, and first and second molar.

Anatomy:
- The crown is visible and the root is attached to the bony walls by periodontal membrane fibres. The crown is covered with enamel and the root with cementum. The junction is the cervical line. Under enamel and cementum is the dentin. In the centre is the pulp chamber. The pulp tissue supplies nerve and blood vessels to the tooth through apical foramen.
- *Nerve supply:* lower teeth supplied by the inferior alveolar branch of the mandibular division of the trigeminal nerve. The upper teeth are supplied by the maxillary division of the trigeminal nerve which divides into the posterior superior alveolar branch from the pterygopalatine portion and the middle and anterior superior alveolar branches from the infra-orbital nerves.

Development:
- Get primary (deciduous) and secondary (permanent) dentition. At birth the maxilla and mandible contain the partially formed crowns of 20 deciduous teeth. All erupt in the first 2 years, starting with central incisors, then first molars, then second molars. The first permanent teeth erupt at age 6 and take 6 years to complete.
- All will be replaced by teeth of the same type except the primary molars which are replaced by bicuspids and the permanent 1–3 molars, which are posterior to the second primary molar. The third molars (wisdom teeth) erupt at cessation of jaw growth (17–21 years).
- *Missing teeth:* the most common congenitally missing tooth is the third molar. Several missing teeth (oligodontia) or anodontia is often associated with ectodermal dysplasia and oral–facial–digital syndrome.

Trauma: the most common tooth injury is fracture. A root fracture is most favourable if in the apical 1/3. Subluxed teeth can be intruded or extruded. If intruded they need repositioning. If extruded it should be replaced and splinted.

Occlusion: See Angle classification.

Terminology:
- *Mesial:* toward the midline.
- *Distal:* away from the midline.
- *Lingual:* toward the tongue.
- *Buccal:* toward the cheek.
- *Mesial:* surface facing central incisor.
- Crossbite: an abnormal buccolingual relation of the teeth. Anterior crossbite is lingual crossbite of the upper incisors. Posterior crossbite is buccal crossbite of the maxillary premolars and molars.
- *Overbite:* vertical overlap of the incisors, where the upper incisors are in a lower than normal position.
- *Overjet:* horizontal overlap of the incisors, where the upper incisors are positioned anterior to their normal position.
- *Open bite:* lack of contact between teeth in the mouth-shut position.
- *Tooth vitality:* sensate tooth with an intact pulpal nerve supply. (A tooth may have an adequate blood supply, but is non-vital if a nerve supply is not present.)
- *Curve of Spee:* curvature of the occlusal plane.
- *Centric occlusion:* position of the mandible where there is maximal intercuspation of the maxillary and mandibular teeth.
- *Centric relation:* the most retruded position of the mandible, where the condyles are comfortably seated in the glenoid fossae.
- *Centric occlusion and centric relation:* May be the same in a normal patient but may differ in cases of malocclusion. (Centric relation can exist in the absence of teeth.)
- *Ankylosis of a tooth:* solid fixation of a tooth resulting from fusion of the cementum and alveolar bone with obliteration of the periodontal ligament. (The tooth is 'locked' in bone and cannot be moved orthodontically.)
- *Retrogenia:* the chin is not necessarily small, but is positioned posterior to its desired location.
- *Retrognathia:* posterior positioning of the mandible.

- *Microgenia:* a small chin is present with an overall deficiency of bone, generally in all three planes.
- *Micrognathia:* the entire jaw is small.
- *Macrogenia:* the chin is large.
- *Mandibular prognathism:* anterior positioning of the mandible.

See Orthognathic surgery.

Telangiectases
- *Generalized essential telangiectasia:* onset varies widely, but is most common in adults. F:M 2:1. Get groups of pin-sized, vascular puncta in the lower extremities. The lesions extend proximally to form sheets of telangiectasias. Flashlamp pulsed dye laser therapy is relatively effective.
- Cutis marmorata telangiectatica congenita (Van Lohuizen Syndrome).
- Hereditary haemorrhagic telangiectasia (HHT; Rendu–Osler–Weber Syndrome).
- Ataxia-telangiectasia (Louis–Bar syndrome).

See Vascular malformations.

Telecanthus
Abnormally long distance from the medial canthus to the nose.

Temporalis muscle
Origin:
- *Deep:* temporal fossa calvarium.
- *Superficial:* deep temporalis fascia.

Insertion: coronoid process and anterior ramus of mandible.

Innervation: CN V3 anterior and deep temporal branches.

Blood supply: deep temporal fascia. Middle temporal branch of superficial temporal artery.

Action: anterior fibres are elevators and posterior fibres are retractors of the mandible.

Temporalis muscle flap
Based on the deep temporal vessels. First described by Golovine in 1898. It can be used to reconstruct the maxillofacial region and as a motor in facial nerve palsy when it can be detached from the origin as a turnover flap

with a fascial extension or detached from the insertion on the coronoid process.

See <u>Oral cavity reconstruction</u>.

Temporomandibular joint (TMJ)

- Called a gingylmoarthrodial joint as it has both a hinged and a gliding motion. There is a meniscus separating superior and inferior joint compartments. The articular surface is lined with fibrocartilage.
- Both TMJs function as a single unit – the craniomandibular articulation. The end point is the position of dental occlusion.
- The articular disc separates the joint into two spaces. Hinge occurs in the inferior space and sliding in the superior space. The joint surfaces consist of the mandibular condyle and temporal articular surface. The condyles are elliptical. They are surrounded by the fibrous joint capsule. The disc is a biconcave structure composed of dense fibrous connective tissue. It is anchored anteriorly to the superior head of the lateral pterygoid muscle and the eminentia articularis, inferiorly to the medial and lateral aspect of the mandibular condyle, and posteriorly in two zones.
- The main function of the disc is to distribute load evenly along the joint surfaces, as well as aiding in their lubrication and protection during translatory movements.

Temporomandibular joint dysfunction

- 30% of the Western population may have symptoms. F:M 3:1.
- Patients complain of pain, noise and limitation of movement. Look for asymmetry, dentition, malocclusion, joint movement.
- *Imaging:* XR, arthrography, CT and MRI.

Myofascial pain dysfunction syndrome (MPD): Usually no anatomic abnormalities are seen in the TMJ. The cause is multifactorial and includes bruxism and anxiety and occlusal prematurity, which lead to spasm of the jaw muscles and pain. The aim of management is to break the spasm cycle. Treat occlusion problems with a splint. A splint at night will prevent bruxism. Also use NSAIDs, heat, diathermy and ultrasound.

Trauma: Usually get anterior displacement of the disc trapping retrodisc tissues causing pain. Get premature wear of the articular surface. The management is stage-dependent but in the early stages treat as for MPD.

Ankylosis:
- Classified as true (intra-articular) or false (extra-articular) and bony or fibrous. Most commonly due to trauma, infection and juvenile arthritis.
- Get fibrous then bony fusion. Patients have oral hygiene problems. If the patient is young, mandibular growth will be retarded.
- Treatment with condylectomy or gap and interpositional arthroplasty. In severe cases replacement with costochondral graft harvested from contralateral 5th or 6th rib, and split longitudinally. Temporalis fascia is used between the graft and glenoid fossa.

TMJ dislocations:
- Acute dislocations of the TMJ occur as the condyle extends anteriorly beyond the eminence as a result of hypermobility secondary to trauma or exaggerated mouth opening as in yawning. Spontaneous reduction usually follows, but in some cases the dislocation persists and requires manual reduction.
- With thumb inside and finger outside, push the mandible down and posteriorly. Muscle relaxants may be required.

Infective arthritis:
- Local spread or haematogenous spread with development of osteomyelitis and ankylosis of the TMJ.
- Treat with open drainage, intravenous antibiotics, and sequestrectomy if indicated.

Avascular necrosis:
- After trauma or devascularization at the time of TMJ surgery. The patient will present with the typical symptoms of TMJ syndrome including pain and limited jaw motion.
- Treat by debridement of the necrotic condyle and possible condylar replacement in severe cases.

Surgery treatment of TMJ problems:
- *TMJ arthroscopy:* lavage and debridement may improve symptoms. Long-term benefit has not been demonstrated.
- *TMJ arthrotomy:* through a preauricular incision the inferior border of the disk is incised. Disc displacement requires repositioning by resecting a wedge posteriorly. If there is significant degeneration then a total meniscectomy is performed. Osteophytes are shaved.
- *TMJ implants:* implants in young patients have caused significant problems. Implants are only indicated in severe ankylosis and degenerative disease.

Temporoparietal fascial flap

- Superficial temporal artery runs beneath subcutaneous tissues and within temporoparietal fascia. The vein is more superficial lying on the surface of the fascia.
- Temporparietal fascia (TPF) is a thin fascial sheet covering temporal occipital and parietal scalp which is an extension of SMAS layer. Deep to TPF is the deep temporal fascia and temporalis muscle.
- A deep branch of the superficial temporal artery at the level of the zygoma separates to supply the deep temporal fascia.
- The deep temporal fascia can be dissected as a separate component to increase the size of the flap.
- There is an inconspicuous donor site scar, and the size of the flap can reach 14 × 17cm though usually 8 × 10 cm.
- Dissection may cause alopecia..

Application:
- The tissue may be transferred on an ipsilateral pedicle or as a free flap. It may carry hair-bearing scalp and calvarial bone.
- It can be used to cover auricular cartilage and for a gliding surface in tendon reconstruction in the hand. It is good for facial soft tissue augmentation.

Technique: Isolate artery and vein through a facelift incision 1–2 cm in front of the ear and deep to parotid fascia. Expose fascia through a vertical incision up to $^2/_3$ of the apex of the skull then a horizontal incision to complete the T. Elevate skin flaps immediately deep to hair follicles. Strip temporoparietal fascia from pericranium and deep temporal fascia after the plane of the vascular pedicle has been established. Harvest bone if required with a bur, saw or osteotome.

Tendon

Anatomy: Inelastic fibrils of type I collagen in a ground substance of dermatan sulphate. Fibrils are bundled into fibres. The main cells is the fibroblast. Tendon is covered with paratenon. Endotenon covers the central portions. Blood vessels run in paratenon from muscle and from bone. Also vincula system. Blood flow is low. Tendons within sheaths are covered with synovial fluid which is nutritive. Tendons contain few cells and those present include tenocytes, synovial cells and fibroblasts.

Healing:
- Normally tendons are not very metabolically active. Healing occurs by adhesion from surrounding tissue and intrinsic healing driven by fibroblasts within the tendon. Both normally contribute to healing.
- *Extrinsic healing:* adhesion formation is maximized by immobilization and is similar to healing in other tissues. *See* Wound healing.
- *Intrinsic healing* depends much less on the inflammatory response. Early motion generates more intrinsic healing. Fibroblasts migrate from epitenon into the damaged area facilitated by fibronectin. Neovascularization occurs. Collagen is synthesized by fibroblasts. Early motion gets quicker gain in tensile strength. Extensive injuries are more likely to heal with adhesion. Lunborg showed that tendons heal when wrapped in a semipermeable membrane and placed in the knee joint of a rabbit.

Surgical repair: Careful apposition of ends is important. Reconstructing sheath has not been shown to improve healing.

Tendon harvest
- *Plantaris*.
- Long toe extensors. Make a transverse incision at the level of metatarsalphalangeal joints. Long extensor are isolated proximal

to the hood. Pass a stripper but when it gets stuck make further transverse incision and free the tendon then use the stripper again. Can take long extensor of 2, 3, 4th toes.

See Tendon reconstruction.

Tendon rupture: in rheumatoid arthritis

In *Rheumatoid arthritis* due to attrition over bone, infiltration by synovium, ischaemia due to pressure from synovium. Ulnar subluxation of extensor tendons and PIN compression may cause confusion.

Extensor tendons:

- Get sudden loss of finger extension. Usually painless after trivial injury or activity. May go unrecognized. The factors causing an isolated rupture often lead to subsequent rupture often in order from little to index. Often the tendons are abraided on the distal ulna.
- Tendon rupture can be mimicked by:
  - ○ MCP joint dislocation (but lacks passive extension).
  - ○ Ulnar subluxation of the extensor tendons between the metacarpal heads.
  - ○ Paralysis of the common extensor tendon secondary to posterior interosseous nerve compression by elbow synovitis.

Management:

- *Single:* usually little finger. Amount of extensor lag depends on whether both tendons ruptured. If EDQ is ruptured may get 30° lag. Test EDC by holding other fingers flexed. if the extensor lag increases then EDC is still active.
- End to end repair may be feasible. If not possible suture to adjacent tendon. Perform dorsal synovectomy. Remove bony spicules or ulna head. Transfer dorsal retinaculum deep to tendons if bone exposed. With double ruptures involving little and ring finger it may not be possible to suture the little finger extensor stump to the middle finger. Use EIP or ECU. If more than 2 tendons are ruptured used FDS brought through interosseous membrane. Palmaris longus or if the wrist is fused a wrist extensor can be used as a bridge graft. Put the weave in tight as the muscle will stretch post-operatively.

- *Tendon ruptures with MCPJ disease:* first tackle the joints as unless the joints can be extended passively they won't benefit from tendon reconstruction.

Tendon transfers

General principles:

- Used to restore balance to a hand with impaired function of extrinsic or intrinsic tendons. The transferred donor tendon remains attached to its parent muscle and the neurovascular pedicle remains intact.
- Fractures should be fixed. Flaps may be required. Silicone rods may be required. Passive movement should be maintained.
- *Timing:* can be early, conventional or late. Conventional is performed when there is no reinnervation 3 months after the expected time. Early can be performed at the same time as nerve repair as a temporary substitute which may augment a suboptimal recovery.
- *Surgery:* mobilize the muscle carefully. The tendon should glide through a tunnel. Repair with a *Pulvertaft weave*, carefully tension. Immobilize for 3 weeks then gentle active ROM exercises.

Selection of donor:

- The muscle–tendon (MT) unit should be expendable.
- Consider the strength of the paralysed muscle and that of the antagonist. The maximum force of a muscle is that at its resting length. Should be >grade 3 power to function well.
- Muscle excursion should be adequate to restore function. *See Amplitude.*
- Ideally one tendon should perform one function.
- It should pass in a straight line.
- It should preferably be synergistic to the muscle being replaced. Wrist extension is synergistic to finger flexion and wrist flexion is synergistic to finger extension.
- So, consider – expendable, strength, excursion, line and synergy. Brachioradialis doesn't function well after transfer.

Smith and Hastings algorithm:

- List all muscles that are functioning.

- List all muscles available for transfer, eliminating all that would leave an unacceptable deficit.
- Decide which functions need to be restored.
- Match available muscles with the needed functions.
- Consider other options such as arthrodesis and/or tenodesis.
- Divide the reconstruction into stages according to whether post-operative immobilization will be in flexion or extension.

Radial nerve palsy:

- Inability to extend wrist and fingers and abduct thumb. Biggest problem is the wrist instability. Sensory loss not a problem. Timing is controversial, some advocating early repair with the nerve repair. The more proximal the injury, the less likely is it that innervation will occur. Studies conflict as to the successfulness of repair. Results are less predictable with extensive injury, significant gap and older patients. In this group early transfer is indicated.
- Need to retain a wrist flexor. Preserve FCU as flexion and ulnar deviation is important for power grip, especially in PIN palsy as the ECU activity is lost.
- 3 options. All have PT → ECRB. Two have PL → EPL. Boyes uses FDS for wrist and thumb.

Operations:

- *FCU transfer:* inverted J incision over volar ulnar aspect of forearm. Transect at wrist crease. Mobilize PL, transecting distally. S incision on volar radial aspect of forearm. PT tendon divided from its insertion. ECRB transected at the musculotendinous junction. PT is rerouted to insert onto ECRB. A tunnel is made around the forearm and FCU is passed dorsally to lie across EDC. Perform end to side repair if some function might return. EPL is divided at the musculocutaneous junction and passed to PL. Each EDC tendon is sutured to FCU.
- *FCR transfer:* can be exchanged for FCU.
- *Boyes sublimis transfer:* advocated as the excursion of FCU or FCR is not enough for EDC without using the tenodesis effect. The advantages are simultaneous wrist and finger extension, independent thumb and

index extension and no reduced wrist strength. However, may get reduced grip and swan neck. Use FDS to ring and middle and pass through a window in the interosseous membrane. This window should be at least 4 cm long to allow gliding. EPL and EIP are woven to ring FDS, EDC to middle FDS.

Low median nerve palsy:

Indications:

- If distal to the extrinsics, main problem is loss of thumb *Opposition* and sensory loss. FPB has dual innervation in 70% of patients so loss may be more difficult to detect. Prior to tendon transfers, need to ensure that no contractures develop. Release of the web space may be required. The direction of pull should come from the pisiform and insert into the dorso-lulnar base to produce pronation. The more distal the transfer in the palm, the greater the power of flexion. Perform early transfer in older patients with a poor prognosis for reinnervation. Early transfer will probably not be required if FPB is dual innervated. If not, patients may be able to achieve some abduction with APL if the arm is pronated. These patients would benefit from transfer.

Operations:

- *EIP transfer (Burkhalter):* transect. Repair stump to EDC to prevent extensor lag. Mobilize through two incisions proximal and distal to extensor retinaculum. Further incision in forearm to mobilize muscle. Make incision proximal to pisiform and pass EIP around the ulnar border then obliquely across the palm and woven into APB. By tenodesis, palmar flexion should give adduction.
- *FDS transfer (Bunnell):* isolate ring finger FDS and transect between A1 and A2 pulley. Bring out through distal forearm. Split FCU to create a pulley. Pass through this, across palm and into the radial aspect of MPJ. This is stronger with a greater length. May not be available. May get flexion contracture or swan neck. (Royles–Thompson) FDS ring is passed up the sheath of FPL to attach to superficial head of FPB and opponens pollicis.

- *PL (Camitz):* simple. Provides abduction but little pronation. Good for elderly patients with carpal tunnel syndrome. Dissect a strip of fascia with distal PL and extend into forearm. Fascia can be tubed. Develop tunnel to a mid-axial incision on the radial aspect of the MPJ of the thumb. Suture to APB tendon.
- *ADM (Huber):* in children. Provides little abduction. Transect insertion and raise muscle, preserving NVB. Rotate and suture to APB.

High median nerve palsy:

Indications: Loss of thumb opposition and also flexion to thumb and index. Often the middle finger can flex due to connection with the ring FDP. Functions which need restoring are thumb IPJ flexion and index PIP and DIPJ flexion.

Operations:

- *Thumb IPJ:* brachioradialis to FPL. Divide FPL at the musculotendinous junction and weave to BR. If there may be some recovery, weave end to side. FDP can be sutured to FDP of ring and little. If more power is required, transfer ECRL. ECU can be used as a thumb flexor or wrist pronator, wrist flexor and thumb abductor. Timing can be difficult. If seen late then perform transfers at the same time as nerve repairs.

Low ulnar nerve palsy:

Indications: Distal paralysis results in imbalance between flexors and extensors. Extension at the MCP joint is unopposed and the volar plate is weak. Flexion at the IPJs are unapposed. Grip is weak and flexion asynchronous. Function is improved by static or dynamic means on the MCP joint preventing hyperextension. Also get weak pinch due to adductor pollicis paralysis. Timing of transfers is based on probability of recovery. Consider early transfer if clawing is debilitating

Operations to prevent clawing:

Static: To prevent hyperextension of the proximal phalanx. Volar plate can be advanced to give 20° of flexion. Tendon graft can be attached to TCL, volar to deep transverse ligament then dorsally to radial lateral band.

Tendon transfers:

- Differ as to whether they provide MCP joint flexion or also IPJ extension. If the extrinsic extensors can fully extend IPJ then only MCP joint flexion is needed. So transfer can attach to A1 pulley (Zancolli), A2 pulley or drill hole in proximal phalanx. If central slip is attenuated, put transfer into lateral band. Using FDS does not increase grip whereas using a wrist flexor will.
- *MPJ flexion only:* FDS to ring and little is divided distal to A1. Each is looped around A1 and sutured to itself. For a high palsy, motor the FDS lassos with ECRL or FCR.
- *MPJ flexion and IPJ extension:*
  ○ *Modified Stiles-Bunnell transfer:* FDS to middle finger divided and split into two slips. Each is passed down the lumbrical canal of ring and little and sutured to the radial lateral band. If there is a total intrinsic palsy then FDS to middle and ring is used. The disadvantage is that the FDS is not expendable and may result in swan neck deformity.
    - Divide middle finger FDS proximal to PIPJ through radial mid-axial incision. Withdraw tendon through transverse distal palmar crease incision and split into 2.
    - Find radial lateral bands to ring and little finger through radial mid-axial incision and pass each slip down the lumbrical canal of the ring and little finger.
    - Suture to radial lateral band with MCPJ in 45° flexion and IPJ fully extended.
    - Should get intrinsic plus position with dorsiflexion.
    - Immobilize for 1/12 with dorsal blocking splint – slight wrist flexion, and MCPJ 70° flexion. May need to split into 3 or for 4 fingers use FDS to middle and ring.
    - May get swan necking and, therefore, only use with mild PIPJ contractures.
  ○ *FDS expansion:* split FDS to middle into 4 and through a lateral incision to 3rd, 4th and 5th and medial incision to 2nd suture to lateral bands. Place hand on board with 70° MCPJ flexion to get tension right. Start with 5th then tension index until 5th just moves

o ECRL/B transfers: Paul Brand used ECRL with plantaris through lumbrical canals to the radial lateral bands of middle ring and little and the ulnar lateral band of the index finger. The tendon is rerouted around the radial border of the forearm. Plantaris is divided in half and split to give 4 tendon grafts. Each is sutured to ECRL, passed through lumbrical canals, the slack is taken up and they are sutured to the lateral bands just proximal to the PIP joints. Brand also described a 4-tailed graft with ECRB passing from dorsal to volar through the intermetacarpal spaces.

• *Correction of ulnar deviation of little finger:* detach ulnar half of EDM, pass volar to deep transverse intermetacarpal ligament, suture to radial collateral ligament of the MPJ or loop under A2.

• *Thumb adduction:* ring finger FDS deep to flexor tendons of index and middle into a drill hole distal to adductor insertion. ECRB with tendon graft through 2nd intermetacarpal space, tunnelled beneath AP to its insertion.

High ulnar nerve palsy:
Grip strength can be improved by suturing FDP to adjacent tendons or by transferring FDS to middle. If ulnar deviation of the wrist is required, FCR should be transferred to FCU.

Tennison–Randall repair
Cleft lip repair with a Z-plasty of the cleft lip edges which reconstructs the Cupid's bow, but puts a scar across the philtral column.

Tenosynovitis
• Ligaments, pulleys and septums separate and restrain the tendons. Tendons are covered in tenosynovium. Any condition which changes the volume of the tenosynovium, tendon or canal will lead to stress and friction forces resulting in tenosynovitis with pain and disability. Most commonly occur in APL, flexors, FPL, FCR.

• Treatment is rest, splinting, NSAIDs, steroid injection and release.

Suppurative tenosynovitis:
• Usually caused by a penetrating injury especially over the volar joint creases where skin

and sheath are close. Also secondary spread from felons, palmar space infections and haematogenous spread. Most commonly seen in index middle or ring finger.

• Clinically test for *Kanavel's signs*. Pain on passive extension is the most reliable sign. Treat surgically if there is no improvement after 24 hours. Perform sheath aspiration, but have a low threshold for exploration.

• Perform tendon washout with post-operative irrigation. If the tendon is necrotic the entire tendon sheath is opened and delayed tendon reconstruction performed.

Rheumatoid tenosynovitis:
• The incidence is 50% with chronic *Rheumatoid arthritis*. Tendon attrition is caused by irregular bony prominences. 50% of patients undergoing prophylactic tenosynovectomy have been found to have tendon invasion.

• Because of the risk of tendon rupture and the difficulty of predicting it, tenosynovectomy is recommended if the tenosynovitis persists after 4 months of medical treatment. It will also treat the carpal tunnel syndrome which is as high as 65%. It also treats restricted movement and triggering.

Specific tenosynovitis:
• *Trigger thumb and finger.*
• *De Quervain's disease.*
• *Intersection syndrome.*
• *Extensor pollicis longus tenosynovitis.*
• *Flexor carpi radialis tendonitis.*
• *Flexor carpi ulnaris tenosynovitis.*

Tensor fascia lata

Origin: Outer surface of anterior iliac crest between tubercle of the iliac crest and anterior superior iliac spine.

Insertion: Iliotibial tract (anterior surface of lateral condyle of tibia).

Nerve: Superior gluteal nerve (L4,5, S1).

Blood supply: Lateral circumflex femoral.

Action: Maintains knee extended and abducts the hip.

Tensor fascia lata flap

One of the earliest described free flaps, now mainly used pedicled.

Indications: Good option for abdominal wall and pressure sores of the trochanteric area.

Blood supply: Type I muscle supplied by lateral circumflex femoral vessels, which pierces the medial aspect of the flap 8–10 cm below the ASIS. Can be sensate. Cutaneous paddle reliable up to 5–8 cm above the knee. Fascia and skin can be transferred with minimal donor defect.

Procedure: The pedicle is found 10 cm distal to the ASIS. The flap is outlined laterally, with the anterior border being the line, which joins the ASIS to the patella. Develop the plane between TFL and sartorius. Incise the medial border of the fascia and expose the pedicle. See <u>Abdominal wall reconstruction</u>.

Tenzel flap

- Rotation flap based high above outer canthus based superiorly for upper eyelid reconstruction and inferiorly for lower eyelid reconstruction.
- Cut semicircular flap of skin and orbicularis muscle which is high arched. Keep incision within the peri-orbital skin. Incision should not extend beyond the lateral part of the eyebrow. The orbital septum is freed, the conjunctiva mobilized and the lid pulled medially. Resuspend new lateral canthus to intact limb of lateral canthal tendon.

See <u>Eyelid</u> reconstruction.

Terry Thomas sign

Gapped tooth sign. Widening of the scapholunate interval >3 mm. Also <u>Cortical ring sign</u>. See <u>Carpal instability</u>.

Tessier classification of craniofacial clefts

Classification of <u>Craniofacial clefts</u> by Paul Tessier.

- The orbit, nose and mouth are key landmarks.
- Clefts are numbered 0–14. 0–7 represent facial clefts and 8–14 the cranial extensions. Can have multiple and bilateral clefts.

- Broadly can be grouped into:
  - *oral-nasal clefts:* those that disrupt the nose and lip, Tessier 0, 1, 2, 3;
  - *oral ocular clefts:* those that disrupt the lip and orbit, Tessier 4, 5, 6;
  - lateral facial clefts: lateral to mouth and orbit, Tessier 7, 8, 9;
  - *cranial clefts:* affect the cranium, Tessier 10, 11, 12, 13, 14.
- If a cleft traverses both hemispheres then they generally follow the same pattern which adds up to 14 – 0–14, 1–13, 2–12, 3–11 and 4–10. This is because 8 is the most lateral and subsequent clefts move medially.

Oral nasal clefts:
Cleft 0:

- Also called median craniofacial dysraphia. Midline cleft before nasal halves have fused. Severity depends on how much has developed. May have midline lack of fusion or midline agenesis. May have bifid columella, nasal tip, septum etc. There may be a median cleft of the lip. Get diastasis between the central incisors. Orbital hypertelorism may occur or there may be absence of the nose and hypotelorism with associated brain malformation.
- The median cleft can extend cephalad as a 14 cleft or caudad as a cleft mandible called by Tessier cleft 30. May be associated with encephalocoeles.

Cleft 1:

- Nasoschizis or cleft of the lateral nose – paramedian craniofacial dysraphia.
- Extension cephalad gives a no 13.
- Originates at the lateral Cupid's bow and progresses into the nose. May be dysgenesis or a true cleft. If dysgenesis may get absent half of nose. Milder cases may have hypoplastic nose.

Cleft 2:

- Very rare. Paranasal cleft.
- The cleft originates at the lateral margin of Cupid's bow and extends to the middle third of the nostril as a deficiency and flattening of the soft tissue of the nose. There is absence of a true cleft.
- It may extend cephalad as a no. 12. It doesn't enter the orbit.

Cleft 3:
- Relatively common. Nasal ocular cleft or oblique facial cleft. Unilateral or bilateral.
- It can continue above the orbit as nos 10 or 11.
- The lip portion begins at the lateral margin of Cupid's bow. It then extends across the base of the nasal ala into the region of the normal union between the medial nasal process and the maxillary process.
- The nasolacrimal duct is blocked. Also have <u>Colobomas</u>. The cleft passes through the alveolus between lateral incisor and canine tooth. The frontal process of the maxilla may be absent.

Operations:
- Treatment of O is usually staged. The central lip defect is closed in a straight line or with a rotation. The nose cleft is opposed. If there is aplasia reconstruction is more difficult. Severe defects may require total nasal reconstruction.
- Repair of cleft 1 and 2 involve a hemirhinoplasty.
- 3 need to preserve vision. The upper eyelid is usually not severely involved. Local flaps can be used to close defects. Perform osseous reconstruction later with split calvarial grafts. requires wide mobilization of lateral tissue. Lacrimal reconstruction usually fail. Multiple secondary surgeries are required.

Oral ocular clefts: The integrity of the nose is not disrupted. Also called oblique facial clefts.

Cleft 4:
- One of the most disruptive and complicated. Begins lateral to Cupid's bow between commissure and philtrum. It passes on to cheek lateral to the ala and goes to the lower eyelid, ending medial to the punctum.
- There are varying degrees of eye deformity. There is significant osseous and soft tissue disruption but less extensive than a no 3 cleft. Always medial to the infra-orbital nerve. It may be bilateral and associated with other clefts.
- Treatment principles are similar to a no 3. Discard the labial tissue between the ipsilateral philtral ridge and the cleft otherwise the lip is excessively wide. Use interdigitating

flaps to increase the separation between the medial canthus and the nose

Cleft 5:
- The rarest of the ocular clefts. The lip cleft is medial to the commissure and extends to the lateral third of the lower eyelid. There are varying degrees of ocular involvement. The skeletal deformities are lateral to the canine and extend lateral to the infra-orbital foramen. It enters the orbit in the lateral half. Much bone may be missing.
- Correct the soft tissue defect by increasing the distance between the mouth and the lower eyelid. Use local transposition flaps. The osseous restoration consists mainly of building an orbital floor and an anterior wall of the maxilla and filling the alveolar cleft with bone.

Cleft 6:
- Includes the incomplete form of <u>Treacher Collins</u>. Patients with Nager syndrome possess the same cleft features.
- It is a transition form between the oral ocular and lateral facial clefts. The soft tissue deformity is more subtle than in Treacher Collins. It extends from lateral to the oral commissure to terminate in a coloboma of the lower lid in the lateral third. The ear is normal. There is usually a hypoplastic malar area. The palpebral fissures have an antimongoloid slant.

Operations: Difficult and multistage. Emphasis is on preservation of the globe. Correction becomes urgent to save vision. The coloboma requires correction and the inferiorly dislocated lateral canthus requires repositioning. Extensive soft tissue mobilization is required. Tissue expansion can help. Multiple Z-plasties. Perform bone grafting at the age of 8.

Lateral facial clefts:
Cleft 7:
- The most common craniofacial cleft also called Hemifacial microsomia.

Cleft 8:
- Rare and usually exists with another rare cleft. Isolated to the orbital area. The cleft extends from the lateral canthus to the temporal region. The bony component is centred at the frontozygomatic suture. The soft

tissue may just show a lateral canthal irregularity and a dermoid.

- Usually associated with _Goldenhar syndrome_. Reconstruction of the lateral commissure is achieved with local flaps.

Cleft 9:

- A transition from lateral clefts to orbital cranial clefts. Very rare. It involves the superolateral orbit dividing the eyelid into the lateral third and frequently the brow. Osseous defects occur in the superior orbital rim and temoral bone. It may be accompanied by encephalocoeles.
- Treatment consists of constructing a superior orbital rim, orbital roof and forehead. Local flaps are used for the soft tissue.

Treacher Collins **syndrome 6,7,8:**

Operations: A wide variety of operations. The lateral oral cleft of 7 is best repaired early by reapproximation of oral structures. Z-plasties are used. Lateral orbital clefts usually require proper positioning of the lateral canthus at the lateral orbital rim. Bone grafts may be required. The coloboma requires flaps from upper lid or rotation flaps. Most surgeons operate at age 6–8. Multidimensional distraction osteotomies should help correct these defects.

Cranial clefts:

These extend superiorly from the lateral orbit to midline and traverse the frontal bone, and into the vault. May be isolated or with lower clefts. The larger the defect the greater the cerebral herniation and the more pronounced is the hypertelorism.

Cleft 10:

- Corresponds to no. 4. It is positioned in the centre of the upper lid, brow and orbit. The upper lid has a coloboma. The osseous component divides the superior orbital rim, cranial base and frontal bone. Associated encephalocoele will cause hypertelorism.
- An intracranial approach will be required to correct the asymmetric hypertelorbitism.

Cleft 11:

- Usually if not always with no. 3. Get a cleft of the medial eyebrow and lid with soft tissue irregularity of the forehead. The osseous deformity extends through the cranial base

and into the ethmoid sinuses. Get orbital hypertelorism.

- Local flaps are used for the soft tissues and peri-orbital osteotomies for the hypertelorbitism.

Cleft 12: Extension of no. 2. Get an encephalocoele and disruption of the eyebrow medially. The bony cleft is severe and accompanied by hypertelorism.

Cleft 13: Cranial extension of no. 1. It extends through the olfactory groove giving a widened cribriform plate. Large defects may lead to massive encephalocoeles especially when bilateral. Get an irregular medial eyebrow with displacement into the orbit.

Cleft 14: Midline facial clefts with CNS abnormalities. The cranial extension of the no. 0 cleft but can occur alone. Produced by dysgenesis or agenesis. The holoprosencephalic malformations fall into this group. When a true cleft exists, herniation of the intracranial contents results in morphokinetic arrest of normal migration of the orbit. They remain in the embryonic position giving hypertelorism and cranium bifida. The nose may be widely separated. In severe cases, may get cyclopia or cebocephaly. Life expectancy is limited.

Operations: Preserve brain function, re-establish the cranial vault and reposition facial structures. Correct the cleft early before rupture of meninges occurs.

Tessier classification of hypertelorism

Classifies _Hypertelorism_ based on the interorbital distance:
- _Type I:_ 30–34 mm.
- _Type II:_ 35–39 mm.
- _Type III:_ >39 mm.

Tessier, Paul

Plastic surgeon in Paris, considered the father of craniofacial surgery, being the first to mobilize and reposition the orbits. Head of the plastic surgery and burns department at the Hôpital Foch (Suresnes, Paris) from 1946 to 1983.

TGF-β

_See _Cytokines and growth factors__.

Thalidomide

Used in 1950s and 1960s in early trimester nausea. One cause of limb malformations. Stopped in 1961. Cause intercalated _Transverse arrest_.

Thatte and Thatte classification

Classification of _Venous flaps_.
- _Type 1:_ supplied by a single venous pedicle.
- _Type 2:_ venous flow-through flaps supplied by a vein, which enters one side of the flap and exits from the other.
- _Type 3:_ arterialized venous flaps.

Thenar flap

Vascularized pedicle flap from thenar skin which can be used in the reconstruction of _Fingertip injuries_. Base is perpendicular to thumb MP flexion crease. Divide after 2 weeks. Keep as high as possible on thenar eminence, as radial as possible. Minimize PIPJ flexion, release pedicle as soon as possible. More useful in children as the position of the finger leads to significant stiffness in the adult hand.

Thigh lift

Excision of lax thigh skin usually due to weight loss. If there is still a lot of fat they benefit less as it is difficult to fix the skin into position. Medial thigh lift usually only benefits the upper inner thigh. Lateral thigh lift will benefit the buttock and thighs. Abdominoplasty can benefit anterior and medial thighs. Most patients will benefit from inner and outer thigh lift.

Markings: Mark normal underwear. Make a transverse line just below the upper border which will be the planned eventual scar. Mark width of excision, laterally usually around 10–12 cm, 75% below the reference line. Medially 4–6 cm. Correct any mons descent.

Operation: Place patient in the lateral position and infiltrate. The depth of incision is more superficial over the femoral triangle to leave some lymphatics intact. Suture superficial fascial system to Colles' fascia.

Thoracic outlet syndrome

Examination:
- _General:_ look at posture – kyphosis, slumping of shoulders, angle of root of neck, colour and temperature of upper limbs, examine brachial plexus.
- _Vascular tests:_
  ○ _Adson's test. (adduction):_ arm is adducted and neck extended and chin turned to affected side;
  ○ _Wright's hyperabduction test. (right answer):_ arm maximally abducted;
  ○ _Falconer's test (falcon diving):_ military brace position;
  ○ _Roo's test_ (I surrender).
- _Neurological tests:_
  ○ _Morley's compression test:_ pressure over the plexus;
  ○ _Tinel's test:_ percussion over the nerve.

Other tests:
  ○ _Cervical rotation lateral flexion test:_ test for first rib costotransverse joint dysfunction; the head is turned away from the side being examined and the neck is flexed; if the neck is not able to flex due to a bony block, this is positive; the block may be costotransverse joint subluxation;
  ○ _Spurling's test:_ tests for cervical disc involvement.

Assessment:
- Vascular or neurological presentation. Brachial plexus and subclavian artery come through interscalene triangle bordered by anterior and medial scalene muscles and first rib. Symptoms are vague.
- Neurology is most commonly with ulnar nerve symptoms.
- Pulse obliteration may occur. Elevate arms above head while flexing digits for 3 minutes but also common in normal subjects.
- EMG does not help.
- Classic person is obese woman with large breasts.

Treatment:
  ○ Postural correction, breast reduction, psychological help.

○ Surgery is the last resort – rib resection through transaxillary approach – not very successful, combine with scalenotomy.

○ Operation technique: lateral decubitus, axillary approach, remove correct rib which can be difficult – use XR if necessary. Do scalenotomy from 2nd rib. Remove first rib (or cervical rib if present). Incidence of cervical rib is 0.5%. Similar symptoms from cubital tunnel and cervical disc.

Thrombus

• Exposure of collagen fibres is a trigger for platelet aggregation and degranulation. Releases ADP and thromboxane.

• These stimulate further platelet aggregation.

See _Coagulation cascade_, _Heparin_, _Dextran_, _Aspirin_, _Microsurgery_.

Thumb duplication

6% of congenital upper limb abnormalities. Aetiology is unknown, but rarely syndromic (Carpenter's).

Classification: _Wassel_ classification. The most common level is duplication of the proximal and distal phalanges (type IV). It occurs sporadically and unilaterally, though type VII (triphalangial thumb) may be hereditary and associated with big toe polydactyly. The ulnar digit is more developed and is the one preserved.

Treatment principles: Neither thumb is normal, all tissues are involved. The remaining thumb will be thinner and stiffer. The operation is not ablation of one of the thumbs but attempts to create the best possible thumb from the 2 abnormal digits.

Treatment options:

• Remove one duplicate and reconstruct the other. Use for Wassell type 4 (most common). Need to reconstruct the radial collateral ligament. Usually perform with a periosteal flap from the amputated digit.

• Remove equal parts of both and combine the remaining to form a single finger. Usually for more distal duplications. An example is the _Bilhaut–Cloquet_ operation.

• Remove unequal parts and combine.

See _Congenital hand anomalies_. See _Polydactyly_.

Thumb hypoplasia

• This is a radial longitudinal failure of formation.

• Associated with ring D chromosome abnormalities, Holt–Oram syndrome, trisomy-18 syndrome, Rothmund–Thompson syndrome and thalidomide.

• A completely absent thumb is almost always associated with an absent radius except in Fanconi's syndrome when the thumb is present even though the radius is absent.

Classification: _Blauth_.

• _I:_ minor hypoplasia, normally functioning.

• _II:_ thumb small and less stable. Get adduction contracture of web space, lack of thenar muscles and laxity of UCL.

• _III:_ type II elements with skeletal hypoplasia, CMC vestigial, absent intrinsics, rudimentary extrinsics:

  ○ III-A has intact CMC;
  ○ III-B has basal metacarpal aplasia.

• _IV:_ floating thumb – pouce flottant.

• _V:_ total absence.

Treatment principles:

• Type I do not require treatment.

• Type II and III with stable CMC joints (IIIA) are candidates for reconstruction. Web space needs deepening, extrinsic tendon corrections and opponensplasty (Huber).

• Type IIIB, IV and V require pollicization. Shorten.

See _Congenital hand anomalies_.

Thumb-printing/copper beaten sign

XR appearance of skull with raised intracranial pressure seen in _Craniosynostosis_.

Thumb reconstruction

• _Pollicization_.

• _Toe to hand transfer_.

Thyroglossal duct cysts

• A remnant from the descent of the thyroid from the base of the tongue. It usually reaches the final position by 8 weeks of gestation and the duct disappears. It may remain at any point on the path.

- Commonly present in the 20s and in the midline at the level of the thyrohyoid membrane.
- Excision of the tract is required which may involve resection of hyoid bone. Thyroid scans should be performed to confirm the presence of other thyroid tissue. Usually present as a slow-growing mass in the midline. Often present when they are infected. They move up and down on swallowing. Image the neck and assess thyroid preoperatively.

Operation: Horizontal skin incision. Retract strap muscles. Transect infrahyoid strap muscles to clear the junction of greater cornu and body of hyoid to enable the tract to be excised from the pharyngeal wall in continuity with the midpoint of the hyoid. As the tongue is approached, a finger is placed in the foramen caecum at the base of the tongue to find the tissue to be removed with the tract.
See Head and neck.

Thyroid nodule

- First determine TSH and thyroxine levels. If the patient is hyperthyroid, a scan will distinguish a hot from a cold nodule. A hot (hyperfunctioning) nodule does not require further investigation. If TSH is normal, do FNA. Around 5% of FNAs are suggestive of malignancy. Solitary benign nodules are treated with thyroid suppression therapy. In patients over 50 with atypia of follicular epithelium thyroidectomy is recommended as the risk of malignant change is high.
- Prognostic factors predicting outcome are age, size, histology, spread, nodes and metastasis.

Tibia

- Blood supply is from nutrient artery, which is from the posterior tibial artery, metaphyseal vessels and periosteal vessels.
- The nutrient artery penetrates the tibialis posterior then follows the nutrient channel on the posterior surface of the tibia. It traverses intracortically. Once in the medulla it

divides into proximal and distal branches, which supply the inner 2/3 of the cortex.

- Metaphyseal arteries anastomose with proximal branches.
- Periosteal vessels branch from major limb vessels and course perpendicular to the axis of the tibia thus both sides of a fracture may derive the majority of their blood supply via these vessels as the other sources may be compromised by the fracture.

TILT

Triquetral impingement ligament tear.

- Ulnar wrist pain involving triquetrum.
- Triad of localized triquetral pain, hyperflexion injury and normal radiographs.
- Cuff of fibrous tissue becomes detached from ulnar sling mechanism and chronically impinges on triquetrum.
- Get synovitis, bony eburnation and pain. Find point tenderness on triquetrum just distal to ulnar styloid.

Tinel's sign

- Percussion over a nerve eliciting a tingling sensation.
- Commonly elicited at sites of suspected nerve compression or in the assessment of nerve repair where tingling represents the leading edge of regeneration.
- A Tinel's sign which does not advance may represent misdirected extra epineurial growth cones.
- Can get a Tinel's sign in motor nerves such as the facial nerve, probably due to proprioreceptor fibres.

Tissue-cultured skin

Human epidermal cells grown *in vivo*, stable enough for grafting.

- Whole skin is enzymatically digested with trypsin to produce a single cell suspension of keratinocytes which are grown as a monolayer on irradiated mouse fibroblasts. From a section of skin 2 cm^2, a 1 m^2 sheet can be made in 3–6 weeks.
- Used for areas of large skin loss such as burns or non-healing areas such as leg ulcers.
- A disadvantage is hyperkeratosis for long periods. It may be that the epidermis is

hyperproliferative without the checks of the dermis. There may be a potential risk of malignancy as they are cultured in mitogens. They are also expensive and fragile.

Tissue expansion

- First performed by Charles Neumann who expanded preauricular skin in 1956. Then popularized by Chedomir Radovan in 1984.
- An expander is inserted subcutaneously and filled gradually over weeks until the desired degree of skin expansion has occurred.

Mechanism of expansion

- 70% stretch, 30% growth. In the short term get interstitial fluid forced out giving greater expansion. Viscoelastic deformation (creep) and recruitment of adjacent mobile soft tissue occurs along with growth with increased collagen and ground substance.
- Mechanical creep refers to elongation of skin under constant load over time. Collagen fibres stretch and realign, elastin fragments, water is displaced. All occurs during intraoperative expansion.
- Biological creep refers to the generation of new tissue due to a chronic stretching force.
- Stretch-relaxation describes reduction in the resistance of skin to stretching force with time

Histology:

- *Epidermis*; thickens due to hyperplasia with increased mitoses.
- *Dermis:* thins, collagen realigns to become more parallel, elastin fibres rupture.
- *Adipose tissue:* cells atrophy with some permanent loss.
- Vascular supply is increased with increased VEGF.
- *Capsule:* Paysk described 4 zones within the capsule surrounding an expander:
  - Inner zone is a fibrin layer within the capsule surrounding the expander
  - Central zone contains elongated fibroblasts and myofibroblasts
  - Transitional zone of loose collagen fibres
  - Outer zone contains blood vessels and collagen.

Principles:

- Expansion provides tissue that is most like the lost tissue and is sensate. The donor defect is minimal, there is good contour and it is not a major procedure.
- May be a remote incision, or an incision orientated radially to the edge of the expander. Place incisions in stable tissue which will heal. start injections one week after insertion if the wound is stable.
- To gauge the degree of expansion needed, measure the arc and subtract the width to give the amount of advancement. 20% of measured expansion is lost so over expand. Capsular scoring may improve advancement.
- It is limited by the amount of relaxation and growth of tissues. Irradiation and scar make it more difficult or impossible.

Complications:

- Migrations, extrusion, infection, rupture, wound dehiscence.
- It is contraindicated near malignancy, under skin graft, under tight tissue, near an open wound and in an irradiated field.

Rapid intra-operative tissue expansion:

- Uses cyclical loading or temporary expanders for 3–5 min of stretch and 2 min of relaxation.
- This takes advantage of the viscoelastic skin properties of mechanical creep and stretch-relaxation to cause incremental increase in length of the loaded skin. This is partly due to extrusion of fluid from between collagen fibres. Also due to recruitment of adjacent skin. May get 40% increase in surface area and flap length. At each expansion the end point is tautness of skin, not blanching. With larger expanders each inflation can last 20 minutes with 10 minutes rest.

Tissue plasminogen activator (t-PA)

- Second generation plasminogen activator with activity specific for fibrin. Fibrin posesses t-PA binding sites close to the plasminogen binding sites and therefore t-PA promotes plasminogen activation and lysis of clot.
- It has no antigenicity and no febrile or allergic reactions. It is more effective than streptokinase in acute limb ischaemia.

Titanium

Unalloyed it is very maleable. Titanium alloy (titanium-aluminium-vanadium has a tensile strength like vitallium and has a high biocompatibility. It is the least corrosive with the least artifact on CT/MRI.
See *Alloplasts*.

Toe to hand transfer

- The first toe to hand transplant was performed by Nicoladoni in 1898 by attaching a pedicled toe to the hand for 3 weeks in a 5-year-old boy.
- Note the level of amputation and the dominance. Length, strength of grasp and sensation is more important for the non-dominant hand as it grasps objects for the dominant side.
- Reconstruction is more difficult when there is agenesis as other structures will be abnormal. They are easier with constriction rings.
- The 2nd toe can be used for congenital absence as it hypertrophies. It is a preferable donor loss. Great toe atrophies to some degree. Attempts to improve size mismatch have been made and in particular the wrap-around though there is a functional loss.
- Great toe is the best option unless metacarpal is also required in which case 2nd toe can be used or big toe with 2nd metatarsal.
- Homotransplantation is possible, but problematic as skin provokes the strongest immune response.

Anatomy: Many variations to the blood supply. The most common main supply is from the dorsalis pedis to the superficial first metatarsal artery. Next is the plantar first metatarsal artery either from plantar system or dorsal via a perforating branch. The ideal system is the dominant dorsal system. A long vascular pedicle can be mobilized, which can reach mid forearm if needed.

Intra-operative drugs: Heparin in saline 100 units/ml is used to irrigate the operative field. Dextran can be used. Papaverine 60 units/ml is used after anastomosis. For spasm, papaverine 6 units/ml can be used. Streptokinase can be used to flush out clots. Dilute to 5000 units/ml and infuse 25 000–50 000 into the flap.

Technique: Mark the pedicle on the upper surface to prevent a twist. Rotation can easily happen and is disastrous. First fix the bone. Vasospasm is more severe in children and women.
See *Thumb reconstruction*.

Tongue carcinoma

- Mainly in 60s, but also young and even adolescent.
- It is the most common site for intra-oral malignancy and most tongue cancers are in the anterior two-thirds on the lateral borders or the ventral surface.
- It usually presents as a lateral chronic non-healing ulcer and spreads locally to the floor of the mouth.
- It usually presents as a T2 lesion.
- It contains a rich lymphatic supply so that 40% have nodal involvement and 20% have bilateral nodes.

Treatment:
- T1: surgery or RT. Wedge resection under LA or *Brachytherapy*.
- T2 lesions will require partial glossectomy and possibly mandible if involved.
- ELND for T2 and T3 N0 necks. Give RT as well.

Results: 5-year survival rate is 50%.
See *Head and neck cancer*. See *Glossectomy*.

Tonsil carcinoma

- Can be exophytic or deeply invasive.
- Tend to present late with 76% of patients having nodal involvement at presentation.
- Anterior tonsillar pillar lesions tend to have a better prognosis. Tonsillar fossa tumours tend to be more common and all are more radiosensitive than other sites.

Treatment:
- Most T1–T3 tumours can be cured with RT.
- Stage I and II are resected, and neck dissection performed. Stage III and IV have resection, neck dissection and radiotherapy.
See *Head and neck cancer*.

Torre's syndrome

See *Sebaceous adenoma*. See *Muir–Torre syndrome*.

Torticollis

- 'Twisted neck'. Secondary to fixed shortening of sternocleidomastoid. The head tilts towards the affected side with the chin towards the opposite side.
- The incidence is 0.3%, rarely bilateral. M = F, Lt = Rt. Higher incidence in breech.
- The aetiology is unknown. Theories include muscle injury and haematoma at birth, venous occlusion, intrauterine malposition causing ischaemic fibrosis.
- *Pathology:* fibrous tissue, no muscle degeneration, no evidence of haematoma.

Classification:

- Congenital: muscular, vertebral.
- Acquired: 2° to muscle (trauma, infection), ocular, spasmodic (usually >40 years), psychogenic.

Clinical presentation:

- Usually a small tumour is felt in the first few weeks of birth, and the SCM feels short, stiff and cord-like.
- The head is tilted and rotated to the affected side with chin up and away to the opposite side. The shoulder may be higher on the affected side.
- The tumour may increase for some weeks then remain static then slowly resolve by 8 months.
- If it doesn't resolve scoliosis capitus results. The mastoid, ear, jaw, maxilla and orbit can be growth restricted and pulled down giving facial asymmetry.

Treatment:

- *Non-operative:* reassurance, physiotherapy, stretching, botox.
- *Operative:* if it persists after 1 year. Options:
  ○ perform total excision of the SCM (may leave a hollow);
  ○ tenotomy;
  ○ *Foelderl's lengthening:* clavicular head divided in middle ⅓ and transposed to cranial end of sternal head;
  ○ *LaFerte lengthening:* vertical split and slide.

Outcome: From surgery excellent results. Best if <4 years. Beware spinal accessory nerve, recurrence, diplopia and instability.
See Craniosynostosis.

Tourniquet time

- Tourniquet nerve damage will result in lower motor neuron damage with reduced pin prick, reduced vibration sense and reduced movement.
- MDU recommends:
  ○ apply in healthy limbs;
  ○ TQ size 10 cm arm and 15 cm leg;
  ○ *pressure:* arm 50–100 mmHg above systolic and leg double systolic or arm 200–250 mmHg, leg 250–350 mmHg;
  ○ time absolute maximum 3 hours (recovers in 5–7 days), generally do not exceed 2 hours. Document duration and pressure.

Toxic Shock Syndrome (TSS)

- A systemic illness, which can occur following _Burns_ due to colonization of the burn with toxin producing strains of *S. aureus*.
- Enterotoxin is the most common toxin and is produced by up to 20% of strains of *S. aureus*. It works by over-stimulating the immune system.
- It usually start 3 days after a burn and can occur even in minor burns.
- The incidence in childhood burns is not known, but it is estimated that 2.5% of burns admissions in children develop TSS.
- Get fever, myalgia, pain, nausea and DandV followed by hypotension.

Tracheostomy

Emergency: Perform cricothyroidotomy. Make an incision through the cricothyroid membrane which lies superficially. The superficial tissue is relatively avascular apart from the anterior jugular veins. Emergency low tracheotomy is performed through a tracheal incision below the 2nd tracheal ring.

Elective: Incise below the thyroid isthmus in the 2nd–3rd or 3rd–4th tracheal ring. Place sheet under patient to extend head and push back the shoulders. Incise transversely 4 cm, 2–3 cm above the suprasternal notch directly over the sternal opening. Incise vertically in the midline between the strap muscles. The isthmus may need to be ligated and divided. Place hooks in the trachea and incise once the balloon is deflated. Incise trachea vertically between the 3rd and 4th tracheal ring. Remove the ETT and insert the tracheostomy tube.

TRAM flap

Transverse rectus abdominus myocutaneous flap. Most frequently used for _Breast reconstruction_. Rectus is taken with overlying fat and skin. It may be pedicled on one or both superior epigastric arteries or free on the inferior epigastric artery.

Anatomy:

- _Vascular anatomy:_ there is some confusion with the description of zones. I and II are served by perforators from deep inferior epigastric artery (DIEA) and superficial inferior epigastric artery (SIEA). III and IV is served through communications between SIEA and superficial circumflex iliac artery. Superior skin island receives its blood supply from above.

Risk factors: Obesity, smokers, abdominal scars, RT. Systemic diseases such as diabetes, heart disease.

Pedicled:

- Design the flap higher in the abdomen than a free flap because of the reduced vascularity.
- The flap can be made more reliable by:
  - _delay:_ ligate inferior epigastric artery 2 weeks prior to raising the flap;
  - _supercharging:_ anastomose the inferior epigastric vessels to the thoracodorsal vessels.

Free: Dissect from side opposite to where the vessels are planned to be used first so that the position of the perforators can be assessed, then when doing the contralateral side they can be divided. Anastomose to thoracodorsal vessels or internal thoracic. Better vascularity and less muscle taken than with a pedicled TRAM.

Complications: Fat necrosis, partial loss and skin necrosis, abdominal hernias, wound dehiscence, size mismatch.

Contraindications: Previous abdominoplasty, abdominal scars suggesting division of the superior epigastric artery would be a contraindication to a pedicled TRAM flap.

Alternatives: Gluteal flap, latissimus dorsi flap, lateral thigh flap, Ruben's flap.

Tranquili–Leali flap

See _Atasoy volar V-Y flap_:

Transcyte

Human fibroblast-derived temporary skin substitute.

- Transcyte provides a temporary protective barrier.
- It consists of a polymer membrane and newborn human fibroblast cells. This nylon mesh is coated with porcine dermal collagen and bonded to silicone. As fibroblasts proliferate within the nylon mesh during the manufacturing process, they secrete human dermal collagen, matrix proteins and growth factors. Following freezing, no cellular metabolic activity remains; however, the tissue matrix and bound growth factors are left intact.

See _Biological skin substitutes_.

Transplant immunology

Cells of immune response:

- _Antigen presenting cells:_ of lymphoid origin. Bind antigen and process it. As well as presenting antigens to other cells, some, particularly macrophages, secrete _Cytokines_.
- _B cells:_ produce antibodies.
- _T cells:_ central in coordinating immune response. Divided into 2 subsets determined by the presence of CD4 or CD8. CD4 cells are T-helper cells, and CD8 are T-cytotoxic cells. CD4 cells secrete cytokines. CD8 cells bind cells of particular antigen type and kill them. Natural killer cells respond without requiring presensitization. They have a role in tumour surveillance and they can detect cells not expressing self-antigens.

Graft rejection:

- _Hyperacute rejection:_ almost immediately. Due to preformed abs, e.g. blood group. This is a major obstacle to xenotransplantation.
- _Acute rejection:_ days to weeks after transplantation. T cell-mediated.
- _Chronic rejection:_ Months to years after transplantation. Multifactorial and may be slowed by immunosupression.

Immunological testing: As well as blood type, HLA −A,B and Dr should be matched. A heterozygous individual with all matching would have six-antigen match. See MHC.

Clinical immunosupression:

- Unless the immune system is partially suppressed, all tissue except in identical twins will eventually be rejected. Combinations are given.
- *Steroids:* downregulates all T-cell functions. Complications include hypertension, hyperglycaemia, osteoporosis and peptic ulcer.
- *Azathioprine:* interferes with nucleic acid synthesis. Inhibits differentiation and proliferation of lymphocytes. Can result in severe leucopenia. Also hepatic toxicity.
- *Methotrexate:* folic acid antagonist. Inhibits DNA and RNA synthesis.
- *Cyclosporine:* provides immunosuppresion without marrow depression. Inhibits IL-2 and therefore T-cell differentiation. Nephrotoxic.

Allotransplantation of tissues:

- *Bone:* frozen bone allograft is now common practice for reconstructing long bone defects. Either to bridge a gap or provide articular surface. They are devoid of living cells and become replaced by host bone. Immunosuppressants are not required though replacement is slow, starting at a year. Bone is removed in a theatre, soft tissue and marrow is removed and bone is frozen in a glycerol solution. Can also be freeze-dried. Also gamma-irradiated. They have been used for craniofacial procedures. Hand surgery patients treated for enchondromas with allograft compared favourably to autograft from iliac crest. Good results have been obtained in children with congenital hand problems. Avascular necrosis of scaphoid has been treated successfully with allograft – allograft being used to replace the proximal fragment and union being obtained.
- *Cartilage:* used for facial skeleton but high rate of resorption. It may be useful to resurface joints.
- *Skin:* primarily for burn victims. Risk of disease transmission. Rejection in around 14 days. Immunosuppression has been tried

for children. Attempts to reduce the antigenicity of skin by exposing to UVB, stripping epidermis, and preserving in glycerol. Dermal scaffolds with all cellular elements removed have been produced. Alloderm is acellular dermis. Dermagraft is human neonatal dermal fibroblasts seeded onto a synthetic mesh.

- *Nerve:* has not been used much and immunosupression is required for a short period.

Transposition flap

Rectangular flap, which rotates about a pivot point laterally into an adjacent area. Because it becomes shorter in length as it rotates, it is made longer than the defect. The pivot point is at the base distal to the defect. A backcut will reduce tension but will narrow the pedicle. See Rotation flap.

Transverse arrest: congenital hand

Complete: At any level, but most commonly at the junction of the proximal third and the middle third of the forearm. Treatment is usually non-surgical and involves the fitting of a suitable prosthesis.

Intercalated:

- Phocomelia is an intercalated deficiency of the upper limb. It was linked to thalidomide use. Thalidomide is still used for treatment of leprosy.
- Phocomelia is divided into:
  ○ *complete phocomelia:* the hand on the torso;
  ○ *proximal phocomelia:* normal forearm and hand on torso;
  ○ *distal phocomelia:* hand attached to upper arm and elbow.

Treatment:

- *Upper 1/3 forearm:* fit prosthesis by 6 months. Surgery to lengthen is not indicated. The Krukenberg procedure may help.
- *Carpus, metacarpus, phalanges.* Absence of digits may be transverse absence, cleft hand, constrict ring or symbrachydactyly. Range of treatment is the same for all. Most have a normal wrist joint so palpate for skeletal parts. If the thumb metacarpal is present

check the basal joint. Treat with distraction manoplasty – to lengthen skin envelope and toe phalangeal transfer. They survive well if performed before 15 months. Take periosteum and repair collateral ligaments. Bony distraction is performed for 4th or 5th metacarpal remnant. Toe transfer – function difficult to achieve as tendons and nerves are rudimentary.

Transverse carpal ligament

- The flexor retinaculum is a fibrous band arching over the carpus. Forming the roof of the carpal tunnel. See *Carpal tunnel syndrome*.
- Medially it is attached to the pisiform and hamulus of the hamate and laterally to the tubercle of the scaphoid and ridge of trapezium.
- Palmaris longus and flexor carpi radialis are partly inserted into it, and the short muscles of the thumb and little finger take their origin from it.

Trapeziectomy: operative

- Incision from base of metacarpal curved towards FCR. Preserve radial artery and superficial branches of radial nerve.
- Establish position of CMC joint with needle and incise capsule to expose trapezium and base of metacarpal.
- Remove trapezium with combination of osteotome and rongeur. Preserve FCR in base.
- Expose area of metacarpal base and drill with a 2.3 mm rosehead burr.
- Through short transverse incisions expose FCR and place slings around. Pass prolene suture through one third of the tendon proximally. Strip down distally. Divide proximally. Pass through the line of FCR into the CMC space.
- Pass wire through hole in metacarpal base and hook suture tied to tendon. Bring tendon through, then back around intact FCR. Suture tendon to metacarpal and onto intact FCR. Wrap twice and leave any remaining tendon as spacer.
- Close capsule, skin. K wire MCP joint and apply a POP backslab. Change in 4 days for a full plaster, leave for a further 5 weeks then

apply a thermoplastic splint for a further 3 weeks.

Trapezium: fracture

- 5% of carpal bone injuries. Either through the body or the ridge. Fractures of the ridge are typically caused by a fall on the outstretched hand.
- Mechanism is either a direct blow or avulsion of TCL. Get volar point tenderness.

Classification: Ridge fractures classified by Palmer.
- *Type I:* through base, heal well with immobilization.
- *Type II:* through tip. High incidence of nonunion.

Treatment:
- Ridge fractures are treated conservatively.
- Body fractures are treated by open reduction if displaced.

Trapezius

Origin: External occipital protuberance, ligamentum nuchae, spinous processes of C7–T12.

Insertion: Into clavicle, spine of scapula and acromion.

Blood supply: Based on the superficial transverse cervical artery. Type II muscle with minor pedicles from the dorsal scapular artery, posterior intercostals and a branch of occipital artery.

Nerve supply: Spinal root of accessory nerve (motor) and cervical nerves (C3 and C4) (pain and proprioception).

Action: Elevates, retracts, depresses and rotates scapula.

Trapezius flap

- Can be a lateral or lower musculocutaneous flap.
- Useful for midline defects of the upper spine and occiput. It may be used for *Intra-oral* reconstruction. Only the muscle under the skin and around the pedicle is raised.
- Shoulder strength can be preserved as long as the upper portion of muscle and the

spinal accessory nerve are preserved. The lower region is functionally and aesthetically dispensable.

Technique:

- The flap pivots on the descending branch of the transverse cervical artery which runs along the deep aspect of the muscle and enters 5–7 cm lateral to the midline at the level of C7 spinous process.
- Mark C7 to T12 and the acromion. This triangle contains the trapezius.
- An extended flap can be used, but should be delayed.
- The skin island should be 8 cm wide. The larger the segment the more likely it is to contain perforators and to survive.
- Skin is incised down to muscle and lateral border is identified. Muscle is separated from paraspinous muscle. The vascular pedicle is found and the flap raised.

See *Trunk reconstruction*.

Trapezometacarpal joint

- A biconcave saddle joint.
- The proximal surface is concave radioulnar and convex dorsopalmar.
- Base of metacarpal is saddle shaped centrally with volar and dorsal peaks. The volar beak has no ligament.

Ligaments: intra- and extra capsular.

- *Anterior oblique ligament:* the most important. Also call the beak ligament. From the palmar tubercle of trapezium to palmar tubercle of 1st metacarpal base (beak). Gets weak in OA leading to subluxation.
- *Posterior oblique ligament:* strong dorsal ligament running from dorsoulnar tubercle of trapezium to palmar tubercle of metacarpal. Tight in opposition and abduction.
- *Dorsoradial ligament:* intracapsular from dorsoradial tubercle of trapezium to metacarpal. Tight in adduction. Gets attenuated in OA.
- *First intermetacarpal ligament:* strong extracapsular ligament attached to the base of first and second metacarpal. Stretched in CMC OA allowing radial subluxation of the base of metacarpal.

- *Ulnar collateral ligament:* extracapsular from TCL to ulnar tubercle of base of 1st MC. Tight in extension, abduction and pronation

Movement:

- Simple movements such as abduction, extension and complex movements, such as opposition and retroposition.
- Simple movement occurs in the saddle joint but complex movements also involve the articulation between the convex spheroidal surface of the trapezium and the radial slope of the base of first metacarpal. With adduction get internal rotation which helps pulp-to-pulp pinch of the thumb.

Trauma

Tissue damage due to the energy exchange between the patient and the environment. Classify by:

Aetiology:

- *Mechanical:* blunt, penetrating, blast.
- *Thermal.*
- *Chemical.*
- *Electrical.*
- *Electromagnetic.*

Degree of energy exchange: Low, medium or high.

Setting:

- Iatrogenic.
- Civilian trauma (RTA, industrial, etc.).
- Armed conflict (GSW, mine, chemical weapons, etc.).

Traumatic dystrophy

- Minor traumatic dystrophy: the most common clinical form of <u>RSD</u>. Initiated by an injury which doesn't involve nerve damage, such as crushed fingers or sprains.
- *Major traumatic dystrophy:* involves major trauma to the hand, such as Colles' fracture, but no specific nerve injury.

Treacher Collins

Described by Treacher Collins in 1900. Also called Francheshetti syndrome and mandibulofacial dysostosis.

- Autosomal dominant. Gene on chromosome 5. See *Craniofacial genetics*.
- Incidence 1:25 000, M = F.
- *Tessier* cleft 6, 7 and 8 with malformation of structures derived from the first and second pharyngeal arches and pouch.
- Facial abnormalities are symmetric and bilateral.
- Get *Coloboma* of the lower eyelid with no. 6, absence of zygomatic arch with no. 7, absence of the orbital rim with no. 8.
- Hypoplasia of the supra-orbital area and zygoma.
- The face is narrow with depressed cheekbones, receding chin and large downturned mouth. Described as bird-like with anti-Mongoloid slant, hypertelorism.
- 35% have a cleft palate. Also micrognathia.
- The external ears are absent, malformed, or malposed.
- Hearing is impaired due to variable degrees of aural atresia.
- The degree of deformity at birth is fairly stable.
- The airway may be compromised with constricted nasal passages secondary to maxillary hypoplasia resulting in choanal stenosis or atresia. It may be worsened by cleft palate repair. Feeding and swallowing may also be affected.

Treatment summary:
- A tracheostomy may be required.
- *Zygoma and orbit:* bone graft.
- *Mandible:* rib grafts, advancement, distractions, bimaxillary procedures.
- *Ear:* reconstruction.

Reconstruction:
- *Zygomatic and orbital reconstruction:* calvarial bone grafts. Expose through a coronal (scalp) incision. Also vascularized cranial bone transfers for zygomatic reconstruction but injury to the frontal branch of the facial nerve is likely. Usually perform at age 7, when bony development is nearly complete.
- *Maxillomandibular reconstruction:* get an Angle Class II anterior open-bite malocclusion. Reconstruction is performed in early skeletal maturity when orthodontic treatment can also be performed.

- *Nasal reconstruction:* The bridge is wide with a mid-dorsal hump, with a long nose and a drooping tip. Perform rhinoplasty with osteotomies, but first perform orthognathic surgery.
- *Eyelid reconstruction* has not been too successful. Transposition of upper eyelid to lower eyelid skin has been performed. Also FTSG used, but get a patchy look.
- *Ear reconstruction.*
- *External ear canal and middle ear reconstruction:* most of the hearing loss is due to the middle ear malformations though atresia or stenosis of external auditory canal may contribute. Surgery is not very successful. Patients usually require a bone-conduction hearing aid so middle ear reconstruction is rarely indicated. The hearing aid may be a traditional unit, a modified amplification system, or a bone-anchored conduction unit.

Triangular fibrocartilage
Anatomy:
- **TFCC:** articular disc that is 1–2 mm thick originating from the base of the ulnar styloid and inserting into the sigmoid notch of the radius, the ulnocarpal ligament, the UCL and dorsal and palmar radioulnar joint. It is the major stabilizer of the *DRUJ*. It is a load-bearing structure between the carpus and ulna. 20% of load is transmitted across it, the rest is across the radiocarpal joint.

Clinical: With tear patient gets ulnar-sided wrist pain following a twisting injury. May get popping or catching. Assess stability of radioulnar joint. Traumatic peripheral tears can heal, central tears cannot.

Investigations:
- XR: look for ulna minus variance, ulnar styloid fracture which may disrupt the attachment of the TFCC. In *Pseudogout* get calcification of TFCC.
- Triple injection arthrogram, MRI.
- *Arthroscopy:* trampoline test – during arthroscopy the centre is balloted. It should feel firm. If not, a peripheral tear is suspected.

Classification: by Palmer, two types – traumatic and degenerative.

- *Class I:* traumatic TFCC tears:
  - *type A:* central perforation (most common);
  - *type B:* avulsion from ulnar attachment;
  - *type C:* avulsion from ulnocarpal ligaments;
  - *type D:* avulsion from sigmoid notch.
- *Class 2* – degenerative tears:
  - *stage 1:* TFCC wear;
  - *stage 2:* wear with lunate/ulnar chondromalacia;
  - *stage 3:* TFCC perforation, chondromalacia;
  - *stage 4:* TFCC perforation, chondromalacia, lunotriquetral ligament perforation;
  - *stage 5:* all above with ulnocarpal arthritis.

Treatment:
- For traumatic based on type of tear and length of ulna:
  - A: debride;
  - B: open or arthroscopic reattachment;
  - C: debridement or open repair;
  - D: as B.
- If positive ulnar variance do shortening ulnar osteotomy, see _Ulnocarpal impaction syndrome_.
- As long as the dorsal and palmar radio-ulnar ligaments are preserved, debridement of the central portion of the horizontal disc does not compromise stability of the radioulnar joint.

Triangular ligament
- Formed by the transverse fibres, which connect the lateral bands of the _Extensor tendons_ at the level of the proximal part of the middle phalanx, which may limit volar and lateral shifting of the lateral bands during flexion.
- It is attenuated in _Boutonnière deformity_ contributing to volar subluxation of the lateral bands.

Triangular space
- Teres minor superiorly, teres major inferiorly, long head of triceps laterally.
- Through this space emerges the circumflex scapular artery.
See _Scapular flap_. See _Quadrilateral space_.

Trichiasis
Eyelashes turned into the globe. Often associated with entropion.

Tricho-epithelioma
- Solitary or multiple lesions, generally benign and do not metastasize. Can be confused with BCC.
- Best described pathologically as a highly differentiated keratotic basal cell epithelioma.
- The multiple form is inherited as an autosomal dominant disorder.
- 2–5 mm diameter firm flesh-coloured papules developing early in life especially on the nose, nasolabial folds, forehead, upper lip and eyelids.
- Treatment is excision.

Trichofolliculoma
- Hair follicle naevus on the face or scalp.
- Skin-coloured papule with central pore containing white hairs.
- Resemble BCCs, but contain keratin-filled macrocysts.
- Treatment is excision.

Tricholemmal cyst
Also called Pilar cyst.
- 90% in the scalp. Derived from the outer hair sheath.
- They are true cysts consisting of a cell wall. The cyst content often has focal calcification.
See _Epithelial cysts_.

Tricholemmoma
- Solitary facial papule. Rarely multiple papules occur as part of _Cowden disease_.
- Get buds of follicular sheath-type epithelial cells which show pallisading.
- It is benign, usually occurs on the scalp and is treated by excision.

Trichloro-acetic acid peels (TCA)
- A type of _Chemical peel_. Unlike phenol which is all or none response, the concentration of TCA can be varied. Light peel 10–25%, intermediate 30–35%, deep 50–60%. There is less toxicity than phenol. The desired degree of peel can be chosen.

- TCA has less effect on melanin metabolism so it may be better in darker patients and for regional peels. But the degree of penetration and neocollagen formation is less. It is, therefore, not so effective for coarse wrinkles.
- Skin is pretreated with tretinoin and hydroquinone. Retinoic acid effects the epidermis by decreasing the stratum corneum and increasing permeability. Hydroquinone suppresses melanocytic activity.
- Depth is judged by the appearance of the skin, the turgor and the time taken to return to normal colour after TCA application. A deeper peel is associated with frosting. If it is too deep the frosting becomes grey/white. Apply TCA with a gauze, leave for 30 seconds to 2 minutes after which it is neutralized.

Trigger thumb and finger

- Stenosing tenosynovitis of thumb or finger at the level of the A1 pulley resulting in hand pain with triggering or locking. Difficulty flexing or extending the finger depends on whether the tendon is caught distally or proximally to the A1 pulley.
- Most common in middle-aged women. Also secondary to RA, DM, gout when multiple digits may be affected. The ring and middle fingers are most commonly involved.
- Get fibrocartilaginous metaplasia of the inner layer of the pulley or synovial proliferative changes in the tendon. Rucking at the site of constriction leads to development of a nodule, which is aggravated by further movement. The primary lesion is in the sheath and Notta's node is a secondary phenomenon.

Treatment:

- *Conservative:* steroid injection and NSAIDS.
- *Operative:* percutaneous or open release of the A1 pulley. If the flexor tendon is enlarged then it may need to be reduced by excising a central portion of the tendon. Cut A1 pulley of thumb on the radial border as oblique pulley inserts into A1 on ulnar border and may also get cut if pulley is cut on ulnar border. In the rheumatoid patient try to avoid cutting the A1 pulley to prevent ulnar drift or cut finger pulley on the radial side. Also

but try to in the rheumatoid patient. Perform synovectomy, flexor tenoplasty, or decompress the sheath by excising one or two slips of FDS.

Congenital trigger thumb:

- Clinically similar to adults. 25% present at birth, 25% bilateral. 30% of congenital trigger thumbs seen at birth resolve spontaneously by one month but only 12% of those seen at 6 months resolve. The only known association is with trisomy-13 – Patau's syndrome.
- Clicking is difficult to elicit in a child. A nodule (Notta's node) may be palpable over tendon of FPL proximal to A1 pulley.
- Surgical treatment involves release of A1 pulley.

Complications: Digital nerve injury.

Triphalangeal thumb

- *Wassel* Type 7 – duplication or isolated.
- Maybe autosomal dominant. M = F, most bilateral. Related to thalidomide.
- Associated with:
  - *Holt-Oram syndrome*;
  - *Fanconi's anaemia* is always associated with triphalangeal thumb;
  - trisomy 13–15;
  - Juberg–Hayward syndrome.
- 3 types – delta phalanx, short rectangular phalanx, normal length rectangular phalanx.
- The thumb is long and may be supinated with hypoplastic thenar muscles – may be extra finger, rather than a thumb.

Surgery:

- Often indicated for 5 problems:
  - associated malformations;
  - narrow web – *4 flap* Z-plasty;
  - abnormal shape extra phalanx – if small remove, in older child fuse to either distal or proximal phalanx;
  - digits in same plane requires pollicization;
  - thenar muscle deficiency – perform Huber opponensplasty.
- Complete operations by 6–24/12.

Tripier flap

Pedicled flap take from upper lid which can be uni or bipedicled to reconstruct the lower lid. See *Eyelid reconstruction*.

Triquetrum fracture

- Second most common carpal bone to fracture (15%) usually due to a fall on the dorsal or palmar flexed wrist or avulsion of the radiotriquetral ligament. Isolated fracture more uncommon. Most fractures are associated with other carpal injuries, such as lunate injuries.
- Get dorsal cortical fracture due to avulsion of dorsal extrinsic ligaments and the body fracture caused by shear force on the ulnar styloid. Get point tenderness dorsally over the triquetrum. Check of VISI deformity or a break in _Gilula's lines_.
- Treat by splinting for 6 weeks.
See _Carpal instability_.

Triscaphe OA
Scapho-trapezium-trapezoid.

Surgery: Arthrodesis of the triscaphe articulation. If there is pantrapezial arthritis then resect trapezium and reconstruct beak ligament along with arthrodesis of the scapho-trapezoid articulation.

Trunk reconstruction
Indications:
- _Pressure sores_.
- Irradiation.
- Tumour.
- _Spinal bifida_.

Management: divide into thirds.
- Upper ⅓ _Trapezius_.
- Middle ⅓ _Latissimus dorsi_.
- Lower ⅓ _Gluteus maximus_.
- Also use _Scapular/parascapular flap_ and paraspinous flaps.

Tubed pedicle flaps

- Method of transporting tissue from distant sites in multiple stages often with the wrist as carrier, but seldom used now.
- First delay a flap, turning it into a tube. Once it has matured it is sutured to an intermediate carrier. After a delay, the base is detached and brought to final destination still attached at the wrist. Once healed it is separated.

Tuberous breast
See _Mastopexy_. Also called a constricted breast. Characterized by a deficient breast-base dimension, a tight and elevated inframammary fold, an elongated thin breast, herniation of the NAC and stretching of the areolar.

Classification: By Heimburg.
- _Type 1:_ hypoplasia of the inferior medial quadrant.
- _Type 2:_ hypoplasia of both inferior quadrants.
- _Type 3:_ hypoplasia of both lower quadrants and subareolar skin shortage.
- _Type 4:_ severely constricted breast base.

Surgery: a difficult problem. The principles include reducing the size of the areola, dividing constrictions in the breast parenchyma, lowering the inframammary fold, insert implant or expander. A circumareolar mastopexy may also be required. Skin may need to be imported via a medially based thoracoepigastric flap.
- _Type 1:_ augment with submammary implant.
- _Type 2:_ augment with internal flap – unfurling of breast tissue on chest wall. Perform through inferior areolar incision.
- _Type 3 and 4:_ augment, internal flap, skin importation with Z-plasty, thoracoepigastric flap or tissue expansion.

Tuberous sclerosis
- Autosomal dominant condition with triad of mental retardation, epilepsy and facial skin rashes. Also get cardiac and renal tumours.
- Skin signs:
  - angiofibromas in butterfly distribution;
  - hypomelanotic macules;
  - forehead fibrous patches;
  - shagreen patches – thickened discoloured skin in lumbar region;
  - fibromas from nails of hands and feet;
  - profuse skin tags.

Tufted angioma
Or angioblastoma of Nakagawa.
- A rare vascular tumour that can be mistaken for a _Haemangioma_.
- An ill-defined, tender, purple indurated patch, several centimetres in size.

- More common in the upper trunk.
- Microscopically see cellular lobules ('tufts') throughout the dermis.
- The tumour may grow slowly and should be excised.

Tumescent anaesthesia

- Used in liposuction.
- Large volumes of dilute LA with adrenaline are injected to give good anaesthesia with reduced blood loss.
- Use 0.05% lignocaine with adrenaline 1:1 million NS. Add sodium bicarbonate. Inject twice as much as the amount of fat aspirated.
- High concentrations of lignocaine from 33 to 55 mg/kg have been reported. Lignocaine lasts longer in the tumescent technique than normal.

See Local anaesthetics.

Tumour necrosis factor

See Cytokines.

Tumours

Bone. Soft.

Turner syndrome

- *Sex differentiation defect* with 45,X karyotype.
- Short stature, high arched palate, webbed neck, shield-like chest, cardiac and renal anomalies, inverted nipples.

Turricephaly

Towering of the skull seen in severe *Craniosynostosis*.

Two-point discrimination

- Method of *Sensation testing*. Over 6 mm is abnormal.
- Value varies with most patients having a normal static value at the pulp of 2–3 mm, reduced to 5–6 mm with heavy labour and 1–2 mm with blindness.
- The disk-Criminator is an easy way of testing this. Move prongs from distal to proximal. 7/10 consistent results are required to give a 2PD value.
- Dynamic 2PD has normal value of 2 mm. This returns before static 2PD.
- 2PD is the last sensory modality to return.

U Ulna, distal: arthritis to Urbaniak classification

Ulna, distal: arthritis

Painful rotation. Treat by:
- Excision distal end ulna (*Darrach*).
- modification of Darrach.
- Hemiresectio interposition arthroplasty.
- Resection and replacement (Swanson).
- Arthrodesis and pseudoarthrosis (*Sauve–Kapandji*).
- Arthrodesis.

Ulna variance

- The length difference between the radius and the ulna is measured with the wrist in neutral (90° shoulder and 90° elbow flexion).
- Positive variance may be associated with wrist pain.

- It becomes more positive with forearm pronation or power grip.

Ulnar artery

Lies radial to FCU, passes superficial to TCL in Guyon's canal. A deep branch joins deep branch of nerve under FDM. It passes between transverse and oblique part of AP to lie dorsal to AP. A deep branch joins the radial artery to form the deep palmar arch, it then becomes the superficial palmar arch.

Ulnar artery flap

- Although the main blood supply to the hand, it can safely be raised as a flap and is less hair-bearing than the radial side. First perform an Allen's test.

• The pedicle lies within the fascial septum of FCU and FDS. It can be made sensate by including the medial anti-brachial cutaneous nerve. It can also include PL and FCU.

Operation: Incise border of flap through fascia. Elevate medial and lateral edges of flap to the septum. Artery is ligated proximally. A distally based flap may occasionally get venous congestion and require anastomosing of a vein to a recipient vein in the hand.

Ulnar club hand

• ¹/₁₀th as common as *Radial club hand*.
• Can get a spectrum of abnormalities ranging from slight hypoplasia of the ulnar digits to total absence of the ulna.
• It differs from radial club hand as:
• the hand is stable at the wrist, but unstable at the elbow;
• it is associated with abnormalities of the musculoskeletal system;
• partial absence is the most common finding.

Classification:
• *Type 1*: hypoplasia.
• *Type 2*: partial absence.
• *Type 3*: total absence.
• *Type 4*: fusion of radius to humerus – radiohumeral synostoses.

Treatment: Depends of severity of deformity. Surgical treatment involves release of the fibrous anlage and realignment of the carpus and forearm.
See *Congenital hands*.

Ulnar collateral ligament

Anatomy: See *Thumb MPJ*.
• Range of motion of thumb MCP joint variable. Spherical heads have greater ROM. Little intrinsic stability.
• Strong proper collaterals run from metacarpal lateral condyles to volar third of proximal phalanx. Accessory collaterals(ACL) run more volar and inset into volar plate and sesamoids. Proper collaterals are tight in flexion and loose in extension and ACLs are the opposite. 3-sided ligament box differs from PIP joints as there is no flexor sheath and, therefore, no check rein

ligament. Intrinsics insert into sesamoid bones embedded in distal volar plate.

Injury:
• Acute UCL injury – distal tears 5 times more common than proximal.
• Stener lesion – adductor aponeurosis interposes between distally avulsed ligament and its insertion.
• Important to distinguish between partial and complete tears. If there is 30° laxity more than the other side in extension and 30° of laxity in flexion there is probably a complete rupture. Also assess if the joint can be opened with no clear end point.

Treatment:
• Partial tear treat with splint for 4 weeks and protect for 3 months.
• *Complete tear*: treat by repair.
• *Chronic UCL injury*: use tendon graft to reconstruct.

Operative technique:
• Lazy S incision on ulna border of thumb overlying MCP joint. Incise adductor aponeurosis 3 mm volar to ulnar border of EPL. Examine joint.
• Suture ligament or use mitek or pull-out suture.
• If there is a bony fragment it can be fixed with a small screw or a pull-out wire.
• After ligament repair:
  ○ suture distal ligament to volar plate;
  ○ repair dorsal ulnar capsule;
  ○ test stability with radial stress;
  ○ K wire in flexion and ulnar deviation, suture extensor expansion to adductor aponeurosis.

Ulnar dimelia
• Also called mirror hand.
• Very rare (only exceeded by multiple hands)
• 7 digits occur, but only the medial two are obviously little and ring.
• The forearm contains two ulnae, but no radial bones. The thumb is missing and there is an excess of fingers.
• The elbow is stiff and the forearm rotation reduced. The contralateral hand is usually not affected.

Treatment:
- Excise olecranon to increase elbow mobility.
- Excise excess fingers and policize. The finger to be pollicized will depend on observation.
- All fingers have their complement of tendons and these can be used in the pollicization and to rebalance the wrist.

Ulnar nerve
- In the forearm ulnar nerve travels between FDS and FDP supplying FDP to ring and little finger.
- The ulnar nerve gives off a dorsal cutaneous branch 5–7 cm proximal to styloid process of ulna. It winds around the ulnar aspect of the forearm to supply the dorsum of the hand.
- The ulnar nerve divides into deep and superficial branches at the level of *Guyon's canal.*
- Superficial branch supplies palmaris brevis then splits into two branches to little and half of ring finger.
- The deep branch passes under the fibrous arch of the origin of FDM. It accompanies the *Deep palmar* arch passing between ADM and FDM, giving branches to the hypothenar muscles. It runs radially deep to palmar interosseus fascia and ends by passing between the two heads of AP. It supplies the *Interosseous muscles* and the 2 ulnar lumbricals. The interosseous branches enter the muscles on the palmar side and the lumbricals on the dorsal side.

Ulnar nerve compression
See *Cubital tunnel syndrome*. See *Guyon's canal.*

Ulnar nerve palsy

Motor loss: by muscle.
- Lumbrical: *Duchenne's* sign – ring and little finger clawing, also *Bouvier's* manoeuvre, *Andre–Thomas* sign. Loss of normal flexion, which starts at MCP joint, instead curl from distal to proximal.
- Interosseus: *Pitres–Testut* sign – inability to abduct and adduct as well as cross the fingers, digital Froment's.

- Hypothenar muscles: *Masse's* sign of hypothenar wasting and *Wartenberg's* sign of the abducted little finger.
- Adductor pollicis: *Jeanne's* sign – loss of lateral pinch and *Froment's* sign with IPJ flexion.
- *FDP 4th and 5th finger: Pollock's* sign.
- *FCU:* partial loss of wrist flexion.

Sensory loss: To ulnar 1 ½ fingers.
See *Tendon transfers.*

Ulnar translocation of the carpus
Carpal instability, which occurs after radiocarpal dislocation and commonly in rheumatoid arthritis.

Classification: by Taleisnik.
- *Type I:* entire carpus displaced ulnarly with widened radioscaphoid articulation.
- *Type II:* scapholunate interval is widened. So scaphoid stays in place.

Ulnocarpal impaction syndrome
- Ulnar-sided wrist pain with ulnar positive *Variance.* Get erosion of carpus, synovitis, thinning of TFCC, and disruption of ulnocarpal ligaments.
- Caused by congenital or acquired positive variance – usually due to a malunion of a distal radius fracture or radioulnar instability (*Essex–Loresti* injury).
- Treat by decompressing the ulnar side with *Darrach*, shortening osteotomy, or arthroscopic excision.
See *TFCC.*

Ultraviolet radiation (UV)
- Harmful effects are due to electron excitation in the absorbing atoms and molecules, which induces damage in DNA and may be responsible for cell death and neoplastic transformation. Also get production of oxygen-free radicals, which damage cell membranes and nuclear DNA.
- Also may have an immunosuppressive effect with depletion of Langerhan's cells.
- Adverse effects are reduced by hair, thick stratum corneum and melanin.
- Though most of the radiation reaching the human skin is UVA, UVB causes most of the problem with sunburn and neoplasia.

UVA: 320–400 nm.
- Contributes to erythema, carcinogenesis and photo-aging.
- This is emitted by most sunbeds.
- Exposure is thought but not proved to increase the risk of developing <u>Melanoma</u>.

UVB: 290–320 nm. Causes sunburn, tan, pre-cancer and cancer.

UVC: 200–290 nm. Mostly filtered out by the ozone layer.

Umbilical sculpting

Technique: Defat umbilicus and the reduce length of the pedicle by resecting upper portion of umbilicus. Suture edge of umbilicus to fascia. Mark position of new umbilicus on abdomen with some tacking sutures to skin edges. Excise a horizontal ellipse. Resect a core of fat. Lift skin flaps and cut an ellipse of fat away particularly from inferior margin. Put stay suture into edge of umbilicus to enable it to pull through opening. Once the abdomen is sutured pass stitch through and stitch with non-absorbable suture.

Unicameral bone cyst
- A cavity fills with yellow serous fluid.
- Occurs in long bones, 90% in proximal femur and proximal humerus.
- Present in 10s–20s after a pathological fracture.

- Early lesions occur in the metaphysis abutting the physeal plate. Older lesions have moved away.
- They become multiloculated.
- *XR:* an eccentric radiolucent cyst of variable size in the metaphysis of tubular bone.
- They don't undergo malignant degeneration.
- Treat by intralesional aspiration and injection with methylprednisolone.
- Larger lesions can be curetted and bone grafted. The natural history is spontaneous healing in adulthood.
See <u>Bone tumours</u>.

Upton classification
See <u>Apert's hands</u>.

Urbaniak classification
Classification of <u>Ring avulsion</u> injuries. relates to microsurgical management.
- *I:* circulation adequate.
- *II:* circulation inadequate and microvascular reconstruction will restore circulation and function:
  - ○ *IIA:* requires repair of digital arteries alone;
  - ○ *IIB:* arteries, bone and tendon;
  - ○ *IIC:* only the veins.
- *III:* complete degloving of skin. Microvascular reconstruction will restore circulation, but with poor function. Amputation is recommended.

V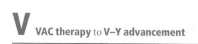
VAC therapy to **V–Y advancement**

VAC therapy
Vacuum-assisted closure.
- Developed by Louis Argenta in 1997.
- Used intermittent or continuous vacuum through a sealed foam dressing to stimulate granulation tissue and speed healing.
- The principles are to remove exudates, provide a moist environment, remove oedema, increase blood flow, increase granulation, encourage epithelialization.

- It can be used over SSG at a lower pressure (50 mmHg) or on chronic wounds – 125 mmHg, higher pressures collapse blood vessels.

Action:
- Removes chronic oedema which improves O_2 delivery.
- Wound fluid also inhibits fibroblasts and keratinocyte activity and matrix metalloproteins break down collagen.

- Encourages granulation tissue.
- Increases blood flow.
- Decreases infection.
- Encourages contraction.

VACTERL syndrome
- *V*ertebral.
- *A*nal atresia.
- *C*ardiac anomalies.
- *TOF*.
- *E*sophageal atresia.
- *R*enal disorders.
- *L*imb anomalies.
See *Radial club hand*.

Vaginal agenesis
- Known as Mayer–Rokitansky–Küster–Hauser syndrome.
- 1:4000 live female births.
- Results from failure of development of the paramesonephric duct (see *Embryology*).
- 50% associated with abnormalities of the urinary tract. Ovaries are usually normal. A vestigial vaginal dimple may be present. If no uterus, present with amenorrhoea, if uterus present, present with haematocolpos.

Investigation: Examination may reveal a vaginal dimple. USS and IVP to assess upper urinary tract. EUA, chromosomal abnormality.

Vaginal reconstruction
For:
- Females born without a vagina. (Mayer–Rokitansky–Küster–Hauser syndrome). Most have no uterus, but normal ovaries.
- After excision for neoplasm.
- Male to female gender reassignment.

Surgery:
- *McIndoe procedure:* cavity developed between rectum and bladder, which was lined with SSG. A stent was required. Complications were stenosis, and fistulae. A mould was sutured in and left for 6 months.
- *Bowel:* vascularized ileum or colon. Disadvantage is the mucus and trauma during intercourse.
- *FTSG:* similar to McIndoe procedure. Graft from either groin sutured together. Stent made with foam and condom. Postoperatively a candle is used covered in con-

dom to stent the neovagina. Graft doesn't constrict.
- *Pedicled colon:* one of the best methods of reconstruction.
- *Dilatation:* if a dimple is present it can be dilated progressively.
- Also use flaps of labia minora and gracilis.

Van der Meulen hypospadias repair
- *Hypospadias* repair, a modification of the Duplay technique.
- It involves transposition of a flap based on the adjacent penile skin to form a neourethra followed by wrap around of the preputial skin. This moved the meatus distally, but did not sink it into the glans.

Van der Woude's syndrome
Lip pit-cleft lip syndrome.
- Autosomal dominant.
- Lower lip pits that are accessory salivary glands are present in 80% of patients.
- Missing central and lateral incisors, canines and bicuspids.
- Associated with cleft lip and palate or cleft palate.
- The gene for this condition is localized to the long arm of chromosome 1.
See *Craniofacial genetics*.

Van Lohuizen Syndrome
See *Telangiectases*.

Vascular injuries: upper limb

Anatomy: *Ulnar artery, Radial artery*.
- Aneurysms.
- *Arteriovenous fistulae*.
- *Buerger's disease*.
- Emboli.
- *Thrombosis:*
  - *Hypothenar hammer syndrome*;
  - it can also occur in the radial artery – particularly following cannulation. atherosclerosis is rare, digital ischaemia secondary to thrombosis of a persistent median artery has been described.
- *Vasospastic disorders*:
  - *Raynaud's*.

Vascular leiomyoma
Or dermal angiomyoma.

- A small tumour that arises from the tunica muscularis of small vessels and presents as a painless enlarging mass.
- They are located in the dermis or subcutaneous layer.
- They are well encapsulated white lesions.
- Histologically they have bundles of smooth muscle surrounding vascular channels.

Vascular malformations

Pathology:
- *Haemangioma* has increased endothelial turnover in the proliferative phase.
- *Malformation* describes a vascular anomaly with a normal endothelial cycle. These are inborn errors of vascular channel morphogenesis formed by a combination of abnormal capillary, arterial, venous or lymphatic channels. It is present at birth and neither proliferates or involutes, but grows with the child. Some grow after a triggering factor.
- *Ectasia* are lesions with normal endothelial turnover but vascular dilatation. These are vascular anomalies, such as cherry angioma and spider angioma.

Classification: See *Mulliken and Glowacki*.
- Divided into slow and high flow lesions.
- *Capillary malformation* (port wine stain).
- *Telangiectases.*
- *Lymphatic malformations.*
- *Venous malformations.*
- *Arteriovenous malformations.*
- *Complex combined vascular malformations.*

Pathogenesis:
- Errors of embryonic development.
- The genes are known for two recessive enzymatic deficiency disorders that present with cutaneous vascular papules: autosomal fucosidosis and X-linked Fabry disease.
- One of the genes responsible for hereditary hemorrhagic telangiectasia (Rendu–Osler–Weber disease) is on chromosome 9q.
- Several defective genes cause ataxia-telangiectasia (Louis–Bar syndrome).

Associated syndromes:
- *Bonnet–Dechaume–Blanc.*
- *Sturge–Weber.*
- *Parkes–Weber syndrome.*
- *Klippel–Trenaunay syndrome.*

- *Rendu–Osler–Weber disease.*
- *Maffuci's syndrome.*

Treatment:
- 3 indications for treatment – cosmetic, functional impairment and life-threatening consequences.
- *Surgery:* excision may be combined with sclerotherapy or embolization. Small haemangiomas may be excised. Nasal tip lesions should be treated more conservatively. Excision before pregnancy has been recommended because of the growth potential. Embolization can trigger involution. AV malformations are difficult to treat. Recurrence often occurs in the tissue around the resection margin. Never ligate feeding vessels proximal to an AV malformation. Treatment with selective angiography and embolization with excision within 24–48 hours gives the best results. Prupesku suturing is used to compartmentalize a vascular malformation prior to excision.
- *Steroid therapy:* not effective for cavernous haemangiomas in adults, AV fistulas, portwine stains and lymphangiomas. Systemic or intralesional (though intralesional have reported complications of cavernous sinus thrombosis and globe rupture when treating ocular lesions).
- *Chemotherapy:* all capillary haemangiomas contain oestrogen receptors. Vascular malformations don't have any hormonal markers. Cyclophasphamide and α-inteferon have been used for massive haemangiomas. α-inteferon is given at 3 million U/m2/day for 4–9 weeks. It has lowered the mortality of intrahepatic haemangiomas and has been successful with Kasabach–Merritt phenomenom.
- *Pressure therapy:* compression of haemangiomas is non-invasive, safe and effective. It may act by ischaemia and necrosis.
- *Thermal therapy/cryotherapy:* most result in extensive scarring.
- *Radiation therapy:* though used extensively there is no evidence for any benefit.
- *Laser therapy:* pulse-dyed laser can be used in the proliferative phase to treat superficial small haemangiomas, but will not penetrate deep enough to treat larger lesions.
- *Embolization and sclerotherapy.*

Vasculitis

- Get general malaise, high ESR, CRP, low complement.
- Need immunosupression with steroids and cyclophosphamide.
- Classify according the size of vessels and the organs involved:
  - large vessels are involved in periarteritis nodosa and temporal arteritis;
  - small vessel involvement occurs in Henoch–Schönlein purpura, Waterhouse–Friderichsen syndrome and Wegener's syndrome.
- Get ischaemic lesions that are slow to heal due to increased coagulability of the blood.

Vasospastic disorders

- Get cold intolerance (occurs in 20% of pre-menopausal women) due to vasospasm or occlusion with inadequate microvascular perfusion.
- Primary vasospasm is _Raynaud's_ disease.
- Normally less than 10% blood flow goes through nutritional capillaries. Blood flow is dependent on vascular integrity and appropriate control mechanisms.
- Cutaneous circulation is controlled by alpha adrenergic receptors via the sympathetic system.
- Primary Raynaud's has abnormal responsiveness of catecholamine receptors.
- Secondary Raynaud's has abnormal vessels.

Clinical:
- Repetitive trauma, drugs, smoking.
- Perform Allen's test, vascular studies. Stress test especially in collagen disease with vascular occlusion. The difference between thermoregulatory flow and nutritional flow is difficult to distinguish. Vital capillaroscopy is one way of doing this by looking at finger with microscope.

Vastus lateralis flap

Anatomy: Origin is the lateral surface of greater trochanter and inserts into the rectus femoris and upper lateral patella.

Blood supply: Descending branch of the lateral circumflex femoral artery from the profunda femoris. Runs from medial to lateral coming from under rectus femoris. Enters the anterior belly 10 cm inferior to the ASIS. The distal third is supplied by perforating branches of the superficial femoral artery. Only the proximal two-thirds can be reliably elevated.

Reconstruction: Perform through a lateral incision. Get significant weakness with knee instability.
See _Pressure sores_.

Vaughn–Jackson syndrome

Ulnar prominence can lead to rupture of ulnar-sided extensors.
See _Caput ulna syndrome_.

VEGF

Vascular endothelial growth factor.
- An endogenous stimulator of angiogenesis and vascular permeability. It is expressed in developing blood vessels.
- It includes VEGF A, B, C, D, E and placental growth factor.
- VEGF-A is the most predominant protein. Experimentally it is found to be upregulated in flap ischaemia and administration may improve flap survival.
See _Growth factors_.

Velocardiofacial syndrome

Shprintzen's syndrome. VCF, CATCH 22.
- Most are sporadic, some are inherited.
- 83% of individuals have a deletion of chromosome 22q11.2.
- Have velopharyngeal insufficiency, cleft palate, cardiac anomalies, unusual facies and learning difficulties.
- The facial feature includes a long face both physically and in expression, epicanthic folds, pinched nasal tip.
- Anomolous internal carotid arteries are seen in 25% of patients with VCF. Pulsations in the posterior pharyngeal wall may influence the choice of surgery for VPI.
- Also called CATCH 22.
  - Cardiac;
  - abnormal face;
  - thymic aplasia;
  - cleft palate;
  - hypocalcaemia;
  - 22 chromosome.

See Craniofacial genetics.

Velopharyngeal incompetence (VPI)
See Cleft palate.

- Inability of the soft palate to make contact with the pharyngeal wall during *Speech*, which is essential for intelligible speech.
- Develop hypernasality, misarticulation, nasal emissions and aberrant facial movements.

Anatomy:

- Closure relies on raising and tensing the velum and also the size of the pharynx and tension in the pillar of fauces. Firm closure allows negative pressure and this back pressure assists in vocal cord closure.
- With VPI consonants lack clarity, there may be nasal snorting and glottal sounds.

Causes:

- *Idiopathic insufficiency.*
- *Congenital palatal insufficiency:* velum too short or pharynx too large.
- *Submucous cleft palate:* muscles don't unite. Have bifid uvula. Can have occult submucous soft palate.
- *Post-palate repair:* there may be a shortened soft palate, or inadequate lateral wall movement or central defect.
- *After pharyngeal flap or pharyngoplasty:* due to inadequate flap width.
- *After adenoidectomy:* usually resolves as palate moves more up to 1 year after.
- *Enlarged tonsils:* the weight may inhibit velar elevation.
- *After midface advancement:* especially after palate repair.
- *Neurogenic:* give weakness, incoordination and fatigue. E.g. hemifacial microsomia.
- *Lack of VPI movement:* immobile for speech, but normal for swallowing. Not helped by pharyngoplasty.
- *Functional/hysterical hypernasality:* common in the deaf due to inappropriate use of sphincter.

Operations:

- All aim to produce partial obstruction by:
  ○ lengthening the palate by pushback, intravelar veloplasty, or double-opposing Z-plasty;
  ○ reduction of the opening by subtotal central obstruction (pharyngeal flap) or a posterior port reduction (sphincter pharyngoplasty).
- All risk causing airway obstruction.

Pharyngeal flap:

- The most common method. Tissue from the posterior pharynx is attached to the soft palate to create a midline obstruction with two lateral openings which remain open for respiration and close for oral consonants.
- It was first described by Schoenborn in 1876.
- Correct width is important. A superiorly based flap is transversely incised inferiorly and raised to the level of the palatal plane which usually corresponds to 1–2 cm above the tubercle of the atlas. An inferiorly based flap is incised just below the adenoid pad. The flap is usually inset with turn back flaps on the nasal side of the uvula, with or without opening the midline palate repair.
- Flap contracts on healing and contraction is reduced by lining the flap with turnover flaps. The final flap width is, therefore, difficult to judge. Some have advocated assessing the amount of lateral wall movement pre-operatively. No difference has been shown between superior and inferiorly based flaps but superior-based flaps are more popular. The inferior-based flap has a length limitation and attachment tends to tether the flap in an inferior direction.

Sphincter pharyngoplasty:

- Aims to tighten the central orifice.
- Originally described by *Hynes* and modified by others, such as *Ortichochea* and Jackson.
- Involves the construction of palatopharyngeus myomucosal flaps from the posterior tonsillar pillars, which are sutured to the posterior pharyngeal wall. There have been no studies validating its use.
- The height of insertion of the flaps appears to be critical for success.

Palatal lengthening:

- Used in attempts to eliminate small gaps. This would appear to be more physiologically normal. The V–Y pushback has never been validated.

- Pushback with a flap may be helpful in some patients. The significant mucoperiosteal stripping may affect facial growth. Get high rates of fistula formation.
- The _Furlow_ double-opposing Z-plasty has gained popularity. Improvements have been shown for primary palatoplasty, as well as secondary management. May be particularly good for a subgroup of patients with a small central velopharyngeal gap.

Posterior wall augmentation:
- Many substances have been tried such as silastic, Teflon, proplast, paraffin and have been abandoned because of unpredictable results. Autogenous material has been tried. Use of these is restricted to small velopharyngeal gaps.
- Advantages are no alteration in nasal airway, safe in children who are at risk of airway problems, relatively simple and reversible.
- Studies of augmentation do not show improvement in speech.

Prosthetics: A palatal prosthesis, velar lift or velopharyngeal obturator may be used, particularly when there is adequate tissue but poor control of coordination and timing.

Complications: Acute obstructive sleep apnoea: is 13% after sphincter pharyngoplasty. Most improve with time without requiring revision of flaps.

Venkataswami flap
Sensate advancement digital flap based on the neurovascular bundle.

Venous flaps

Classification: _Thatte and Thatte._
- Based on venous rather than arterial pedicles. Many have small arteries running alongside them, e.g. the _Saphenous flap_.
- Venous flaps become very congested postoperatively and have not become universally accepted.

See _Flaps_.

Venous hypertension
Causes 80% of _Leg ulcers_. Occurs with long standing elevation of venous blood pressure.

Caused by incompetent valves, most commonly due to previous thrombophlebitis.

Anatomy:
- Deep veins are paired and run with the artery with crossing branches. Superficial veins don't travel with arteries and are not paired. Both systems have valves and connect via perforating veins.
- Perforating veins are principally found between the long saphenous and posterior tibial system. Perforator contribute to ulceration when the valves don't work.

Investigations:
- *Venogram:* invasive assessment now rarely formed.
- *Duplex scanning:* assesses anatomy and function.
- *Photoplthysmography and air plethysmography:* used to assess backward flow of blood.

Venous malformations
See _Vascular malformations_. Present at birth, but not always evident. They are slow flow and appear as a faint blue patch or a soft bluish mass. They can occur internally. They are usually solitary but multiple hereditary forms occur.

Familial glomangiomatosis:
- Rather common autosomal dominant syndrome of high penetrance.
- Multiple, often tender, blue nodular dermal venous lesions that can occur anywhere on the skin.
- Histologically, these differ from typical VM by the presence of numerous glomus cells lining the ectatic venous channels.

Familial cutaneous-mucosal VM: inherited in an autosomal dominant mode.

Blue rubber bleb nevus (Bean syndrome):
- Sporadic combination of cutaneous and visceral VMs.
- The skin lesions are soft, blue and nodular; they can occur anywhere.
- Typically located on the hands and feet.
- The gastrointestinal lesions are sessile (submucosal–subserosal) or polypoid, located in the oesophagus, stomach, small and large bowel, and mesentery.

- Recurrent intestinal bleeding can be severe, requiring repeated transfusions.

VMs are easily compressible and swell if dependent. They are often painful. Thrombosis and phleboliths occur. Limb VM rarely causes growth discrepancy. MRI is helpful. A coagulation profile can be performed as with extensive VM there is a risk of localized intravascular coagulopathy which is different than Kassabach–Merritt phenomenom as platelets are only minimally decreased, but fibrinogen is low.

Treatment: for functional problems.
- Small cutaneous VM in any location can be injected with a sclerosant. A large VM, cutaneous or intramuscular, requires general anaesthesia and 'real-time' fluoroscopic monitoring during sclerotherapy. Sclerosis of a large VM is potentially dangerous. Compression and other manoeuvres prevent passage of the sclerosing agent into the systemic circulation. Local complications include blistering, full-thickness cutaneous necrosis, or neural damage. Systemic complications include renal toxicity and cardiac arrest. Multiple sclerotherapeutic sessions may be necessary, often at several-month intervals.
- Venous anomalies have a propensity for recanalization and recurrence.
- Surgical resection is considered, after completion of sclerotherapy, to reduce tissue mass for functional or cosmetic indications.
- Elastic support stockings.
- Low-dose aspirin (75 mg od) seems to minimize the occurrence of episodic, painful phlebothrombosis.
- Subtotal (contour) resection can be beneficial for VM of the hand/foot, particularly in the digits.
- Intramuscular VM in the thigh or calf can diminish function and require resection.
- VMs of the gastrointestinal tract have been managed by banding via the endoscope, sclerotherapy, and bowel resection.

Venous ulcers

Pathogenesis: Not completely clear. Loss of valvular competence, raised venous blood pressure, extravasation of protein and blood cells into subcutaneous tissues, pericapillary fibrin cuff acts as a diffusion barrier, inflammation leads to scarring and lipodermatosclerosis (brawny oedema). This tissue is poorly vascularized and easily traumatized, and slow to heal.

Position: Gaiter region between maleoli and gastrocnemius. Possibly due to excessively high pressures in the perforating veins on contraction of gastrocnemeus.

Conservative treatment:
- Elastic compression, bed rest, elevation.
- Skin grafting has recurrence rates of 45%.
- Compression enhances fibrinolysis, reducing fibrin deposition. Unna boot – (4-layer bandaging) – compression bandaging with various pastes.

Surgery:
- Varicose vein stripping, perforator ligation, valvuloplasty (demonstrates good results with primary valvular incompetence).
- These do not address the problem of the lipodermatosclerosis.
- _Linton flap._
- Superficial venous ulceration may benefit from skin grafting.
- _Free flaps:_ may provide long-term cure by replacing lipodermatosclerotic bed with healthy tissue. In several series there was no venous ulceration in the flap though some wound-healing problems at the margins. Use for deep venous insufficiency with scarred tissue. The free flap has normal microvalvular system.

See _Leg ulcers._

Verruca vulgaris
- Caused by papavovirus, transmitted by direct contact or auto-inoculation.
- Get hyperkeratosis, acanthosis and parakeratosis.
- Treat with topical irritants, cryotherapy, excision or laser ablation.
- The basal epidermal layer is not invaded so re-epithelialization occurs rapidly.

Vicryl
- Braided synthetic suture composed of polyglactin 910 (90% glycoside, 10% L-lactide).

- It loses its strength in 3 weeks, it is absorbed in 3 months.
- It may be more prone to bacterial colonization due to its braided nature.
- It may provoke an inflammatory reaction.

Vincula
- Folds of mesotendon which provide connective support to the FDS and FDP tendons.
- The blood supply passes through these vincula via transverse communicating branches of the common digital artery. Each tendon is supplied by a short and long vincular, which enter the dorsal portion of each tendon.
- The short vincular are located close to the insertion point. The vinculum longum of FDP pierces superficialis close to PIP joint. Vessels run on the dorsum of tendons.

See *Flexor tendons*

Vitallium
Cobalt-chromium-molybdenum alloy. High tensile strength so can be low profile.
See *Alloplasts*.

Vitamin A
- Deficiency affects all stages of *Wound healing*.
- Counteracts the impairment in wound healing due to steroid administration by the labialization of lysosomes within inflammatory cells.
- Clinical use has been variable and definite improvements in healing have not been demonstrated.

Vitamin C
A cofactor required for the hydroxylation of proline and lysine. Deficiency causes cross-linking deficiency of collagen and impairment of *Wound healing*. Treat vitamin C deficiency with 100–1000 g/day.

Vitamin E
A membrane stabilizer. Deficiency may inhibit healing.

Voice restoration
Alaryngeal voice may be produced by air-flow induced vibration of the pharyngooesophageal mucosa by ingested air (oesophageal speech) or shunted air (fistula or tracheooesophageal speech).

Oesophageal speech: Only 25% of patients can manage this. Only small amounts of air can be ingested and only 4–5 words can be expressed. Air must be able to pass freely through the neopharynx. Get a low-pitched voice with a lot of jitter (cycle to cycle pitch perturbation and shimmer (cycle to cycle amplitude perturbation). A radial forearm flap may give more successful oesophageal speech than a jejunal flap.

Artificial larynx:
- This is a crude vibrator, which produces a focused tone electronically or pneumatically that mimics the vocal cords.
- When applied firmly to the neck or along the cheek, a penetrating signal enters the mouth. It is this new signal or voice that is used for speech.
- The user must learn to articulate vowels clearly with considerable exaggeration of mouth and tongue position. Only indicated when surgical reconstructive results are poor. It may be used while waiting for tracheo-oesophageal puncture (TEP) reconstruction.

Tracheo-oesophageal puncture and voice prosthesis placement:
- The addition of pulmonary air supply brings acoustic quality closer to normal. This is achieved with a TEF. The addition of a voice prosthesis allows for fluent speech.
- Developed in 1980, a one-way valve allows air to enter the oesophagus when the patient exhales with the tracheostoma occluded, but stops liquid and food entering the trachea when the patient swallows. Skin reconstruction gives better speech results.
- First the reconstruction is performed, preferably with a radial forearm flap. The Blom-Singer prosthesis can be inserted at the same time or as a separate procedure. With the neck extended a TEP is created by inserting a needle through the posterior wall of the tracheostoma just superior to the lower anastomosis. This hole is dilated to allow a size 14 catheter to be inserted as a stent.

A week later the Blom–Singer voice prosthesis is inserted. This acts as a one-way valve, directing air into the oesophagus when a finger occludes it. The neooesophagus acts as the new vibratory segment. The frequency of voice is low.

Volar plate
- A thick ligament on the volar surface of the joints of the finger which resembles a swallow's tail. The space between allows the passage of the vincula.
- Distally the volar plate blends with volar periosteum of the middle phalanx, the strongest attachments being laterally.
- There a 3 layers. The dorsal layer has a proximal membranous portion and a distal meniscoid portion. The middle layer contains fibres which form the check rein ligament. The volar layer contains transverse fibres, which anchor the flexor sheath to the volar plate.
- A small recess separating the meniscoid portion from the middle phalanx allows the plate to hinge open with joint flexion.

See *Proximal interphalangeal joint*.

Volkmann's ischaemic contracture
- Occurs after a *Compartment syndrome* in the upper limb, often following a supracondylar fracture with a contracted functionless arm.
- The forearm is fixed in pronation, wrist flexed, MCP joints are hyperextended, PIP and DIP joints are flexed. The hand is insensate. Due to muscle necrosis, fibrosis and shortening.
- If only one compartment has been injured then tendon transfers may be possible. A flexor slide may be indicated or free muscle transfers for severe cases. A delayed amputation may be required.

Vomer flap
Used in *Cleft palate* repair, closure of the hard palate can be achieved using a superiorly based flap of nasal mucosa from the vomer. In a bilateral cleft they can be taken from each side.

Sommerlad lip and vomer flap:
- Mark and score lip incisions. C flap extends onto premaxilla to meet line of oral and nasal mucosa at commencement of vomer.
- Laterally the incision along mucosal margin extends down to between inferior turbinate and palatal shelf.
- Incise laterally in buccal sulcus to bone and elevate periosteum until infra-orbital nerve becomes visible. Score periosteum just below origin of nerve to free and mobilize lateral lip.
- Now move to inside mouth with gag in place. Incise along vomer to posterior spine. elevate vomer along its length – bone is fragile! On lateral side elevate oral layer off palatal shelf for just a few millimetres. Release inferior turbinate and save bone to graft lateral segment.
- Suture vomer flap under oral mucosa on lateral side. Then move to lip repair, starting with nasal floor. Inferior turbinate sutures to inferior part of vomer flap.

Von Graefe
1818: introduced the term 'plastic'. He wrote a book on nasal reconstruction called *Rhinoplastik*, describing the Italian and Indian method and the new German method. He used a free skin graft. He also described blepharoplasty and palatoplasty.

Von Langenbeck repair
Cleft palate repair described in 1859. The cleft palate is repaired using large mucoperiosteal flaps raised from the hard palate. Approximation in the midline is achieved by lateral releasing incisions.

Von Recklinghausen's disease
Multiple *Neurofibromatosis*.

V–Y advancement
- A type of *Advancement flap* with forward advancement of a V without rotation and closure as a Y.
- Useful for lengthening the nasal columella, correcting whistle tip deformity of the lip, fingertip tissue loss and closure of cheek defects.
- An extended V–Y flap adds a transposition element to the side.

W-plasty

- Used for reorientating the direction of a linear scar. Triangles of equal size are outlined on either side of the scar with the tip of the triangle on one side placed at the midpoint of the base of the triangle on the other side. At the ends of the scar the excised triangles should be smaller with the limbs of the W tapered.
- The main disadvantage is that the scar is not lengthened. The tension on the tissue is increased as tissue is sacrificed. Mainly used for scar revision. Limbs should not exceed 6 mm.

Wallace rule of 9s

- Used for the assessment of surface area in *Burns*. In adults:
  ○ head and neck, 9%;
  ○ arm, 9%;
  ○ trunk anterior, 18%;
  ○ each leg, 9%;
  ○ genitalia, 1%.
- For children
  ○ head and neck, 18%;
  ○ each leg, 14%;
  ○ for each year over 10, take 1% of head and neck and add to combined leg measurement.

Wallerian degeneration

The process of degeneration of the distal segment in nerve injury. Get ground-glass appearance of degenerated myelin and axonal material. These are phagocytosed by macrophages and Schwann cells and the space becomes occupied by columns of Schwann cell nuclei and their basement membranes. The collapsed columns of Schwann cells have a band-like appearance – the bands of Büngner.

Wardill–Kilner–Veau repair

For *Cleft palate* repair. V–Y advancement of the mucoperiosteum of the hard palate with the intention of lengthening the hard palate. Bone is left exposed and re-epithelialize,

but this scar may contribute to maxillary growth disturbance.

Wart

See *Verruca vulgaris*.

Wartenberg's sign

- Clinical sign in *Ulnar nerve palsy*.
- Abduction of the little finger with inability to adduct.
- EDM has 2 bundles, radial bundle passes over centre of axis of MCP joint, the ulnar bundle passes ulnar to axis and also has an attachment to ADM. Therefore, EDC pulls on proximal phalanx and if unopposed will abduct the little finger.

Wartenberg's syndrome

- Radial nerve divides into posterior interosseous nerve and superficial radial nerve 4 cm distal to lateral epicondyle. Superficial branch travels under bracioradialis and becomes superficial in the distal forearm.
- Superficial branch of radial nerve may be compressed under brachioradialis in mid-forearm or it may be compressed at the wrist by bracelets or watches.
- Get pain in distribution of radial nerve, radiating proximally. Numbness and tingling on pronation with Tinel's over nerve. Forceful pronation against resistance useful test.

Treatment: Free throughout its length. It may be entrapped by tendinous margin of brachioradialis, ECRL or the intervening fascia.

Washio flap

Transfer of retroauricular tissue on a temporal pedicle. It provides thin skin and cartilage with a hidden donor site. It is an axial pattern flap. It can be used for nasal reconstruction. Also described for columellar reconstruction.

Wassel classification for thumb duplication

- Bifid distal phalanx.

- Duplicated distal phalanx.
- Bifid proximal phalanx.
- Duplicated proximal phalanx.
- Bifid metacarpal.
- Duplicated metacarpal.
- Triphalangia.
Thumb duplication.

Waterlow score

- Used to assess patents according to their risk of developing *Pressure sores*.
- The categories are:
  ○ weight for height;
  ○ continence;
  ○ mobility;
  ○ sex and age;
  ○ appetite;
  ○ special risks – tissue condition, neurology, major surgery, medication.
- The score in each section is summated to give the overall score, which indicates the relative risk.
  ○ 0–9 low risk;
  ○ 10–14 – at risk;
  ○ 15–19 – high risk;
  ○ 20+ – very high risk.

Watson test

Scaphoid shift test.

- Test for scapholunate ligament incompetence.
- Put wrist in ulnar deviation, stabilize the scaphoid in extension. Grip left hand of patient with left hand.
- Bring wrist to radial deviation and resist scaphoid flexion with the thumb on volar surface, which forces the scaphoid dorsally.
- If the ligament is lax the scaphoid shifts dorsally. An audible painful clunk may occur.
- Many patients have mobility (36%), but clear instability with pain is a positive result.
See Carpal instability.

Weber–Ferguson incision

Paranasal incision for access to the oral cavity.
See Oral cavity reconstruction.

Weber 2-point discrimination

Test with callipers – 7 out of 10 should be correct. Normal pulp values are 2–3 mm, but can be 5–6 mm in manual labourers and less in congenital blindness.

Webster operation

- Used for *Lip reconstruction*, a modification of *Bernard operation*.
- In this modification skin only is excised in *Burow's triangles*.
- The triangular excisions are further lateral, placing the scar in the nasolabial fold.
- Paramental Burow's triangles are created to ease inferior advancement of cheek tissue.
- Vermilion is advanced.
- Get improved sensation.

Werner's syndrome

- Adult *Progeria*.
- Autosomal recessive.
- *Scleroderma*-like skin changes, baldness, ageing, hyper/hypopigmentation, cataracts, diabetes, muscle atrophy, neoplasms.
- Plastic surgery is contraindicated due to microangiopathy.

Wet leather sign

Crepitus with tendon movement suggestive of an inflammation-induced change in synovium or synovitis.

Whitlow

See Herpes.

Whitnall's ligament

- A condensation of the superior sheath of levator which is a check ligament.
- This attaches medially to the pulley of superior oblique muscle and laterally to the lacrimal gland.
- It functions as a pulley to facilitate the change in direction of the levator action from horizontal to vertical.

Windblown hand

- Flexion and ulnar deviation of fingers and fixed flexion of thumb.
- Associated with craniocarpotarsal dystrophy and arthrogryphosis.
- Typically bilateral and worsens as the child grows.
- Most patients have 1st web space contracture and flexion deformity of the MPJ.

- Windblown hand is a manifestation of many processes. Different processes may be responsible for a similar appearance such as thumb abnormalities, PIP joint changes, tendon subluxation. It may represent a combination of persistent intrinsic muscles with a disturbance of normal limb rotation.

Treatment:
- Try splintage initially.
- Correct skin contractures and splint. This may be all that is required and is needed before tackling other structures.
- Release at base of PIP joint and also release abnormal fascial bands.
- Subluxed extensors may require centralizing.
- Also the 1st web space contractures may require release and flexor and intrinsic muscles.

Wood
1862: performed a groin flap.

Wound
A defect/wound is an interruption in the anatomical and/or the functional integrity of a tissue.

Wound closure

Primary or first intention: Where the wound edges are approximated directly such as a surgical wound. Collagen metabolism provides strength and epithelialization produces a thin scar.

Delayed primary: In a contaminated wound first allow a few days for the host defences to debride the wound. Healing is as for primary.

Secondary: Where the wound is left open and spontaneous re-epithelialization occurs, such as in a burn wound either from remaining epithelial elements or from the epithelial margin. The key processes are contraction and epithelialization. Myofibroblasts appear at day 3 and are gone by the time contraction is completed.

Tertiary: A wound not closed primarily and closed with imported tissue, such as a flap or graft.

Partial thickness: Mainly epithelialization with minimal collagen deposition.

Wound healing
- Wound healing is the restoration of anatomical integrity to a traumatized tissue.
- Wounds heal by a combination of epithelialization, connective tissue deposition and contraction.
- Also describe healing by the surgical process as either primary intention, secondary intention or delayed primary closure. *See Wound closure.*

Phases of wound healing:
- *Haemostasis:* exposed collagen causes platelet aggregation. Get clot, thrombus and vasospasm. Platelets initiate healing by releasing growth factors (PDGF, TGF-β). Fibrin is produced.
- *Inflammatory:* At the beginning, lasts 24–48 hours. Platelets release _Growth factors and cytokines_, which are chemo-attractant for macrophages and neutrophils. Monocytes are called macrophages once they pass through the vessel wall. These remove necrotic debris. Neutrophils are the first to enter the wound and establish acute inflammation. Pro-inflammatory cytokines amplify the response. Monocytes are attracted to the wound especially by TGF-β. These are converted to macrophages, which continue to destroy bacteria and debride the wound. They also produce a lot of cytokines. The matrix is initially composed of fibrin.
- _Proliferative_: By day 3 fibroblasts arrive, attracted by _TGF-β_ released from macrophages. They are usually located in perivascular tissue and migrate along networks of fibrin fibres. Collagen is produced. Also glycosaminglycans (GAGs) and elastin. GAGs become ground substance when hydrated. Also new capillaries
- *Remodelling:* Starts 2–4 weeks after the injury and lasts up to a year. Randomly laid down _Collagen_ is cross-linked and orientated to increase strength. A well-healed wound reaches 70–80% of unhealed strength. After 21 days there is ongoing synthesis and degradation, and ECM is remodelled. Fibronectins are matrix molecules

that are involved in wound contraction, cell–cell and cell–matrix interaction, cell migration, collagen matrix deposition, and epithelialization. They act as a scaffold for collagen deposition. They bind a wide variety of molecules. Their main function during repair is to promote cell–cell and cell–matrix interaction.

- *Epithelialization:* after a wound is created, basal cells flatten and hemidesmosomal attachments are lost allowing them to migrate. The leading epithelial cells phagocytose clot. Migration stops once another front is reached. After 2 days get basal cell proliferation. If the basement membrane is intact can get complete healing in 4 days. The epithelium comes from the edge and from hair follicles. Several growth factors modulate epithelialization. Epidermal growth factor (EGF) is a potent stimulator of epithelial mitogenesis and chemotaxis. Other factors, including basic FGF and keratinocyte growth factor (KGF), also stimulate epithelial proliferation.
- *Angiogenesis*: new capillaries originate as outgrowths from venules. Get endothelial cell migration. Vascular connections with other capillaries. Neovascularization remodels after flow established. Lots of angiogenic factors. O_2 tension is a potent stimulus.
- *Open wound contraction:* contraction is due to movement at the wound edges. Caused by myofibroblasts. Contain actin.

Delayed wound healing:
Systemic and local factors:

Systemic:
- *Congenital: Pseudoxanthoma elasticum, Ehlers–Danlos syndrome, Cutis laxa, Progeria, Werner's syndrome, Epidermolysis bullosa,* Sickle cell.
- *Acquired – systemic factors.*
  - *Nutrition:* deficiency of *vitamin A, Vitamin C, Vitamin E, Iron, Zinc* and copper. Albumin is an indicator of malnutrition. Low levels are associated with poor healing, but malnutrition only affects healing when severe.
  - *Pharmacological: Steroids,* NASIDs, (decrease collagen synthesis), chemotherapy.
  - *Endocrine: Diabetes.*

- *Ageing:* wounds take longer to heal with age. Connective tissue deposition is reduced. More fibroblasts in younger people. Macrophage function is reduced.
- *Smoking:* no proven relationship between smoking and delayed healing. _Nicotine_ is vasoconstrictive and increases platelet adhesion and thrombus. CO competes with O_2. Cessation of smoking for 2 weeks give normal rates of healing.

Acquired – local factors:
- *Infection:* contamination does not necessarily impair healing and *Staph. aureus* accelerates healing. Infection alters every stage of the healing process. They prolong the inflammatory phase and interfere with epithelialization, contraction and collagen deposition.
- _Radiation._
- *Hypoxia:* stimulates angiogenesis, but reduced O_2 tension impairs healing. Below 4.6 pKa fibroblasts can't replicate. In arterial disease reduced O_2 is due to reduced inflow and in venous disease due to reduced diffusion.
- *Trauma:* neoepidermis is disrupted by trauma.
- *Neural supply:* denervated tissue heal slowly.
- *Pressure.*
- *Foreign material.*
See Skin.

Wright's hyperabduction test
- Clinical test in _Thoracic outlet syndrome_.
- Palpate radial artery with arm maximally abducted. Change in pulse or neurological signs is a positive test.
- Remember as student in classroom knowing the **right** answer.

Wright's ligaments

Interosseous: join adjacent bones.
- Lunate to triquetrum and scaphoid. They are short as the bones move in unison.
- Joining 4 bones of distal row – palmar and dorsal.
- Joining forearm bone to proximal carpal row. On palmar surface radioscapholunate and ulnolunate ligament. Dorsally is the radiocarpal ligament.

Transosseous: cross bones. Mainly tie radius to carpus on palmar side and attach radius to ulnar side of the carpus.
- Radioscaphocapitate.
- Radiolunatotriquetral.
- Triquetrohamitocapitate.

Wrist OA
90% involve the scaphoid in 3 patterns – *SLAC*, *triscaphe* (scapho-trapezium-trapezoid) and a combination of the two.

Wucheri bancrofti
A principal cause of lymphoedema in the tropics. Treated with dimethylcarbazine, but the lymphoedema is usually irreversible.

X Xanthelasma palpebarum to Xeroderma pigmentosa

Xanthelasma palpebarum
- The most common kind of xanthoma, occurs on the eyelids, usually near the inner canthi.
- Soft, thin, yellowish, slightly raised, elongated plaques, often symmetrically distributed.
- 50% have associated hyperlipoproteinemia.
- Also biliary cirrhosis and in histiocytic disorders such as reticulohistiocytoma cutis, Hand–Schüller–Christian disease and xanthoma disseminatum.
- Treatment for cosmesis is excision, diathermy or trichloro-acetic acid.
- Recurrence occurs in 40% of the patients who undergo excision.

Xanthogranuloma
- Juvenile xanthogranuloma are self-limiting benign papules which occur in early infancy into adulthood.
- The typical lesion is papular and red to yellow, <1 cm diameter.
- They occur as single or multiple lesions in the head and neck.
- They usually involute spontaneously.
- 10% have visceral involvement with occasional eye involvement.

- Histologically they show an accumulation of histiocytes with a granulomatous infiltrate, which may contain foam cells, foreign body giant cells and Touton giant cells.

Xanthoma planum
Resembles xanthelasma, but may involve extensive areas beyond the eyelids, especially the palmar creases, axillae, flexor areas of the extremities, neck, inner thighs, trunk and shoulders.

Xeroderma pigmentosa
- Autosomal recessive disorder.
- Deficiency of thiamine dimerase.
- Thiamine absorbs light and forms dimmers, which cannot be broken down.
- The build-up of thiamine dimers induces defects in DNA structure.
- Acute sensitivity to sunlight secondary to defective DNA repair mechanism results in multiple epitheliomas with malignant degeneration in the first two decades.
- May get neurological deterioration 'xeroderma idiocy'.
- Treat aggressively with sun protection, topical 5FU, excision and grafts.

See Basal cell carcinoma, Skin.

Y–V advancement flap
A type of *Advancement flap*. Used in serial fashion for release of scar contractures.

The Y limb cuts across the scar contracture and the V advances into it.

Z-plasty
- Described by Fricke in 1829 and William Horner in 1837.
- Two triangular flaps are interdigitated to gain length in the direction of the common limb and a change in direction of the common limb.
- The central limb is usually placed along the direction of the scar or contracture. The limbs are equal length and the angle varies from 30 to 90°.
- If there is tension, get immediate flap transposition. The wider the angle of the flaps the greater the difference between the long and short diagonals and the greater the lengthening so:
  - 30° gives 25% lengthening;
  - 45° gives 50% lengthening;
  - 60° gives 75% lengthening;
  - 90° gives 125% lengthening.
- Less does not produce significant lengthening, greater angles produce too much tension.
- Actual gains may be more or less than theoretical gains and depend on the ability of the skin at the base to fit in the new position.
- Multiple Z-plasties can produce as much lengthening as a larger single Z-plasty. Multiple Z-plasties do, however, produce less transverse shortening. It can also give a better cosmetic result.
- When a Z-plasty is used to change the direction of scars:
  - draw the present scar – this will be the central limb;
  - draw the intended final position of the scar – the same length and crossing the scar;
  - join up adjacent ends;
  - the limbs the same length as the scar will make up the Z-plasty.

See *Four-flap*, *Z-plasty*, *Five-flap Z-plasty* (also called jumping man or double-opposing Z-plasties. Six flap Z-plasty.

Zinc
Required for DNA and RNA polymerase. Deficiency may retard epithelialization and fibroblast proliferation. Deficiency is seen in large burns, alcoholism and GI fistulae. See *Wound healing*.

Zygomatic fractures
Anatomy:
- The zygoma is a pyramidal bone in the midface, which gives prominence to the cheek and forms the inferolateral border of the orbit
- It has frontal, maxillary, temporal and orbital processes.
- It articulates with the frontal, temporal (arch), maxillary (medial orbit) and sphenoid bones (lateral orbit).

Fractures:
- Fractures tend to displace the zygoma downward, medial and posterior.

- Fractures tend to occur in a tetrapod fashion at its junction with:
  - zygomatic process of the frontal bone (ZF suture);
  - greater wing of the sphenoid in the lateral orbit;
  - maxilla in the orbital margin, orbital floor and anterior wall of the maxillary sinus;
  - temporal bone in the zygomatic arch.

Symptoms and signs:
- Bruising and swelling over the zygoma and inside the mouth.
- Malar depression.
- Palpable bony step.
- *Subconjunctival haematoma:* with no posterior limit as the fracture line extends behind the orbital septum. It will be bright red due to transconjunctival oxygenation.
- *Trismus:* when the zygomatic arch abuts the coronoid process of the mandible.
- *Epistaxis:* due to a tear in the mucosal lining of the maxillary sinus.
- *Paraesthesia:* in distribution of *Infra-orbital nerve*.
- *Enopthalmos*.
- *Dystopia*.
- *Diplopia:* usually on upward gaze due to trapping of inferior rectus muscle. Tethering can be detected by the forced duction test. The eye is anaesthetized. Gentle traction is applied to the inferior conjunctiva. Limitation in globe movement indicates tethering.
- *Decrease visual acuity:* due to retinal detachement.

Radiology: use the following.
- PA views.
- Lateral views.
- *Water's views:* demonstrate maxillary sinus.
- Caldwell's views: ZF suture.
- CT and 3D CT.

Classification: by Knight and North.

Management:
- *Conservative:* usually for stable undisplaced fractures.
- *Gilles' lift*: for displaced fractures of zygomatic arch.
- *ORIF:* preferred method for many fractures. Plates are placed over the fracture lines.
  - fractures over ZF suture: lateral brow incision;
  - fractures in the infra-orbital rim: lower eyelid incision;
  - fractures in the maxilla: upper buccal sulcus incision;
  - complex fracture: bicoronal incision.

See *Facial fractures*.

DISCOVERY LIBRARY
LEVEL 5 SWCC
DERRIFORD HOSPITAL
DERRIFORD ROAD
PLYMOUTH
PL6 8DH

Abbreviations

2PD	two-point discrimination	**CDNH**	chondrodermatitis nodularis
5FU	5 fluorouracil		helicis
AA	androgenic alopecia	**CFNG**	contralateral facial nerve grafting
abs	antibodies	**CGRP**	calcitonin gene-related peptide
ACL	accessory collateral ligament	**CIC**	carpal instability complex
ACL	accessory collateral ligament	**CIC**	congenital, involutional, cicatricial
ADM	adductor digiti minimi	**CID**	carpal instability dissociative
ADP	adductor policis brevis		syndrome
AER	apical ectodermal ridge	**CIND**	carpal instability non-dissociative
AIIS	anterior inferior iliac spine		syndrome
AIIS	anterior inferior iliac spine	**CL**	cleft lip
AO	Arbeitsgemeinschaft fur	**CL/P**	cleft lip and palate
	Osteosynthesefragen (from Swiss	**CLAVM**	capillary, lymphatic, arteriov-
	classification system)		enous malformation
AP	adductor pollicis	**CLM**	capillary lymphatic malformation
APB	abductor pollicis brevis	**CM**	capillary malformation
APL	abductor pollicis longus	**CMC**	carpometacarpal
aPTT	activated partial thromboplastin	**CMCJ**	carpometacarpal joint
time		**CMF**	cyclosphosphamide, methotrex-
ASIS	anterior superior iliac spine		ate and 5 fluorouracil
ATLS	advanced trauma life support	**CMN**	congenital melanocytic naevus
AV	arteriovenous	**CN**	chemotherapy
AVA	arteriovenous anastomosis	**CNS**	central nervous system
AVFs	arteriovenous fistulas	**CO**	carbon monoxide
AVM	arteriovenous malformation	**COAD**	chronic obstructive airway disease
AVPU	alert, vocal stimulus, painful	**COHb**	carboxyhaemoglobin
	stimulus, unresponsive	**CP**	cleft palate
BBR	bilateral breast reduction	**CRP**	C-reactive protein
BCC	basal cell carcinoma	**CRPS**	Complex Regional Pain Syndrome
BCNU	carmustine	**CSAG**	Clinical Standards Advisory Group
BDD	body dysmorphic disorder	**CT**	computerized tomography
BEAM	bulbar elongation and anasto-	**CTD**	connective tissue disease
	motic meatoplasty	**CTS**	carpal tunnel syndrome
BEE	basal energy expenditure	**CVLM**	complex combined vascular
bFGF	beta fibroblast growth factor		malformations
BMI	body mass index	**CVM**	capillary venous malformation
BMPs	bone morphogenic proteins	**CW**	continuous wave
BOP	bilateral occipitoparietal flaps	**CXR**	chest X-ray
BP	blood pressure	**CXR**	chest X-ray
BXO	*Balanitis xerotica obliterans*	**DAB**	dorsal abductor
ca	carcinoma	**DandV**	diarrhoea and vomiting
CandL	Cormack and Lamberty	**DBD**	dermolytic bullous dermatitis
CAVF	capillary-arteriovenous fistula	**DCIA**	deep circumflex iliac artery
CAVM	capillary arterial venous	**DCIS**	ductal carcinoma *in situ*
	malformation	**DHT**	dihydrotestosterone
CCF	congestive cardiac failure	**DIEA**	deep inferior epigastric artery

DIEP	deep inferior epigastric perforator flap	**G**	grade
DIP	distal interphalangeal	**GA**	general anaesthetic
DIPJ	distal interphalangeal joint	**GAGS**	glycosaminoglycans
DISI	dorsal intercalated segmental instability	**GCMN**	giant congenital melanocytic naevus
DLE	discoid lupus erythematosus	**GHN**	giant hairy naevus
DM	diabetes mellitus	**GI**	gastrointestinal
DMTA	dorsal metatarsal artery	**GIT**	gastrointestinal tract
DP	deltopectoral	**GSW**	gunshot wound
DPA	dorsalis pedis artery	**HA**	hydroxyapatite
DRUJ	distal radioulnar joint	**Hb**	haemoglobin
DVT	deep vein thrombosis	**HBO**	hyperbaric oxygen
EB	epidermolysis bullosa	**HCL**	hydrochloric acid
EB	Epstein–Barr	**HHT**	hereditary haemorrhagic telangiectasia
ECM	extracellular matrix	**HLA**	human leucocyte antigen
ECOG	Eastern Co-operative Oncology Group	**HS**	hydradenitis suppuritiva
ECRB	extensor carpi radialis brevis	**HTA**	high-tension abdominoplasty
ECRL	extensor carpi radialis longus	**IandD**	incision and drainage
ECU	extensor carpi ulnaris	**IF**	interferon
EDC	extensor digitorum communis	**IGAP**	inferior gluteal artery flap
EDM	extensor digiti minimi	**IGF**	insulin-like growth factor
EDQ	extensor digit quinti	**IgG**	Immunoglobulin G
EGF	epidermal growth factor	**IgM**	Immunoglobulin M
EIP	extensor indicis proprius	**IJV**	inferior jugular vein
ELND	elective lymph node dissection	**ILP**	isolated limb perfusion
EM	extracellular matrix	**IMA**	inferior mammary artery
EMG	electromyelogram	**IMA**	internal mammary artery
EORTC	European Organization for Research and Treatment of Cancer	**IMF**	intermaxillary fixation
		IOD	interorbital distance
EPB	extensor pollicis brevis	**IPJ**	interphalangeal joint
EPL	extensor pollicis longus	**IVP**	intravenous pyelogram
ESR	erythroctye sedimentation rate	**K**	potassium
EUA	examination under anaesthesia	**KGF**	keratinocyte growth factor
FCR	flexor carpi radialis	**KS**	Kaposi's sarcoma
FCU	flexor carpi ulnaris	**LA**	local anaesthetic
FD	fibrous dysplasia	**LCIS**	lobal carcinoma *in situ*
FDM	flexor digiti minimi	**LDH**	lactate dehydrogenase
FDMA	first dorsal metatarsal artery	**LFTs**	liver function tests
FDP	flexor digitorum profundus	**LLS**	levator labii superioris
FDS	flexor digitorum longus	**LM**	lymphatic malformation
FGF	fibroblast growth factor	**LN**	lymph node
FGFR2	fibroblast growth factor receptor 2	**LND**	lymph node dissection
FLPD	flash lamp-pumped pulsed dye	**LT**	lunotriquetral
FNA	fine needle aspiration	**LVM**	lymphatico-vascular malformation
FOM	floor of mouth	**LVM**	lymphaticovenous malformation
FPB	flexor pollicis brevis	**M**	metastasis
FPL	flexor pollicis longus	**MABC**	medial antebrachial cutaneous
F–S	Fasanella-Servat	**MAGPI**	meatal advancement and glansplasty
FTSG	full thickness skin graft	**MC**	metacarpal

MCP	metacarpal joint		PIN	posterior interosseous nerve
MCPJ	metacarpophalangeal joint		PIP	proximal interphalangeal joint
MCR	mid-carpal radial		PIPJ	proximal interphalangeal joint
MCU	mid-carpal ulnar		pKa	acid dissociation constant
MDU	Medical Defence Union		PL	palmaris longus
MESS	mangled extremity severity score		PL	palmaris longus
MHC	major histocompatibility complex		PLLA	poly-1-lactic acid
MPB	male pattern baldness		PMN	polymorphonucleocyte
MPD	myofascial pain dysfunction		PNS	parasympathetic nervous system
	syndrome		POC	presurgical orthopaedic
MPJ	metacarpalphalangeal joint			correction
MRI	magnetic resonance imaging		POP	plaster of paris
MRSA	methicillin-resistant *Staphylo-*		PPT	photodynamic therapy
	coccus aureus		PR	cardiac conduction time
MSH	melanocyte-stimulating hormone		PRC	proximal row carpectomy
MT	muscle–tendon		PSJ	pisotriquetrial joint
MTP	metatarsalphalangeal		Pt	patient
MTP	metatarso-phalangeal joint		PT	pronator teres
MTPJ	metacarpal phalangeal joint		PT	prothrombin time
MUA	manipulation under anaesthetic		PTCH	*Patched* gene
Na	sodium		PTFE	polytetrafluoroethylene (Teflon)
NAC	nipple-areolar complex		PVA	polyvinyl alcohol
NAI	non-accidental injury		PVNS	pigmented villonuclear tenovagino-
NandM	Nahai–Mathes			synovitis
NCS	nerve conduction studies		PZ	progress zone
NGF	nerve growth factor		RA	rheumatoid arthritis
NGT	nasogastric feeding		RADS	radiation absorbed dose (unit of
NS	normal saline			measurement of radiation)
NSAID	non-steroidal anti-inflammatory		RBC	red blood cells
	drug		RhF	rheumatoid factor
NV	neurovascular		ROM	range of movement
NVB	neurovascular bundle		ROOF	retro-orbicularis oculi fat
OA	osteoarthritis		RSD	reflex sympathetic dystrophy
od	every day.		RSTL	relaxed skin tension line
OP	operation		Rt > lt	right greater than left
OPG	orthopantomograph		RT	radiotherapy
ORIF	open reduction and internal		RTA	road traffic accident
	fixation		r-TPA	recombinant tissue plasminogen
ORL	oblique retinacular ligament			activator
PA	palmar aponeurosis		SCC	squamous cell carcinoma
PA	postero-anterior view		SCM	sternocleidomastoid
PAD	palmar adductor		SGAP	superior gluteal artery flap
PCA	patient-controlled analgesia		Shh	*Sonic hedgehog* (gene)
PCD	programmed cell death		SIADH	syndrome of inappropriate ADH
PCL	proper collateral ligament and			(antidiuretic hormone)
PDGF	platelet-derived growth factor		SIEA	superior inferior epigastric artery
PDMS	policlymethylsiloxane		SIMON	single, introverted male, overly
PDS	polydiaxone			narcissistic
PEEP	positive end expiratory pressure		SIPS	sympathetically independent pain
PET	positron emission tomography			syndrome
PGA	polyglycolic acid		SLAC	scapholunate advanced collapse

SLE	systemic lupus erythematosus	**TNF-α**	tumour necrosis factor alpha
SLL	scapholunate ligament	**TNM**	tumour, node metastasis
SLNB	sentinel lymph node biopsy	**t-PA**	tissue plasminogenic activator
SMAS	superficial musculo-aponeurotic system	**TPF**	temporoparietal fascia
		TPN	total parenteral nutrition
SMPS	sympathetically maintained pain syndrome	**Tq**	tourniquet
		TRAM	transverse rectus abdominus muscle
SNAC	schaphoid non-union with collapse		
SNAP	sensory nerve action potential	**TSH**	thyroid-stimulating hormone
SOOF	sub-orbicularis oculi fat	**TSS**	toxic shock syndrome
SP	substance P	**UCL**	ulna collateral ligament
SSG	split skin graft	**US**	ultrasound
STSG	split-thickness skin graft	**USS**	ultrasound scan
STT	scapho-trapezium-trapezoid	**UV**	ultraviolet
T	tumour site	**UVA**	ultraviolet irradiation
TAR	thrombocytopenia absent radius	**VAC**	vacuum-assisted closure
TATA	total anterior tenoarthrolysis	**VCF**	velocardiofacial
TB	tuberculosis	**VEGF**	vasoendothelial growth factor
TBSA	total body surface area	**VF**	ventricular fibrillation
TCA	trichloro-actic acid	**VISI**	volar intercalated segmental instability
TCL	transverse carpal ligament		
TEF	tracheo-esophageal fistula	**VM**	vascular malformation
TENS	transcutaneous electrical nerve stimulator	**VM**	venous malformation
		VPI	velopharyngeal incompetence
TEP	tracheo-oseophageal puncture	**VRAM**	vertical rectus abdominus muscle
TFCC	triangular fibrocartilage	**VVs**	varicose veins
TFL	tensor fascia lata	**WDR**	wide-dynamic range (neurons)
TGF-β	tumour growth factor-beta	**WHO**	World Health Organization
TICAS	trauma-induced cold-associated symptoms	**wt**	weight
		XR	X-ray
TILT	triquetrial impingement ligament tear	**ZF**	zygomatico-frontal
		ZPA	zone of polarizing activity
TMJ	temporo-mandibular joint		